STRENGTHENING
FAMILY RESILIENCE

Also from Froma Walsh

Normal Family Processes, Fourth Edition:
Growing Diversity and Complexity
Edited by Froma Walsh

Spiritual Resources in Family Therapy, Second Edition
Edited by Froma Walsh

STRENGTHENING FAMILY RESILIENCE

THIRD EDITION

Froma Walsh

THE GUILFORD PRESS
New York   London

© 2016 The Guilford Press
A Division of Guilford Publications, Inc.
370 Seventh Avenue, Suite 1200, New York, NY 10001
www.guilford.com

Paperback edition 2017

Printed in the United States of America

This book is printed on acid-free paper.

Last digit is print number: 9 8 7 6 5 4 3

The author has checked with sources believed to be reliable in her efforts to
provide information that is complete and generally in accord with the standards
of practice that are accepted at the time of publication. However, in view of the
possibility of human error or changes in behavioral, mental health, or medical
sciences, neither the author, nor the editors and publisher, nor any other party
who has been involved in the preparation or publication of this work warrants
that the information contained herein is in every respect accurate or complete,
and they are not responsible for any errors or omissions or the results obtained
from the use of such information. Readers are encouraged to confirm the
information contained in this book with other sources.

Library of Congress Cataloging-in-Publication Data

Names: Walsh, Froma, author.
Title: Strengthening family resilience / by Froma Walsh.
Description: Third edition. | New York : The Guilford Press, [2016] |
   Includes bibliographical references and index.
Identifiers: LCCN 2015032032 | ISBN 9781462522835 (hardcover : alk. paper);
ISBN 9781462529865 (paperback : alk. Paper)
Subjects: LCSH: Families--Mental health. | Resilience (Personality trait) |
   Dysfunctional families. | Family psychotherapy. | Family social work.
Classification: LCC RC489.F33 W34 2016 | DDC 616.89/156--dc23
LC record available at http://lccn.loc.gov/2015032032

About the Author

Froma Walsh, MSW, PhD, is the Mose and Sylvia Firestone Professor Emerita in the School of Social Service Administration and the Department of Psychiatry at the Pritzker School of Medicine, University of Chicago. She is also Co-Founder and Co-Director of the University-affiliated Chicago Center for Family Health. Dr. Walsh is a past president of the American Family Therapy Academy and past editor of the *Journal of Marital and Family Therapy.* She has received many honors for her distinguished contributions and leadership in the mental health field, including awards from the Society for Family Psychology of the American Psychological Association, the American Family Therapy Academy, the American Association for Marriage and Family Therapy, the American Orthopsychiatric Association, and the Society for Pastoral Care Research. Among her numerous publications are the edited books *Normal Family Processes, Fourth Edition,* and *Spiritual Resources in Family Therapy, Second Edition.* Dr. Walsh is a frequent speaker and international consultant on resilience-oriented professional training, practice, and research.

Preface

Resilience—the ability to withstand and rebound from crisis and prolonged adversity—has become a valuable concept at the forefront in mental health and human services and in developmental and social science research. While the preponderance of theory, research, and practice has focused on resilience in individuals, there is now a groundswell of attention to the importance of resilience in families. My major work, over more than two decades, has centered on increasing our understanding of family resilience and developing useful practice applications with families facing a wide range of serious life challenges.

Traumatic events, major losses, and highly stressful conditions impact the entire family, rippling through the network of relationships. They challenge the family as a functional system; in turn, key family processes influence the adaptation of all members, their relationships, and the family unit. How do some families overcome adversity—and even grow stronger in doing so—when others falter and splinter? What processes enable family members to rally in teamwork and mutual support through tough times? To live well with an illness that can't be cured or a problem that can't be solved? To rebuild lives after a shattering loss or life-altering transition? To rise above severe trauma or barriers of poverty and discrimination? It's crucial to understand how families can effectively overcome scarring experiences and go forward to live and love well.

Leading scholars have come to see individual and family risk and resilience in terms of dynamic multilevel processes over time, involving an ongoing interaction of biopsychosocial influences across the family life cycle. As families strengthen their resilience, they are better able to nurture the positive development of their children, support loved ones in need, and care for their elders.

This volume presents my research-informed family resilience framework for intervention and prevention to strengthen key family processes in overcoming adversity. This fully updated, revised, and expanded third edition incorporates the latest research and practice advances for clinical and community-based services. It presents core principles of a multilevel developmental systemic framework, addressing the ongoing interplay of individual, family, community, sociocultural, and spiritual influences in risk and resilience. Program applications, practice guidelines, and case illustrations are provided to address a wide range of adverse situations: recovering from crisis, trauma, and loss; navigating disruptive transitions, such as job loss, divorce, and migration; overcoming persistent multi-stress challenges with chronic conditions of illness, disability, ongoing trauma, or poverty; and overcoming obstacles to success for at-risk youth. Expanded coverage is given to resilience-oriented approaches with war-related trauma and collective trauma in major disasters and terrorist attacks. Two new chapters address resilience-oriented family assessment and disruptive transitions and resilience across the family life cycle.

A family resilience framework is especially relevant in clinical and community-based practice because most clients seek help in highly stressful times. It shifts focus from how families have failed to how families, when challenged, can succeed. My research and practice experience have deepened my conviction that even highly vulnerable or troubled families have the potential to strengthen their resilience. In contrast to deficit-focused practice models, the resilience-oriented approach I present in this book draws out and expands each family's strengths and resources for mastering challenges. Beyond coping or problem solving, resilience involves positive adaptation and can yield transformation and growth. In building relational resilience, families strengthen their bonds and become more resourceful in meeting future challenges. Thus, every intervention has preventive benefits.

I've long been interested in the concept of resilience. I grew up in a family challenged by serious hardships, tragic losses, and social stigma. As a young adult, my experience of traditional psychotherapy, after my mother died, dredged up all the negative aspects of my childhood and elaborated on my parents' faults. The longer I was in therapy, the worse my parents got. I was viewed as hardy despite their failings, as if I grew myself up. I only later came to see that those adverse experiences made me stronger than I might have been growing up in a family blessed with every advantage. It took a long time to appreciate my parents' struggles and their remarkable courage, perseverance, and resourcefulness.

My early clinical training, in the late 1960s, taught me how to diagnose and treat disorders but not how to recognize and promote positive functioning. I was drawn to the field of family therapy just as it was flowering, especially engaged by a workshop with Virginia Satir, who saw the healthy strivings in troubled families. It was refreshing to cast off deterministic theories of early-childhood, maternal causality for individual problems—with such pejorative labels as schizophrenogenic and refrigerator mothers. The systemic paradigm expanded the focus of assessment and intervention to address the multiple influences in functioning and well-being through transactional processes over time involving the broad relational network and social context. I was fortunate to benefit from clinical training on an innovative psychiatric inpatient unit at Yale Medical Center based on the philosophy of milieu therapy—a patient–staff community with combined interventions of psychotropic medication and individual, group, family, and multifamily group approaches. My first supervisor, Carol Anderson (who later developed family psychoeducation), involved families respectfully, appreciating their challenges with mental illness. Coming to Chicago, I was fortunate to work as Family Studies Coordinator in a schizophrenia research program funded by the National Institute of Mental Health and directed by the visionary psychiatrist Roy Grinker, Sr. Grinker, who had pioneered the study of combat stress in World War II (Grinker & Spiegel, 1945), was a close colleague of von Bertalanffy (1968), the founder of general system theory. Both programs put into practice a biopsychosocial interactionist perspective.

Yet the mental health field continued to focus on family deficits, reflecting the widespread belief that most families were more or less dysfunctional. When I sought to include a "normal" (i.e., nonclinical) comparison group in the schizophrenia research, some colleagues chided me, saying that I wouldn't find any normal families—and they definitely wouldn't recommend their own! Undaunted, I did include a nonclinical group of families in the community and was impressed by their vitality and diversity. Yet even those families faced tough challenges and worried about their adequacy—one mother asked if she and her family could receive a "certificate of normality"!

That experience led me to pursue doctoral studies in human development at The University of Chicago to expand my understanding of family and social processes in healthy functioning and positive growth. My perspective was enriched by early studies of resilience by my mentor, Bertram Cohler; by studies of creative processes by Mihaly Csikszentmihalyi; and by emerging developments in phenomenology and social constructionism. My clinical teaching, training, and practice became increasingly strengths oriented, and I've striven since then to bridge advances in the social sciences and the mental health field. I look back on those valuable learning experiences as my professional "flight into health."

Two myths about normal families have clouded our understanding. First, the erroneous assumption that healthy families are problem free can overpathologize ordinary families struggling with stressful life challenges or traumatic experiences. Second, the assumption that a single, universal model of the healthy family is essential, fitting an idealized image of families of the past, has led to the faulty presumption that varying family structures are inherently dysfunctional and damage children. With the growing diversity of families in societies worldwide, no single model fits all—or even most—families today. In this volume, *family* is defined broadly, to encompass varied family forms, committed couple relationships, and extended formal and informal kinship networks. Studies of strong families worldwide (DeFrain & Asay, 2007) show that families can thrive and children can be raised well in a variety of kin arrangements. What matters most are effective transactional processes for stable, nurturing, and protective bonds.

Over the past three decades, family systems research has provided empirical grounding to identify many key processes that support effective family functioning (Walsh, 2012d). Drawing together these findings with a growing body of research on resilience, the family resilience framework presented here provides a flexible map to guide practice with a broad diversity of families facing varied situations of adversity. This approach attends to the interplay of individual, family, socioeconomic, cultural, and spiritual influences and affirms many varied pathways in resilience.

The family resilience practice approach described in this volume builds on recent advances in strengths-based, collaborative systemic models, contextualizing distress in highly stressful experiences. The framework and practice applications in this new edition have been developed, refined, and reformulated over many years of clinical teaching, supervision, and direct practice grounded in a developmental systems orientation. Key processes are identified and practical guidelines are offered to foster family empowerment in mastering a wide range of life challenges. Case illustrations draw on many varied examples of family resilience from my professional practice, research, and training of practitioners, as well as from my personal life. Names and details have been carefully altered to protect families' privacy. Throughout this volume, I discuss ways in which couples, families, and helping professionals can identify, affirm, and strengthen ways of forging positive change and growth from adversity.

In Part I of the volume, Chapter 1 presents the foundation for a family resilience approach to practice. It clarifies the concept of resilience, surveys what we have learned from studies of individual resilience, and presents a multilevel systemic view of resilience that integrates ecological and developmental perspectives. Chapter 2 situates family resilience in social context, highlighting trends in the growing diversity and complexity of families and their stressful challenges in our rapidly changing world. This perspective is essential for family assessment and intervention to be attuned to today's families and their varied pathways in resilience.

Part II integrates research findings and practice perspectives to identify key transactional processes that can facilitate effective family functioning and resilience. Because practitioners can be overwhelmed by the complexities of family processes under stressful conditions, I have found it useful to organize these processes into three domains of family functioning: belief systems, organizational processes, and communication processes. Chapters 3–5 describe and illustrate key processes for family resilience in each dimension of functioning. This is not a typology or model of static universal traits. Rather, these are dynamic processes that are recursive and synergistic. They may be expressed in varying ways and to varying degrees depending on cultural differences; on family preferences, resources, and constraints; and on the adverse situations and emerging challenges families face over time.

Part III describes and illustrates assessment and practice principles and programmatic applications of this family resilience framework. This practice approach builds on developments in strengths-based systemic practice. Parallel to a practice focus on common factors (i.e., core processes) in effective family therapy identified by Sprenkle, Davis, and Lebow (2009), practitioners can target these key process components identified in family process research to strengthen family resilience as presenting problems are addressed. Chapter 6 offers useful maps as tools to guide resilience-oriented family assessment and intervention. Chapter 7 provides core principles, practical guidelines, and case examples to facilitate resilience in work with distressed couples and families. Chapter 8 presents program applications and illustrations of family resilience-oriented clinical and community-based training and service projects developed through the Chicago Center for Family Health locally, nationally, and internationally. Practitioners' own resilience and courageous engagement with clients are discussed.

The chapters in Part IV describe and illustrate the application of a family resilience approach in various adverse situations, from crisis events to disruptive transitions to prolonged adversity. Chapter 9 provides a developmental perspective on challenges and resilience over the changing family life cycle. Chapter 10 addresses the profound challenges families face with death and dying and key variables in risk and resilience with loss. Chapter

11 focuses on resilience-building approaches for family and community recovery in the wake of major traumatic events, ranging from community violence to large-scale disasters, terrorism, war-related atrocities, and refugee experience. Chapter 12 tracks the family journey with chronic physical and mental illnesses, offering guidelines to reduce stress and enable families to thrive in the face of illness-related demands and uncertainties. Chapter 13 addresses the persistent challenges faced by multi-stressed, low-income, highly vulnerable families, countering faulty presumptions that they are too dysfunctional and unmotivated to work with. Useful principles, guidelines, and case examples are offered that reveal their deep yearning for a better life and demonstrate ways to engage collaboratively to support their positive strivings. Chapter 14 draws on my own personal experience as well as the efforts of others who have inspired me. It explores possibilities for reconnection, reconciliation, and forgiveness in families, in groups that have suffered oppression, and in parts of our world torn by strife. It challenges common assumptions that those wounded by past trauma or troubled relationships survive best by severing ties to their families and their past, fortifying themselves as rugged individuals.

The family resilience practice approach presented here is grounded in the firm conviction that we human beings survive and thrive best through deep connections with those around us, those who have come before us, and those who will follow us, including all who have been, and could be, significant in our lives. Even experiences of severe trauma and very troubled relationships hold potential for healing and transformation across the life course and the generations. In facing adversity, resilience is nurtured and sustained through strong family, social, community, cultural, and spiritual connections. I see these as "relational lifelines" for resilience.

This book can serve as a valuable resource for all professionals who are interested in fostering human adaptive capacities and supportive social systems, regardless of practice orientation, discipline, or level of experience. A family resilience framework can be applied in the fields of mental health, health care, human services, child welfare, family life education, community organization, the justice system, family law, and pastoral counseling; by practicing professionals, educators, and students; and by marriage and family therapists, social workers, psychologists, psychiatrists, counselors, nurses, and physicians. It has found application in workplace resilience initiatives, family businesses, and faith-based organizations.

The framework presented here has also found wide international application, with culturally attuned adaptation, in mental health and psychosocial training and services, family research, and social policy, from Latin America, Canada, Europe, Australia, and New Zealand to Africa, the Middle East, and Asia. Previous editions have been translated into Spanish, Portuguese, Italian, Chinese, and Korean.

Although the book is written primarily for helping professionals, it is also of value for a general readership—especially for family members who have faced tragedy or hardship and who are interested in understanding how to build relational resources to strengthen their own individual, couple, family, or community resilience. It is encouraging to see the burgeoning interest worldwide in positive mental health, well-being, and the ability to thrive (World Health Organization, 2011). Most heartening is the increasing attention to ways to promote resilience in individuals, families, and communities (e.g., The Road to Resilience initiative of the American Psychological Association, 2010; Delage, 2008; and the United Nations' development of a global resilience tool [IRIN, 2009] to measure the ability of a system to withstand stresses and shocks in an uncertain world).

The need for family resilience has never been more urgent, as families today are buffeted by global economic, social, political, and environmental upheaval. With devastating natural and human-caused disasters, the world around us has become more hazardous and the future insecure. Yet all families have the potential for adaptation, reinvention, and positive growth. A family resilience approach provides a positive and pragmatic framework that guides interventions to strengthen vital family processes as immediate problems are addressed. In this way, families become more resourceful in dealing with unforeseen problems and proactive in averting future crises. For helping professionals, the therapeutic process is enriched as we bring out the best in families and practice the art of the possible.

Acknowledgments

This book is dedicated to the families everywhere who face serious life crises or persistent adversity and forge remarkable resilience. They have inspired my abiding interest in understanding core processes in family life that promote positive adaptation: families who sustain an indomitable spirit in the face of illness, disability, or loss; those who rekindle hope and build connection and renewal out of trauma and tragedy rather than sink in despair; those who transcend barriers of poverty, racism, and discrimination toward a positive vision rather than alienation; and those who respond compassionately to the plight of others. My clinical teaching and practice have been immeasurably enriched by what we have learned from families that rebound and thrive.

Analogous to an understanding of core components in effective therapeutic practice, our ability to help couples and families in distress is informed by our understanding of the vital processes in effective family functioning. I am grateful for the advances in our research, countering the misguided search for a single invariant model or set of traits. As reflected in the cover image for this volume, we have come to appreciate the many colors and strands in resilience that families weave as members come together, forging varied pathways over time, dealing with their challenging situations, drawing on their available resources, and striving toward their future hopes and dreams.

I am grateful to the families I've been privileged to know in my research and practice, who have deepened my understanding of their suffering and struggles and their capacity to adapt and grow stronger. They inspire my best efforts and affirm my conviction in the human potential for healing and positive growth out of scarring experiences. My work in community-based and international settings over the years has greatly enlarged my perspective and my appreciation of the importance of strong kinship and community networks in withstanding harsh conditions. Families with little material wealth have shown me the greater value of relational connections and cultural and spiritual resources through troubled times.

I want to thank the dedicated staff at The Guilford Press for their work in the production of this new edition. I most appreciate the thoughtful feedback provided by Senior Editor Jim Nageotte, the collaborative spirit of Art Director Paul Gordon, and the helpful responsiveness of Senior Production Editor Jeannie Tang. In the face of ongoing turmoil in the publishing environment, I applaud the resilience of my Guilford Press "family" for the continuing high level of professionalism and commitment to first-rate professional books, thanks to the steadfast leadership of Guilford's "founding fathers," Seymour Weingarten and Bob Matloff.

In my labor of love on this new volume, I have been deeply appreciative of my many valued colleagues near and far. As always, my kindred spirits have been there for me; my heartfelt thanks to Celia Falicov, Monica McGoldrick, and John Rolland for their incisive comments, thoughtful reflections, and strong support. I am grateful for the many mentors who have influenced my work. I have treasured the past 25 years of stimulating exchange with the wonderfully diverse faculty and trainees at the Chicago Center for Family Health and with the bright, enthusiastic students at The University of Chicago. I look forward to future contacts, consultations, and collaborations worldwide, to support all who are striving to advance research, practice applications, and social policy to strengthen family resilience.

My family and the kinship of close friends have been a wellspring for meaningful connection, joy, and resilience in my life. I miss, beyond words, my cherished friend and collaborator throughout my career, Carol Anderson, who died this past year, too suddenly and too soon. I thank my husband, John, for his steadfast love. I admire my daughter, Claire, for her "can-do" spirit, compassion, and deep commitment to international humanitarian work. Above all, I am grateful to my parents for their loving support and encouragement despite their own life struggles. I only wish that while they were alive I had learned more about their lives to fully appreciate their courage, perseverance, and resourcefulness. I carry their indomitable spirit in my heart.

Contents

PART I

OVERVIEW

CHAPTER 1

Foundations of a Family Resilience Approach

> In the depths of winter, I found there was, within me,
> an invincible summer. . . . No matter how hard the
> world pushes against me, within me there's something
> stronger—something better, pushing right back.
> —ALBERT CAMUS (in Thody, 1970, p. 169)

We live in turbulent times, on the edge of uncertainty. As the world around us has changed so dramatically in recent years, we yearn for strong and enduring family bonds, yet we are unsure how to shape and sustain them to weather the storms of life. Although some families are shattered by crisis events or multi-stress conditions, what is remarkable is that others emerge strengthened and more resourceful. With widespread concern about family breakdown, we need more than ever to understand the dynamic processes that strengthen family resilience in overcoming adversity. We need useful conceptual tools as much as techniques in order to support and strengthen couples and families in distress and those at risk. This chapter lays the foundations for a family resilience framework for clinical and community-based practice, prevention efforts, research, and social policy.

UNDERSTANDING RESILIENCE

The concept of resilience has come to the forefront in developmental psychology and mental health theory, research, and practice, countering the predominant focus on dysfunction and disorder. Resilience can be defined as the ability to withstand and rebound from serious life challenges. Resilience involves dynamic processes that foster positive adaptation in the context of significant adversity (Bonanno, 2004; Luthar, 2006). Beyond coping or adjusting, these strengths and resources enable recovery and positive growth.

Resilience entails more than merely surviving, getting through, or escaping a harrowing ordeal. Survivors are not necessarily resilient; some survive physically but remain impaired psychologically and interpersonally by posttraumatic stress symptoms, crippling depression or anxiety, and an inability to love well or thrive. Others become trapped in reactive positions as victims, nursing old wounds or blocked from growth. In contrast, resilience processes enable people to heal from painful experiences, take charge of their lives, and go on to live and love well.

In order to understand and promote resilience, it is important to distinguish it from common expectations to "just bounce back" and myths of "invulnerability" and "self-sufficiency." As research documents, resilience is forged through suffering and struggle and is relationally based through our interdependence with others.

Human Vulnerability, Suffering, and Resilience

The North American ethos of the *rugged individual* (Bellah, Madsen, Sullivan, Swidler, & Tipton, 1985) and "macho" images of masculinity in many cultures confuse strength with invulnerability. Early scholars of resilience referred to the "invulnerable child," viewing survivors of destructive childhood environments as impervious to stress because of their own inner fortitude or character armor (Anthony, 1987). Hardy children were likened to "steel dolls" that wouldn't shatter under pressure or maltreatment. The danger in the myth of invulnerability and the image of "super-kids" lies in equating human vulnerability with weakness. As Felsman and Vaillant (1987) note, "The term 'invulnerability' is antithetical to the human condition. . . . In bearing witness to the resilient behavior of high-risk children everywhere, a truer effort would be to understand, in form and by degree, the shared human qualities at work" (p. 304).

Common Misconception: "Just Bounce Back!"

The term *resilience*, originating in the physical sciences, referred to the capacity of an object, when stretched, to return to its original form, like a spring or an elastic band. As the concept of human resilience became popularized, this led to widespread overuse and misuse of the term. Media news stories abound describing resilient individuals. Sports announcers proclaim that a team was resilient by bouncing back from a season of defeat to win the season trophy. "Resilience" is also a brand of face cream purporting to restore aging skin to its original elasticity. However, it is unrealistic to expect people to bounce right back when faced with serious life challenges. More often, suffering and struggle are experienced in forging resilience.

Similarly, the capacity to rebound should not be misconstrued as simply "breezing through" a crisis, unscathed by painful experience. With only two alternatives posed—either to shake off adversity or to "wallow" in it—our dominant culture breeds intolerance for suffering; we avert our gaze from disability, avoid contact with the bereaved, or dispense chirpy advice to "cheer up" and get over it. Well-intentioned friends and loved ones urge us to "bounce back" from defeat and to get rapid closure from devastating losses. Many encourage the bereaved to rush into new lives and relationships on the rebound. Likewise, rapid-fire media shifts in focus contribute to the common wish to put major tragedies quickly behind us—from community disasters to lengthy wars and their atrocities, or legacies of political, ethnic, and racial injustice—without looking back to draw lessons, come to terms with them, and heal as a human community.

The tendency to cut off from painful and conflict-laden experiences is rooted in our intergenerational and cultural heritage, often influencing us out of our awareness. In my mid-20s, I was in a student clinical practicum at Yale when my mother suffered a debilitating illness. I shuttled back and forth, from coast to coast, to spend a few days at a time with my parents and still not miss a beat in my demanding schedule. When my mother died, the day after her funeral I flew right back, hit the ground running, and kept up the pace throughout the year. Everyone praised me for being so strong. But we must be careful not to equate competent functioning with resilience. It was only much later that I faced the full impact of the loss of my mother and the significance of our bond. A holistic view of resilience involves the whole person, including emotional and relational well-being.

Unlike the image of the Energizer Bunny, resilience involves "struggling well": experiencing both suffering and courage, effectively working through difficulties both internally and interpersonally (Higgins, 1994). In forging resilience, we strive to integrate the fullness of the experience of serious crises and stressful life challenges into the fabric of our individual and collective identity, influencing how we go on to live our lives.

From Rugged Individual to a Relational View

Reflecting heroic myths of the rugged individual—from the Greek hero Odysseus to Hollywood's cowboy images—most European and American interest in resilience has focused on the strengths of exceptional individuals who have mastered adversity. Most research has sought to identify the personality traits, coping strategies, and neurobiological endowment that enable a child, adolescent, or adult to overcome harrowing life experiences. Commonly, resilience is seen as inborn, as if resilient persons grew themselves up: they either had the "right stuff" all along—inherent hardiness, like the steel doll—or gained strengths in pulling themselves up by their bootstraps. This view fosters the expectation that we must be self-reliant and fiercely independent in tackling difficult life challenges—and a demeaning view of those who don't succeed on their own as deficient, weak, and shameful. In our understanding of resilience, we must be cautious not to blame those who are unable to overcome adversity by themselves, especially when they are struggling with overwhelming conditions beyond their control.

In contrast to the highly individualized concept of human autonomy centered on the "self" in Western societies, most cultures worldwide view the person as embedded within the family and larger community. This sociocentric view of human experience recognizes our essential interdependence for mutual support in troubled times and the power of collaborative efforts in overcoming life's adversities. We are relational beings, standing on the shoulders of those who came before us, reaching out to give and receive help, and inspiring those to come. It is through our connectedness with others that we grow and thrive throughout life.

Resilience Forged through Adversity

Individuals—and families—vary in the strengths, vulnerabilities, and resources they bring to an adverse situation. Those with more assets are more likely to fare well in troubled times. Yet, my research and practice experience convince me that we all have the potential to gain resilience. (And indeed, some who have never faced serious life challenges may crumble when unexpected crises arise.) As research has found, resilience can be strengthened *through* the experience of adversity, as we discover and build latent strengths within ourselves and as we reach out to others to give and receive support.

In my own life, I grew up thinking that I was resilient *despite* my family's deficiencies and that my own innate hardiness enabled me to overcome the hardships we suffered in my childhood. I later came to realize that I grew stronger *because* of those challenging experiences and that my family's unrecognized resilience made all the difference (see Chapter 14).

Crisis: Threat and Challenge

The Chinese symbol for the word *crisis* is a composite of two characters: "threat" and "challenge" (not "opportunity," a common mistaken translation). Although we would not wish for misfortune, the paradox of resilience is that our worst times can also bring out our best as we rise to meet the challenges. In Higgins's (1994) study, resilient adults reported that because they were sorely tested and endured suffering, they emerged with strengths they might not have developed otherwise. They experienced things more deeply and intensely, and placed a heightened value on life. Often this became a wellspring for social activism, a commitment to helping others; in turn, they experienced further growth through these efforts (also see Lietz, 2011). Such experiences have led many to dedicate themselves to careers in health care and mental health fields.

Studies of strong families (Stinnett & DeFrain, 1985) found that at times of crisis, 75% experienced positive occurrences in the midst of hurt or despair, and believed that something good came out of the ordeal. Many families reported that through weathering crises together, their relationships became enriched and more loving than they might otherwise have been. A crisis can be a "wake-up call," heightening our attention to what really matters in our lives. A painful tragedy may thrust survivors in unforeseen, growthful directions. As the Navaho believe, the end of a path is the beginning of another. Resilience is about that journey.

A SYSTEMIC VIEW OF RESILIENCE

A growing body of research over recent decades has enriched and expanded our understanding of resilience (Masten, 2014). In the last half of the 20th century, the prevailing assumptions in the developmental psychology and mental health fields, rooted in psychoanalytic theory and clinical case experience, held that the impact of early or severe trauma can't be undone. It was widely accepted that adverse experiences inevitably damage people and ruin lives, and that children from troubled or "broken" families are themselves irreparably "broken." However, countering those deterministic assumptions, an array of studies found that no combination of risk factors, regardless of severity, gave rise to significant and long-lasting disorder in most children exposed to them (Rutter, 1987). For instance, clinicians commonly note that parents who abuse their children were themselves abused. However, wider community studies found that over half of individuals who had experienced family abuse in childhood did *not* become abusive parents (Kaufman & Zigler, 1987). What enabled them to overcome similar high-risk conditions and be able to love their children well?

Influences in Individual Risk and Resilience

Most research to date has focused on individual resilience. With concern for early intervention and prevention, experts redirected attention to understand not only vulnerability to risk and disorder, but even more importantly, the protective factors that fortify children's resilience. Early studies focused on children of mentally ill or deficient parents who overcame early experiences of abuse or neglect to lead productive lives (Masten, 2014). Wolin and Wolin (1993) described a cluster of qualities in resilient adults who had grown up in dysfunctional, and often abusive, alcoholic families.

Increasingly, research broadened to the wider social context, examining risk and resilience under devastating social conditions, particularly poverty (Garmezy, 1991) and community violence (Garbarino, 1997). Felsman and Vaillant (1987) followed the lives of 75 high-risk, inner-city men from poverty-stricken, socially disadvantaged families, whose lives were often complicated by substance abuse, mental illness, crime, and violence. Many of them, although indelibly marked by past experience, led courageous lives of mastery and competence. They took an active initiative in shaping their lives, despite occasional setbacks and multiple factors working against them. As the study concluded, their resilience demonstrated that "the events that go wrong in our lives do not forever damn us" (p. 298). In cross-cultural studies in settings ranging from Brazilian favelas and South African migrant camps to U.S. inner cities, Robert Coles (Dugan & Coles, 1989) also found that, contrary to dire predictions of his mental health colleagues, many children did rise above severe hardship without later "time bomb" effects.

Most early resilience research, focused on individual traits and disposition, found assets such as an easygoing temperament and higher intelligence to be helpful, yet not essential, for resilience. Such qualities tend to elicit more positive responses from others and to facilitate coping and problem-solving skills. More importantly, high self-esteem and self-efficacy, with a sense of hope and personal control, make successful coping more likely, whereas a sense of helplessness increases the probability that one adversity will lead to another (Rutter, 1987).

Research on stress and coping (Lazarus & Folkman, 1984) examined the influence of stressful life events in a range of mental and physical disorders to identify character and cognitive styles that mediate physiological processes and enable highly stressed individuals to cope adaptively and remain healthy. Studies of *hardiness* (Maddi, 2002) identified three general characteristics: (1) the belief that they can control or influence events in their experience; (2) an ability to feel deeply involved in or committed to the activities in their lives; and (3) anticipation of change as an exciting challenge to further development.

Antonovsky's (1998) research, now widely replicated, found that a *sense of coherence*—beliefs that one's life challenges were comprehensible, meaningful to tackle, and manageable—enabled mastery and enhanced the quality of life (see Chapter 3). Studies by Werner (Werner & Smith, 2001) found that the core component in effective coping by resilient youth was a feeling of confidence that they could surmount the odds. Even with chaotic households, by their high school years they had developed a sense of coherence, a belief that obstacles could be overcome and that they were in control of their fate. They were significantly more likely than nonresilient youth to have an inner locus of control—an optimistic belief in their ability to shape events. They developed both competence and hope of a better life through their own efforts and relationships.

Murphy (1987) also described the "optimistic bias" of resilient children, noting that many latch on to "any excuse for hope and faith in recovery" (pp. 103–104), actively mobilizing all thoughts and resources that could contribute to their success. In epidemiological research, Taylor (1989) found that people who hold "positive illusions"—selectively positive biases about overcoming such situations as life-threatening illness—tend to do better than others. Such beliefs enable them to retain hope in the face of a grim prognosis. Seligman's (1990) research on "learned optimism" also informs our understanding of resilience. His early studies on "learned helplessness" found that individuals could be conditioned to become passive and give up trying to solve problems when their actions were not predictably linked to rewards. Seligman then showed that optimism can be learned through experiences of mastery, as individuals come to believe that their efforts can yield success (see Chapter 3).

Dynamic Interplay of Multiple Risk and Protective Factors: Biopsychosocial Influences

As studies were extended to a wide range of adverse conditions—impoverished circumstances, chronic illness, catastrophic life events, trauma, and loss—researchers recognized the mutual interaction between nature and nurture in the emergence of resilience (Sameroff, 2010). Increasingly, it became clear that resilience involves the dynamic interplay of multiple risk and protective processes over time, involving individual, interpersonal, socioeconomic, and cultural influences (e.g., Cicchetti, 2010; Garmezy, 1991; Rutter, 1987). More recent resilience research in neurobiology (Cozolino, 2014; Feder, Nestler, & Charney, 2009; Siegel, 2012; Southwick & Charney, 2012) and epigenetics (Kim-Cohen & Turkewitz, 2012; Spotts, 2012) confirms that individual vulnerability or the negative impact of stressful conditions can be counteracted by positive interpersonal and environmental influences, producing neurological, physiological, and even genetic changes.

Relationships Nurture Resilience

Notably, the positive influence of supportive bonds has stood out across studies of individual resilience (Walsh, 1996, 2003). Worldwide, studies of children facing adversity have found the most significant positive influence to be a close, caring relationship with an important adult who believed in them and with whom they could identify, who acted as an advocate for them, and from whom they could gather strength to overcome their hardships (Coles, 1967). Their resilience is greater when they have at least one involved parent, caregiver, or another supportive adult in their extended family or social world (Ungar, 2004). As Werner emphasized, self-esteem and self-efficacy are promoted, above all else, through supportive relationships (Werner & Smith, 2001). All of the resilient children in her seminal longitudinal study (described later) had "at least one person in their lives who accepted them unconditionally, regardless of temperamental idiosyncrasies, physical attractiveness, or intelligence" (p. 512). They knew that there was someone to whom they could turn, who nurtured and reinforced their efforts, sense of competence, and self-worth. Encouraged by their connections with a mentor, many also developed a special interest or skill (e.g., carpentry, art, or creative writing), which enhanced their competence, confidence, and mastery.

A few early studies focused on positive contributions to children's resilience in family organization and emotional climate (Hauser, 1999; Rutter, 1987; Werner & Smith, 2001), stressing the importance of secure attachments, warmth, affection, emotional support, and authoritative parenting with clear-cut, reasonable structure and limits (see Chapter 4). Moreover, studies noted the strong influence of shared belief systems and important information transmitted through family transactions (see Chapters 3 and

5). Parental understanding and communication about crisis events and disruptive transitions mediate children's adaptation by influencing the meaning they make of the experience (Kagan, 1984). If parents are unable to provide this foundation, relationships with other family members, such as older siblings, grandparents, and extended kin, can serve this function.

The importance of social support through troubled times has been amply documented. Friends, neighbors, teachers, coaches, clergy, and other mentors provide encouragement for individual resilience (Rutter, 1987). Resilient children in troubled families often actively recruit and form special attachments with influential adults in their social environment. They learn to choose relationships wisely and tend to select spouses from healthy families.

Taken together, the research on individual resilience has revealed the importance of a relational perspective. Yet most theory, research, and practice has approached the relational context of resilience narrowly, focused on the influence of a significant person in a dyadic relationship. Family studies and intervention programs have tended to focus on parent–child attachment bonds and parenting practices (e.g., Gewirtz, Forgatch, & Wieling, 2008).

For a fuller understanding of resilience, a complex interactional model is required. Systems theory expands our view of individual adaptation as embedded in broader transactional processes in family and social contexts, attending to the multiplicity and mutuality of influences over time. Resilience is woven in a web of relationships and experiences over the life course and across the generations. Both ecological and developmental perspectives are necessary to understand resilience in social and temporal context (see Chapter 9).

Ecological Perspective

With an ecological perspective, we attend to the many spheres of influence in risk and resilience. The immediate and extended family, peer groups, community networks, school and work settings, and larger social systems can be seen as nested contexts for positive development (Bronfenbrenner, 1979). We also consider powerful cultural and spiritual influences (Falicov, 2012; Walsh, 2009d) as well as political, economic, social, and racial climates in which individuals and their families perish or thrive (Rutter, 1987). This multilevel perspective is being advanced in more recent attention to social resilience (Cacioppo, Reis, & Zautra, 2011) and community resilience (Kirmayer et al., 2009; Landau, 2007; Saul, 2013). From a dynamic systems perspective, these are not simply external forces or factors that impact individuals and families. A multilevel systemic view considers the active, ongoing interplay in family transactional processes as members navigate and negotiate their relationship with their social environment (Ungar, 2010).

Certain risks and protective factors tend to co-occur, creating mutually reinforcing "vicious cycles" of risk, such as conditions of poverty in unsafe neighborhoods with inadequate schools, housing instability, and lack of access to jobs and health care, or "virtuous cycles," in safe neighborhoods with better schools, secure homes, and economic, health care, and social resources.

Caution is needed that the notion of resilience is not misused in public policy to withhold social supports or to maintain inequities, rationalizing that success or failure is determined by individual or family strengths or deficits—that is, the presumption that those who are resilient will overcome their hardships and that those who falter simply weren't resilient. It is not enough to bolster the resilience of vulnerable children and families so that they can "beat the odds"; a multilevel approach includes larger systems interventions to improve the odds against them (Seccombe, 2002).

Developmental Perspective

A developmental perspective is also essential to our understanding of resilience (see Chapter 9). Rather than a set of fixed traits, coping and adaptation involve multilevel processes and influences that vary over time (Masten, 2014). Most forms of stress are not simply a short-term, single stimulus, but a complex set of changing conditions with a past history and a future course (Rutter, 1987). Given this complexity, no single coping response is invariably most successful. An adaptive approach that serves well at one point in time may later not be useful in meeting other challenges. It is important to have a variety of coping strategies and the ability to choose among viable options to meet emerging challenges.

Research has increasingly explored coping and adaptation in navigating the unfolding challenges with chronic illness and disability, developmental transitions and role strain, death of a loved one, separation and divorce, stepfamily formation, prolonged unemployment and economic insecurity, maltreatment and neglect, war and genocide, and community disasters (e.g., Lietz, 2013). Stressful life events are more likely to affect functioning adversely when they are untimely and unexpected, when a condition is severe or persistent, or when multiple stressors generate cumulative effects.

A life cycle perspective on individual and family development is needed to understand the dynamic nature of resilience over time (see Chapter 9). The role of early life experience in determining adult capacity to overcome adversity may be less important than previously assumed. Longitudinal studies following individuals throughout adulthood find that resilience cannot be assessed once and for all based on a snapshot of early childhood or one particular time (Vaillant, 2002). People are developing organisms whose life course pathways are flexible and multidimensional (Falicov, 1988).

Werner's longitudinal studies of resilient youth (Werner & Smith, 2001) provide rich evidence for a complex interactional view of resilience, involving multiple internal and external protective influences in lives over time. In a remarkable study of resilience over three decades, they followed nearly 700 multiethnic/multiracial children of plantation workers living in poverty and hardship on the Hawaiian island of Kauai. One-third were classified as "at risk" because of early exposure to at least four additional risk factors, from serious health problems to familial alcoholism, violence, divorce, or mental illness. By age 18, about two-thirds of the at-risk children had done as poorly as predicted, with early pregnancy, mental health service needs, or trouble in school or with the law. However, one-third of those at high risk had developed into competent, caring, and confident young adults, with the capacity "to work well, play well, and love well," as rated on a variety of measures. In later follow-up through midlife, almost all were still living successful lives. Many had outperformed Kauai children from less harsh backgrounds; more were stably married and fewer were divorced or unemployed. Notably, countering assumptions that past trauma experience leaves people more vulnerable to future catastrophic events, fewer suffered trauma effects from devastating Hurricane Iniki, which destroyed much of the island.

They concluded that earlier researchers had focused too narrowly on maternal influence and the damage done by one parent in the nuclear household, missing the importance of siblings and others in the extended family network. Most children got off to a good start through early bonding with at least one caregiver, often a grandmother, older sister, aunt, or other relative who provided care. Yet even a bad start did not determine a bad outcome. The role of a wide variety of supportive relationships was crucial at every age.

Significantly, many overcame early neglect, abandonment, or developmental delays and began to blossom when they benefited from later nurturing care, through adoption or in special mentoring relationships, as with teachers. Throughout their school years, the resilient youth actively recruited support networks in their extended families and communities. Of note, more girls than boys overcame their adversities at all ages. Gender-based socialization may play a role, with girls raised to be more easygoing and to more readily seek out supportive relationships, and with boys taught to be tough and self-reliant. Moreover, often *because* of troubled family lives, competencies were built by assuming early responsibilities for household tasks and care of younger siblings.

Werner and Smith found that nothing is "cast in stone" because of early life experiences. A few individuals identified as resilient at 18 had developed significant problems by age 30. However, the most noteworthy finding was that resilience could be developed *at any point* over the life course. Unexpected events and new relationships often disrupted a negative chain and catalyzed new growth. Of the two-thirds of at-risk children who were troubled and not resilient as adolescents, fully *one-half* had righted themselves by age 30. Delinquent acts had not led to lives of crime, and many had stable marriages and good jobs. In these cases, most reported that some adult had taken an interest in them when they drifted into trouble. They also credited a major turning point: a good marriage, satisfying work, military service, or involvement in a religious group. Such findings support these core convictions in a resilience-oriented approach to practice: (1) people with troubled pasts have the potential to turn their lives around throughout adulthood; and (2) important new relationships and involvements can make the difference.

Werner and Smith's conclusions are echoed by many studies of at-risk children (Luthar, 2006; Masten, 2014), pointing to the beneficial effects of a web of supportive connections. Over the years, positive interactions have a mutually reinforcing effect in positive life trajectories or upward spirals. With multiple pathways in resilience, a downward spiral can be turned around at any time in the life course.

FAMILY RESILIENCE

Family resilience is defined as the ability of the family, as a functional system, to withstand and rebound from adversity (Walsh, 2003). Crucial family processes mediate stressful conditions and can enable families and their members to surmount crises and weather prolonged hardship. Traumatic events and a pileup of stresses can derail these processes. Even members not directly touched by a crisis are affected by the family response, with reverberations throughout the network of relationships (Bowen, 2004). How a family confronts and manages disruptive life challenges, buffers stress, effectively reorganizes, and moves forward with life will influence immediate and long-term adaptation for every family member *and* for the viability of the family unit.

Family resilience involves pathways a family follows as it adapts in the face of stress, initially and over time (Hawley & DeHaan, 1996). Resilient families respond positively to adverse conditions in varied ways, depending on the context, developmental phase, the interaction of risk and protective factors, and the family's shared outlook. McCubbin and McCubbin (1993) first proposed a model of family resilience in which positive adaptation or maladjustment to illness was seen as a function of (1) vulnerability to increased stresses, (2) current family problem-solving capacities, (3) the meaning that the family ascribes to the stress, and (4) the presence of supportive resources. Maladjustment can lead to an intolerable increase in stressors and push a family into a crisis challenging its ability to function.

From Family Damage to Family Challenge

In the mental health field, clinical training, practice, and research have been overwhelmingly deficit-focused. Attention to the family has tended to seek the cause or maintenance of problems in individual functioning. Psychoanalytic and attachment theories, focused predominantly on the role of maternal/caregiver bonds in early childhood, fostered a deterministic and reductionistic view of family influence. Early family systems formulations expanded the lens to the broad network of relationships over time, yet initially tended to focus on dysfunctional family transactional processes. Popular movements for so-called "adult children of dysfunctional families" spared almost no family from accusations of failure and blame and encouraged "survivors" to cut their ties. A narrow focus on individual resilience has led clinicians to attempt to salvage individual survivors without exploring their families' potential, and to write off many troubled families as hopeless. With the clinical field so steeped in pathology and intense scrutiny of family deficits and blindness to family strengths, I noted, only half-jokingly, that a "normal" family might be defined as one that has not yet been clinically assessed.

Systems-oriented family therapists have increasingly rebalanced theory and practice from a deficit-based to a strengths-based perspective (Goldenberg & Goldenberg, 2013; Walsh, 2014b). A family resilience framework builds on these developments and is useful with all strengths-based practice models. What distinguishes a family resilience approach is the focus on *strengths in dealing with adversity*. It shifts our view from seeing distressed families as damaged to understanding how they are challenged.

Strengths in Families Challenged by Adversity

A family resilience approach seeks to understand how all families, in their diversity, can survive and regenerate even under overwhelming stress. It affirms the family potential for self-repair and growth out of crisis and challenge.

My interest in family resilience was sparked in my early research experience in the 1970s with families of psychiatrically hospitalized and "normal" (i.e., nonclinical) young adults (Walsh & Anderson, 1988). The vitality and variations I observed in families in the normal control group— ordinary families living in the community—countered the image of normal families as dull and monotone. Most impressive, a number of parents had experienced serious childhood adversity and yet had grown up able to form and sustain healthy families and to raise their children well to adulthood. Along with other emerging research, these cases cast doubt on traditional clinical assumptions that those who have suffered childhood trauma are wounded for life. Particularly striking were the strengths shown by one family, Marcy and Tom and their five children, whose individual and family resilience was interwoven across the generations.

> Marcy, one of three children in her family of origin, recounted her father's serious drinking problem, repeated job losses, and family abandonment when she was 7. Despite financial hardship and the social stigma of a "broken home," she emerged quite healthy. She attributed her resilience to the strong family unit her mother forged, her strong sibling bonds, and the rock-solid support of her mother's extended family through troubled times.
>
> From her childhood experience, Marcy described her deep determination to build a strong marriage and family life. When asked what had attracted her to Tom, she immediately replied, "First, I knew I wanted a husband who didn't drink. Second, I wanted my children to have a father who would always be there for them." She consciously sought out and married into a strong family. Tom, one of six children from a solid, stable family, was a devoted husband. He was drawn to her "can-do" spirit and admired her family's ability to weather hardship. Together, they raised their children well, keeping valued connections with both extended families, which, in different ways, offered strong parenting models and supportive kin networks.

My research also revealed that resilience could be brought forth even in the clinical cases categorized as "seriously disturbed." A crisis, such as an emotional breakdown of a family member, can jolt the family into awareness of needed changes. In the following case, the son's psychiatric crisis was triggered by reverberations from his father's past trauma at the same age.

> While on a summer trip in Europe, 18-year-old Martin had an acute psychotic episode and was brought home and hospitalized. After a very constrained family interview, his mother asked to meet with me individually. She related the father's past Holocaust experience as a Jewish refugee from Poland. At the age of 18, he had watched as Nazis shot his brother in the head and took his parents away to their deaths. He survived his own concentration camp experience, came to the United States, and became a physician. On their first date, seeing the camp numbers on his arm, she asked him about his experience. He was so visibly shaken that she never asked again. His past was never mentioned as their children were growing up, even though the tattooed numbers were a visible reminder. An implicit family rule, serving to protect him, rendered the unbearable memories and emotions unspeakable. When Martin turned 18, his father's surprising birthday gift was a trip to Europe. Martin went off, but wrote home revealing that he was unable to enjoy himself, aware that terrible things had happened to his father there. The parents didn't reply. Martin attempted to go to Auschwitz, but broke down en route, becoming incoherent and delusional.
>
> This crisis became a turning point. The family taught me that resilience can emerge even in families rigidly governed by long-standing patterns that have become dysfunctional. What had been unspeakable and had gone underground surfaced when Martin reached the age his father had been at the time of his traumatic experience. In following family sessions, the father shared his story, as his wife and children embraced him and comforted him. Family members were commended for their long-standing concern for the father and their wish to spare him pain. He affirmed that he was no longer vulnerable as in earlier years, and their silence was no longer needed. The "gift" was framed as an opportunity to open up communication and to reintegrate old cutoffs. My follow-up with the family a year later found that the parents had made a trip to Poland, to the father's family's town, which was immensely healing for him and deepened the couple's bond. Martin was doing well in college, and, notably, was majoring in communications.

My research experience fundamentally altered the direction of my clinical work, shifting my attention from family deficits toward understanding and facilitating the family processes that generate healing and growth over the life course and across the generations. As therapists, we can help to mobilize new pathways for resilience at whatever point we encounter a family.

Advantages of a Family Resilience Framework

Systems-oriented family process research over recent decades has provided empirical grounding for assessment of effective couple and family functioning (Lebow & Stroud, 2012). However, family scales and typologies tend to be static and acontextual, providing a snapshot of interaction patterns but often not relating them to a family's stressors, resources, and challenges over time and in their social environment. Families most often seek help in crisis periods, when distress and differences from norms are too readily assumed to be signs of family pathology.

A family resilience framework offers several advantages. First, by definition, it focuses on strengths forged under stress, in response to crisis, and under prolonged adversity. Second, it is assumed that no single model of healthy functioning fits all families or their situations. Functioning is assessed in context—relative to each family's values, its structural, situational, and relational resources and constraints, and the challenges it faces. Third, processes for optimal functioning and the well-being of members vary over time as challenges emerge and families evolve over their life course and across the generations.

Although most families might not measure up to ideal models, a family resilience perspective is grounded in a deep conviction in the potential of all families to gain resilience and positive growth out of adversity. Even those who have experienced severe trauma or very troubled relationships can forge healing and transformation across the life course and the generations.

Key Processes in Family Resilience

The family resilience framework shown in Figure 1.1 was developed as a conceptual map to guide practitioners to identify and target key family processes that can reduce stress and vulnerability in high-risk situations; foster healing and growth out of crisis; and empower families to surmount prolonged adversity. This framework is informed by over three decades of clinical and social science research seeking to understand crucial variables contributing to resilience and effective family functioning (Walsh, 2003, 2012a). Based on a survey of the research literature and on my own research and practice experience, I identified nine key processes in family resilience and organized them conceptually in three domains of family functioning: family belief systems, organizational processes, and communication problem-solving processes. The nine key processes are mutually interactive and synergistic, within and across domains.

It is important to stress that this is not a typology or fixed set of traits of a "resilient family." Rather, these are dynamic processes involving

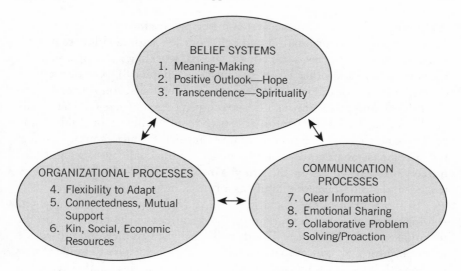

FIGURE 1.1. Key processes in family resilience.

strengths and resources that families can access and gain to increase family resilience. Practitioners can assess and target key processes in intervention and prevention efforts. Various processes may be more (or less) relevant and useful in different adverse situations and in varying social and cultural contexts. Family members may chart varying pathways in resilience depending on their values, resources, challenges, and aims.

This volume attempts to strike a balance that allows us to identify and strengthen core processes, and components, in effective family functioning (see Chapters 3–5), while also being attuned to each family's sociocultural and developmental contexts and the particular strengths needed to meet varied challenges (see Chapters 9–14).

A FAMILY RESILIENCE
ORIENTATION FOR PRACTICE

The family resilience meta-framework presented in this volume can serve as a valuable guide in orienting human services for families facing adversity. A family resilience orientation can be applied usefully with a wide range of crisis situations, disruptive transitions, and multi-stress conditions in clinical and community services. A systemic assessment may be family-centered but include individual and/or group work with youth, parents, or caregivers. Putting a multilevel systemic perspective into practice, interventions may involve coordination and collaboration with health care providers, community agencies, faith congregations, workplace settings, schools, juvenile justice, and other larger systems (see Chapter 8). A systemic view of resilience is essential in all efforts to help individuals, couples, and families to cope and adapt through crisis and prolonged adversity. The family has been a neglected resource in efforts to foster resilience in children and adults—and their communities. A family resilience practice approach fosters a compassionate understanding of family life challenges, searches for unrecognized resources in the broad kinship network—lifelines for resilience—and strengthens the family as a functional unit.

In the field of family therapy, we have realized that successful interventions depend as much on tapping the resources of the family as on the techniques of the therapist. This family resilience framework provides a research-informed, conceptual map and practice principles to guide efforts to strengthen family capacities to deal with serious life challenges. This resilience-based approach is founded on a set of convictions about family potential that shapes all intervention, even with highly vulnerable families whose lives are problem-saturated. Collaboration among family members is encouraged, enabling them to build new and renewed competence, mutual support, and shared confidence that they can prevail under duress. This approach fosters an empowering family climate: Members gain ability to overcome crises and challenges by working together, and they experience success as largely due to their shared efforts and resources. Experiences of shared success enhance a family's pride and sense of efficacy, enabling more effective coping with subsequent life adaptations.

This positive and pragmatic practice framework guides interventions to strengthen family functioning as presenting problems are addressed. This approach goes beyond problem solving to problem prevention; it not only repairs families but also prepares them to meet future challenges. A particular solution to a presenting problem may not be relevant to future problem situations, but in building key transactional processes for resilience, families become more resourceful in dealing with unforeseen problems and averting crises. Thus, in strengthening family resilience, every intervention is also a preventive measure.

The growing body of resilience studies and systems-based research on healthy family processes can inform our efforts to identify strengths and vulnerabilities and target interventions to strengthen key processes for family resilience. In Part II of this volume, Chapters 3 to 5 provide an overview of these core elements, organized in three domains: belief systems, organizational processes, and communication/problem-solving processes. These processes may be expressed in different ways and to varying degrees by families as they fit their values, structures, resources, and life challenges.

To summarize, several basic principles grounded in systems theory serve as the foundations for a family resilience framework:

- Resilience is complex, multidimensional, multilevel, and dynamic in nature. It is best understood and fostered contextually, as a mutual interaction of individual, family, sociocultural, and institutional influences over the life course and across the generations.
- Crisis events and persistent stresses affect the entire family and all its members, posing risks not only for individual dysfunction but also for relational conflict and family breakdown.
- Family processes mediate the impact of adverse situations for all members, their relationships, and the viability of the family unit.
- Maladaptive responses heighten vulnerability and risk of individual dysfunction, relationship distress, and family breakdown.
- Dynamic family processes foster resilience by buffering stress, building strengths, and mobilizing resources to facilitate positive adaptation.
- All individuals and families have the potential to strengthen their resilience; we can maximize that potential by encouraging their best efforts, strengthening key processes, and drawing on resources.

CHAPTER 2

Family Diversity and Complexity in a Changing World

Varied Challenges and Pathways in Resilience

> If we are to achieve a richer culture . . . we must
> recognize the whole gamut of human potentialities, and
> so weave a less arbitrary social fabric, one in which each
> diverse human gift will find a fitting place.
> —MARGARET MEAD, *Blackberry Winter*

Efforts to strengthen family resilience are needed more than ever as families face unprecedented challenges in our rapidly changing world. With profound social, economic, political, and ecological changes over recent decades, families and the societies around them are undergoing major transformation. Our understanding of family functioning and our practice approaches must be attuned to the challenges, constraints, resources, and values of today's families in their sociocultural context.

GROWING DIVERSITY AND COMPLEXITY

Demographic trends reveal increasingly diverse and complex patterns in family life and a more ambiguous and fluid set of categories traditionally used to define the family (Risman, 2010; Walsh, 2012c), including:

- Varied family structures and households.
- Varied and more fluid gender roles, identity, and relationships.
- Growing cultural diversity.
- Vast socioeconomic disparities.
- Varying and expanded family life course.

Although most data reported here are based on demographics in the United States, these patterns are increasingly widespread, especially in developed and rapidly changing societies worldwide.

Varied Family Structures

Over the centuries, in rural settings and preindustrial societies, families have had flexible structures and fluid boundaries with close-knit kinship and social ties, facilitating resilience in weathering harsh and unstable life conditions. With early parental deaths common, children were often raised in stepfamilies and other kin households. Extended networks have become fragmented over recent decades by migration patterns and by the shift to nuclear family households in expanding urban areas (Walsh, 2012c).

The nuclear family structure, which arose with industrialization and urbanization and peaked in the United States in the mid-20th century, became idealized as a self-sufficient household comprised of an intact, two-parent family unit headed by a breadwinner husband and supported by a full-time homemaker wife devoted to household management, child rearing, and elder care. Often, it became a rigid, closed system, isolated from extended kin and community connections—losing relational resources for resilience. The gendered separate spheres of home and workplace, along with unrealistic expectations for couple relationships to meet all needs for intimacy, support, and companionship, contributed to marital discontent and high divorce rates. Women's increasing involvement in the workforce brought changes in gender roles in family life.

Today, a reshaping of contemporary families encompasses multiple, evolving family cultures and structures, as seen in the following trends in the United States.

Dual-Earner Families

Over two-thirds of all two-parent households are dual-earner families (Fraenkel & Capstick, 2012), with two paychecks required to maintain even a modest standard of living. Decades of research clearly show that the vast majority of children do not suffer when their mothers work outside the home. A mother's satisfaction with her situation, the quality of care a child receives, and the involvement of fathers and other caretakers are far more important factors. Still, efforts to navigate multifaceted work and family demands strain everyday family life (Repetti, Wang, & Saxby, 2009). Flexible work schedules and affordable, quality child care are hard to obtain for most American families, in contrast to European societies that provide generous benefits and services to support families with working parents (Cooke & Baxter, 2010). Parents' strategies for organizing breadwinning, child care, and household maintenance are crucial. Flexible arrangements, which allow mothers, fathers, and other caretakers to transcend rigid gender boundaries, help families prevail in the face of unexpected economic and interpersonal crises.

Single-Parent Households

Families headed by an unmarried or divorced parent (predominantly the mother) now account for over 25% of all households. Nearly half of all children, and over 60% of poor, ethnic minority children, can be expected to live for at least part of their childhoods in one-parent households (Anderson, 2012). There has been a decline in unwed teen pregnancy, with its high risk for long-term poverty, poor-quality parenting, and a cluster of health and psychosocial problems. Growing numbers of single adults are choosing to parent on their own if they haven't found a suitable partner to share parenting. Low financial support and involvement with children by nonresidential fathers are the largest factors in child maladjustment. Children generally fare well in financially secure single-parent homes where there is strong parental functioning, especially when supported by extended family and informal kin networks.

Divorce, Remarriage, and Stepfamilies

Divorce rates, after peaking in the 1970s and 1980s, have declined markedly for most first marriages today but remain high for couples with low income and education (Cherlin, 2010). Most divorced individuals go on to remarry, making stepfamilies increasingly common (Pasley & Garneau, 2012). Yet the complexity of stepfamily integration contributes to a higher divorce rate. Claims that divorce inevitably damages children have not been substantiated in large-scale, carefully controlled research on risk and resilience (Greene, Anderson, Forgatch, DeGarmo, & Hetherington, 2012). Fewer than one in four children from divorced families show serious or lasting difficulties (see Chapter 9).

Adoptive, Foster, and Kinship Care Families

Adoptions have been increasing for single parents as well as for couples, both gay and straight (Rampage et al., 2012). Children tend to benefit developmentally in open adoptions, with information about their birth parents, the option for contact, and encouragement to connect with their cultural heritage, especially in multiracial and international adoptions (Pertman, 2011; Samuels, 2010). In foster care, permanency in placement is seen as optimal, keeping siblings together and avoiding the instability and losses of multiple placements. Kinship care by extended family members is preferable, either in legal guardianship or an informal arrangement (Engstrom, 2012). Most often, grandmothers serve as primary caregivers, often with limited financial resources and with health problems that are worsened by being overburdened (see Chapter 13).

Gender Variance, Same-Sex Couples, and Parenting

Conceptualizations of gender identity and sexual orientation have expanded to a broader and more fluid understanding of gender variance including gay, lesbian, bisexual, and transgender persons. Accepting family or social networks has been vital for the resilience of gender nonconforming youth and adults (Oswald, 2002; Sanders & Krall, 2000). Increasing acceptance of same-sex couples and expanding legalization of gay marriage reduce the barriers for the growing numbers of couples and for parents who are raising children through adoption and varied reproductive approaches (Green, 2012). Although stigma and controversy persist, a large body of research over two decades has clearly documented that children raised by lesbian and gay parents fare as well as those reared by heterosexual parents in relationship quality, psychological well-being, and social adjustment (Biblarz & Savci, 2010). Studies of co-mother families find many strengths, including high levels of shared responsibility, decision making, and parental investment. Being reared in gender-variant families involves certain differences, such as family formation and unique social dynamics of having two moms or two dads. Both the commonalities and differences need to be acknowledged. In sum, the research finds that parenting processes are a significant predictor of children's developmental outcomes regardless of the parents' sexual orientations.

Marriage, Childbearing, Cohabitation, and Single Living

Marriage and birth rates have been declining, and the average age of first marriage and childbearing has been rising. Many couples decide not to have children, defining their relationship as family. Cohabitation by unmarried partners is increasingly widespread. Most consider living together as a step toward marriage. Others share a residence and expenses after divorce or widowhood, preferring not to remarry. Couples who drift into cohabitation are more likely to break up within a few years. Childbearing and child rearing by cohabiting couples have become more common. Half of unmarried mothers (i.e., legally single parents) are living with the fathers of their children. Many others live with new partners and have children from current and past relationships who have step- and half-sibling relationships in complex family structures across households. Multipartner fertility and instability in couple relationships and living arrangements increase the risk of child adjustment problems (Fomby & Cherlin, 2007).

More adults are living on their own at some period, although economic strains have led many young adults and older parents to combine residences and resources. An emerging trend for couples is "living apart together" (LAT), where partners in a stable intimate relationship prefer to live separately or live apart at a distance for jobs (Cherlin, 2010). Many adults will marry more than once or form committed partnerships without legal marriage, often in later life. Families with varied structures and different constraints and resources need to organize their lives and role functions to fit their situation. Over two decades of research have provided clear evidence that families and their children can thrive in a variety of kinship arrangements (Lansford, Ceballo, Abby, & Stewart, 2001; Walsh, 2012c).

Varied Gender Roles

Over the centuries (and still today in many traditional cultures) marriage has been viewed in functional terms, with matches made by families on the basis of economic and social position (Coontz, 2005). Traditional patriarchal cultures have regarded wives and children as the property of their husbands and fathers, who held authority and controlled all major decisions and resources. For a husband to be certain of paternity and (male) heirs, the honor of the family required the absolute fidelity of the wife and the chastity of marriageable daughters. The valuing of sons over daughters has had devastating consequences in the maltreatment and very survival of girls in many parts of the world.

In rural settings, the integration of family and work life allowed for intensive sharing of labor. With industrialization and urbanization, family work and paid work became segregated into separate gendered spheres of home and workplace. Rigid gender roles and disparities in power and privilege were detrimental to spousal and parent–child relations (McGoldrick,

Anderson, & Walsh, 1989). Recent decades have seen steady progress in expanding and rebalancing work and family roles so that both parents could share more equitably in the joys and obligations of family life, be gainfully employed, and seek personal fulfillment. Yet gender-based disparities persist in the earnings gap in the workplace and in women's disproportionate burden in household, child care, and elder care responsibilities. Today most men and women share the desire for a full and equal partnership and involvement in family life, yet living out this aim is still a work in progress (Knudsen-Martin, 2012). Studies consistently find that same-sex couples, lacking gender-based differentials, tend to be much more egalitarian in sharing all dimensions of family functioning, including decision making, finances, housework, and child care (Goldberg, 2010; Green, 2012).

Cultural Diversity

One of the most striking features of most societies today is the rapid increase in cultural diversity. In the United States, the proportion of Latino, Asian, and African American families has risen to nearly half of the population and is expected to increase further in coming decades (U.S. Census Bureau, 2014). Although immigrants from a region are often seen as monolithic groups, there are marked differences in country of origin, racial and ethnic identity, language patterns, religious beliefs, education, rural or urban background, and socioeconomic status. Family networks are a complex mix of immigrants and native-born members. Recent economic insecurity and fears of terrorism have heightened racial discrimination and intolerance toward non-European immigrants and minorities, complicating their adaptive challenges.

Recent studies find that immigrant families, especially transnational families, are more resilient in navigating adaptational challenges when they maintain family ties and cultural continuities in both worlds, essentially becoming bicultural (Falicov, 2007, 2012, 2013). Parents are encouraged to raise their children with knowledge of and pride in their kin and community roots, language, ethnic heritage, and spiritual values.

In our multicultural society, growing numbers of children and families are multiethnic and multiracial (Burton, Bonilla-Silva, Ray, Buckelew, & Freeman, 2010; Samuels, 2010). Interracial and interfaith unions are increasingly common and accepted, blending diversity within families (Walsh, 2010). Cultivation of cultural and spiritual pluralism, with mutual understanding and respect for commonalities and difference, can be a source of strength that vitalizes families and society.

Socioeconomic Disparities and Larger Social Forces

Social and economic contexts are vitally important in the success or break-down of marriages and families (Conger, Conger, & Martin, 2010). Many strains and dislocations in families are generated by larger forces in the world around them. Workplace stresses spill over into family life, generating ongoing tensions (Repetti, Wang, & Saxbe, 2009). Conflicting work and family demands create time binds, pressuring lives at an accelerated pace as family members seek elusive "quality time." Many families are exposed to a toxic social and physical environment. Geographic mobility, often due to forces in the job market, has contributed to the fragmentation of families and communities. Many families must repeatedly expand and contract between two-parent and one-parent households to meet demands of distant jobs or military service.

The gap of inequality has widened between the rich and the working class and poor. Harsh economic conditions and job dislocation have a devastating impact on family formation, stability, and well-being. Many struggle anxiously through uncertain times when workers lose jobs. As the economy has shifted from the industrial and manufacturing sectors to services and technology, those with limited education, job skills, and employment opportunities have been hardest hit (see Chapter 8). A new "marriage gap" is increasingly aligned with the growing income gap, with striking racial, ethnic, socioeconomic, and educational differentials (Cherlin, 2010; Fincham & Beach, 2010). Those with bleak earnings prospects are less likely to get married and more likely to divorce. Persistent unemployment and recurring job transitions can fuel substance abuse, family conflict and violence, homelessness, and an increase in poor, single-parent households. Children's life chances are worsened by chronic conditions of discrimination, neighborhood decay, poor schools, crime, violence, and lack of opportunity. Lack of access to good health care and the risks of toxic environmental conditions, neighborhood violence, drug abuse, and HIV/AIDS drastically foreshorten life expectancy.

Yet it is a mistake to equate poor families with problem families. Data for more than 100,000 families from a national survey reveal that, although families in poverty experience socioeconomic disadvantages, they have many strengths, such as the closeness of relationships, and shared meals, outings, and spiritual practices (Valladares & Moore, 2009). Strong extended family bonds foster resilience in low-income families, especially in African American and immigrant families that have struggled to over-come persistent conditions of poverty and discrimination (Boyd-Franklin, 2004; Boyd-Franklin & Karger, 2012).

As Aponte (1994) stresses, the emotional and relational problems in poor, disproportionately minority families must be understood within their socioeconomic and political contexts: they are vulnerable to larger social dislocations and cannot insulate themselves. In harsh economic times, "when society stumbles, its poorest citizens are tossed about and often crushed" (p. 8). Immense structural disparities perpetuate a vast chasm between the rich and the poor, increasing the vulnerability of families struggling to make ends meet. Structural changes in the larger society and its institutional supports are essential for them to thrive.

Instead of individual-level interventions that seek to rescue the most vulnerable children, multilevel systemic approaches are required, with policies and structural changes aimed at narrowing persistent gaps in education, income, and life opportunities.

Varying and Expanded Family Life Course

As societies worldwide are rapidly aging, four- and five-generation families are increasingly common. Two or three committed long-term relationships, along with periods of cohabitation and single living, are increasingly common (Fincham & Beach, 2010; Sassler, 2010). Despite today's high divorce rate, most people remain optimistic; they long for a romantic, committed relationship, and if their attempt fails or their needs change, they try again. Single adults and couples without children forge a variety of intimate relationships and significant kin and friendship bonds within and beyond households.

Our view of the family must be expanded to the varied course of the life cycle: to a wider range of options, life phases, and transitions fitting the diverse preferences and challenges that make each family unique. Many adults and their children experience a variety of family structures as they come together, separate, and recombine. For resilience, they will need to learn how to navigate these transitions and how to live successfully in complex and fluid households and kinship arrangements (see Chapter 9).

Family Complexities

A pluralistic understanding of family functioning is required, mindful that families in the distant past and in cultures worldwide have had multiple, varied structures, and that effective family processes and the quality of relationships matter most for the well-being of children. Families with varied configurations have different structural constraints and resources for functioning. With changing role relations, two-earner families must organize their households and family lives to fit their situation. Single parents must organize differently from two-parent households. Stepfamily constellations need to bridge households and complex extended family networks.

An outdated or unrealistic model of the ideal family can compound a sense of deficiency and failure for families. Despite the growing involvement of fathers and the active contributions to family life by grandparents and other caregivers, there is a lingering presumption that they "help out" or stand in for a working or absent mother, who is still expected to have primary responsibility for the well-being of children. Our language and preconceptions can pathologize or stigmatize relationship patterns that don't conform to the intact nuclear family model.

It is commonly presumed that a single-parent family is inherently deficient and damaging. Often, problems of a child are reflexively attributed to "a broken home" or the absence of a father figure in the home. Even the term "single-parent family" can obscure the important role of a nonresidential parent or a caregiving grandparent and kin network. The pejorative label "deadbeat dad" writes off many fathers who care deeply about their children and could potentially become more involved and responsible than in the past.

Strong bonds forged by stepparents or adoptive parents are unacknowledged, and may legally be threatened, when they are regarded as not being the "real" or "natural" parent. The belief that stepfamilies are inherently deficient often leads them to emulate the intact nuclear family model—sealing their borders, cutting off ties with nonresidential parents, and feeling they have failed when they don't immediately blend.

The strong body of family process research can inform practice, documenting that a variety of family structures can function well; none is inherently healthy or pathological. Research also sheds light on the processes families can strengthen for resilience, as we will see in the following chapters. Key issues concern the quality of relationships within and beyond household borders, whether members feel abandoned, harmed, or cared for by those who are important in their lives, and how positive bonds can be strengthened. A resilience-based approach taps into each family's resources and builds on its potential.

The Yearning for Home

Like Dorothy in *The Wizard of Oz*, we find in life's journeys that there's no place like home. The poet Maya Angelou (2004) remarked on this powerful ache for home in all of us. Yearnings for "family," "home," and "community" are stronger than ever, heightened by continuing threats of global instability. In our turbulent times, our challenge is to expand the relational meaning of "home" and construct new maps to find our way home, from the past and into the future. In today's mobile societies, migrations, and environmental disruptions, many can't return to former homes. Some take flight from unsupportive homes or communities. Most do their best to forge new pathways.

The challenge in our times is to reconstruct a vision of home and make a place where all of us can live and love well into the future: where we can feel "at home" and that we belong, with nourishing bonds and resourceful connections in our social environment. By expanding the concept of home-maker, we can become *home builders,* conserving or creatively refashioning valued elements from our past along with our emerging priorities, either in an old or new setting. This idea of home building extends to a sense of community beyond the immediate family and intertwined in meaning and experience. All concepts of the self and constructions of the world are fundamentally products of relationships, and it is through our interdependence that meaningful lives are best sustained (Bellah et al., 1985). "Community, like the sacred, is an idea that becomes reality because we believe in it" (Bateson, 1994, p. 42). We must then act on this belief, reaffirming it in practice.

FAMILY TRANSFORMATIONS:
FORGING RESILIENCE

Families today are in transformation, with growing diversity and complexity in structure, gender roles and sexual orientation, cultural and socioeconomic influences, and life cycle patterns. As family scholars have stressed, no single model should be used as the standard against which various family forms are measured. Our growing diversity requires an inclusive pluralism, going beyond tolerance of difference to respect for many varied ways to be a family, recognizing both their distinctiveness and their commonalities. In fact, families in our distant past and in most cultures worldwide have constructed multiple, varied kinship arrangements to fit their needs and values.

What remains constant is the centrality, and the fundamental necessity, of relatedness. Most people still view loving, committed bonds as the most important sources of happiness and fulfillment in life. Many, in uncharted territory, are unsure how to build and sustain healthy families that function well and are resilient under stress. Despite concerns, most adults are optimistic about the future of families. The vast majority regard their own family as the most important and satisfying element in their life, and as close as or closer than their childhood family.

Most families today are showing remarkable resilience, making the best of their situations and creatively reconfiguring family life. As they construct varied household and kinship arrangements, they are devising new relational strategies to fit their resources and challenges, and inventing new models of human connectedness. Most are sustaining strong extended family connections across distances and finding kinship with close friends. Many are seeking community and spirituality outside mainstream institutional structures, weaving together meaningful elements of varied traditions to fit their lives (D'Amore & Scarciotta, 2011; Walsh, 2010).

In Stacey's (1990) ethnographic study of working-class families, particularly impressive were bold initiatives to reshape the experience of divorce from a painful, bitter schism and loss of resources into a viable kin network involving new and former partners, multiple sets of children, step-kin, and friends—into households and support systems collaborating to survive and flourish. It is ironic that such families are termed "nontraditional," as their flexibility, diversity, and community recall the resilience found in the varied households and loosely knit kinship of the past.

With tumultuous conditions in our world today, our lives can seem unpredictable and overwhelming. Many families are experiencing actual and symbolic losses with alterations in their family arrangements and environmental context. The many discontinuities and unknowns can generate considerable tension. Yet rather than collapsing under these pressures and threats, humans are surprisingly resilient, as Robert Lifton (1993) contends. He compares our predicament and response to those of the Greek god Proteus: just as Proteus was able to change shape in response to crisis, we create new psychological, social, and familial configurations, exploring new options and transforming our lives many times over the life course. Similarly, Mary Catherine Bateson (1994) observes that adaptation "comes out of encounters with novelty that may seem chaotic" (p. 8). An intense multiplicity of vision, enhancing insight and creativity, is necessary. Although we can never be fully prepared for the demands of the moment, Bateson affirms that we can be strengthened to meet uncertainty:

> The quality of improvisation characterizes more and more lives today, lived in uncertainty, full of the inklings of alternatives. In a rapidly changing and interdependent world, single models are less likely to be viable and plans are more likely to go awry. The effort to combine multiple models risks the disasters of conflict and runaway misunderstanding, but the effort to adhere blindly to some traditional model for a life risks disaster not only for the person who follows it but for the entire system

in which he or she is embedded, indeed for all other living systems with which that life is linked. (1994, p. 8)

If we knew the future of a particular family, therapists and other helping professionals might be able to prepare that family with all the necessary skills and attitudes. But such stability or certainty has never existed. Instead, ambiguity is the essence of life; it cannot be eliminated. We must help families to find coherence within complexity. In Bateson's apt metaphor, "We are called to join in a dance whose steps must be learned along the way. Even in uncertainty we are responsible for our steps" (1994, p. 10).

Gergen (1991) observes that when we become aware of the multiplicity in diverse human experience, we begin to see that each ethnic community, political group, and economic class has its own limited, partial perspective and frames the world in its own terms. We may lose the safe and sure claims to truth, objectivity, and authority—and the idea of self as the center of meaning. Yet, he contends, we may gain something scarcely known in Western culture: the reality, the centrality, and the fundamental necessity of relatedness.

Amid the swirling confusion and upheaval, we can help families to prevail by sustaining continuities along with change and by gaining coherence in the midst of complexity and uncertainty. In the process of small victories, families build competence and confidence. Also, as Bateson (1994) urges, families must be encouraged to carry on the process of learning throughout life in all they do—"like a mother balancing her child on her hip as she goes about her work with the other hand and uses it to open the doors of the unknown" (p. 9). The ability to combine multiple roles and to embrace new challenges can be learned. A family resilience approach to practice encourages such vision and skills. Crisis and challenge are part of the human condition; how we respond can make all the difference for family well-being and successful adaptation.

Defining the Family: A Broad, Pluralistic Perspective

Families comprise a complex web of kinship ties within and across households and generations, evolving and changing over time. Family systems encompass the entire multigenerational network, and may be defined by blood, legal, and/or historical ties; formal and informal kinship bonds; residential patterns; and future commitments (see Chapter 6 on mapping family systems). Many indigenous cultures don't make distinctions between formal and informal kin or "natural" family members and those inducted by marriage or adoption (Robbins, 2015). A sister-in-law is a sister; brothers of a grandfather may be called grandfathers. Family processes support the integration and maintenance of the family unit and its ability to carry out essential tasks for the growth and well-being of its members, especially the nurturance, guidance, and protection of children, elders, and other vulnerable members.

As helping professionals, we need to be aware of implicit assumptions about family normality, health, and dysfunction we bring to our work from our own world views, based in our cultural standards, personal experience, and clinical theories. Our views of normality and health are socially constructed (Walsh, 2012c). Widely held cultural ideals of the "normal" family become standards by which families are judged—and judge themselves—to be healthy and successful. When nonconforming families are viewed as pathological and are stigmatized, it makes their adaptations more difficult. In my research experience with nonclinical families, many worried about how well they were doing; others declined involvement, expressing concern that they would be found inadequate. This gave me perspective on what is commonly labeled as "resistance" in clinical practice. Families often don't come for help because they fear being judged dysfunctional or deficient. They may have had such blaming or shaming experiences in the past. Through these filtered lenses, we and our clients, together, construct the problems and deficits we "discover" in families, and we risk setting therapeutic goals tied to faulty preconceptions about healthy functioning. This makes it imperative to examine our own beliefs, which influence family assessment, how we define and explain problem situations, success or failure, and therapeutic goals.

Helping Families Meet the Challenges of Our Times

In the public rhetoric on "family values" we need to keep in mind that despite cultural and structural differences, the vast majority of families hold strong traditional values of commitment, responsibility, and mutual support. Yet today's families are struggling in the face of overwhelming challenges, from pressures in meeting job and home-front demands to economic dislocations affecting job security, medical coverage, and retirement benefits. Parents worry about the impact of larger forces on their children, from war and terrorist attacks to the cultural transmission of violence, sexism, and racism. For individual and family well-being, quality-of-life issues are at the fore, including a desire for more community involvement, spiritual meaning, social justice, and a concern for the environment.

As we create more viable approaches to family life in our times, our families and society can experience new growth and transformation for greater individual and family well-being. Such attempts must overcome tremendous institutional resistance. To support family resilience, we must press for larger systemic changes and creative strategies for workplace security and flexibility; adequate, affordable health care; and quality day care for children and frail elders. Our challenge is to craft social and economic policies as well as clinical and community services that are responsive to the new family realities and challenges.

When families face serious life crises and challenges, the concept of family resilience affirms their potential for survival, repair, and growth, and offers a valuable framework for strength-oriented approaches to practice. Because families have varied resources, challenges, and adaptive strategies, there are many pathways in family resilience. Clinicians and community-based professionals equipped with an understanding of key processes can mobilize resilience-building resources in distressed families and in those at risk. Distilling the large body of research conducted over recent decades, Chapters 3–5 describe and illustrate these core dynamic processes in resilience.

PART II

KEY FAMILY PROCESSES IN RESILIENCE

CHAPTER 3

Belief Systems

The Heart and Soul of Resilience

Deep in my heart I do believe
We shall overcome someday!
—Anthem in U.S. Civil
Rights Movement

Belief systems are at the heart of all family functioning and are powerful forces in resilience. We cope with crisis and prolonged adversity by making meaning of our experience: linking it to our social world, to our cultural and spiritual beliefs, to our multigenerational past, and to our hopes and dreams for the future. How families view their problems and their options can make all the difference between coping and mastery or dysfunction and despair. This chapter draws on research and practice knowledge to identify key beliefs that facilitate resilience in families facing serious life challenges.

In the empirically based Western world view, it is often said that "seeing is believing." Evidence is required for proof. Native Americans would say, "We must believe in something to see it" (Walsh, 2009d). Beliefs are the lenses through which we view the world as we move through life, influencing what we see or do not see and what we make of our perceptions (Wright & Bell, 2009). Beliefs are at the very heart of who we are and how we understand and make sense of our experience. Our core beliefs, whether secular or sacred, anchor us in the vastness of the unknown, defining our reality.

Belief systems broadly encompass values, convictions, attitudes, biases, and assumptions, which coalesce to form a set of basic premises that trigger emotional responses, inform decisions, and guide actions. Facilitative beliefs increase options for problem resolution, healing, and growth, whereas constraining beliefs perpetuate problems and restrict options (Wright & Bell, 2009). Affirming beliefs—that we are valued and have potential to succeed—can help us to rally in times of crisis. Beliefs that our own needs are "selfish" or unimportant can lead to selfless caregiving or relentless accommodation, leaving us depleted, guilty, or resentful. Some beliefs are more useful than others, depending on our situation. Some are more socially desirable or acceptable within a particular culture. Beliefs and actions are intertwined: our actions and their consequences can reinforce or alter our beliefs.

SHARED BELIEF SYSTEMS

Our beliefs are socially constructed, evolving in a continuous process through transactions with significant others and the larger world (Gergen, 1991; Hoffman, 1990). We experience commonalities not only because of similar events, but also when we construe and interpret the implications of events in a similar way. In living and being together we influence each other's beliefs. We develop our identities within our families, professions, and communities by the belief systems that we share. We live our lives barely aware of many beliefs that powerfully influence us.

Each family's shared beliefs are anchored in cultural values and influenced by its position and experiences in the social world over time (Hess & Handel, 1959). Families construct shared beliefs about how the world operates and their own place in it (Reiss, 1981). These paradigms, or schemas (Dattilio, 2005), influence how family members view and interpret events and behavior. Family belief systems provide coherence and organize experience, enabling members to make sense of crisis situations. They provide a meaningful orientation for understanding one another and approaching new challenges. Shared beliefs develop and are reaffirmed or altered over the course of the family life cycle and across the multigenerational network of relationships.

In well-functioning families, members share a congruent set of beliefs and yet maintain openness to differing viewpoints, approaching human experience as subjective and unique for each person and situation. Because the family, its members, and their environment vary over time, not all beliefs will be shared. Siblings, for example, may have different perspectives arising from nonshared experiences and also influenced by genetic predis-position, birth order, gender, family roles, relationship dynamics, and the timing of critical events. Still, the dominant beliefs in a family system—and its culture—most strongly influence how the family, as a functional unit, will deal with adversity.

Family Norms and Identity

These shared beliefs shape family norms, expressed through patterned and predictable rules that organize interactions and guide family life. These rules, both explicit and implicit, provide expectations about relationships, roles, actions, and consequences. Core beliefs are fundamental to family identity and coping strategies, expressed in such rules as "We never give up when the going gets rough" or "Men don't cry." Over time, mutual expectations are reappraised and rules altered in light of changing needs and constraints, such as the disruption of a parental role as breadwinner by a disability. Family rituals and routines affirm and convey family iden-tity and beliefs (Imber-Black, 2012). They maintain a sense of continuity through disruption, linking past, present, and future through shared tradi-tions and expectations (see Chapter 4).

The deep social and cultural roots of our beliefs often make it diffi-cult to step outside our own context to notice and comment on them. My experiences while living and working in Morocco not only immersed me in a culture vastly different from my own; they also brought new perspec-tives on my social world upon reentry, as I noticed and questioned fam-ily patterns and gender constraints taken for granted. As Bateson (1994) observed, seen from a contrasting point of view or through the eyes of an outsider, one's own familiar patterns can become accessible to choice and change.

Constructing Belief Systems: Storytelling and Narrative Coherence

Meaning-making occurs through the narratives we construct to make sense of our world and our position in it (Freedman & Combs, 1996). Storytelling has served in every time and place to transmit cultural and family beliefs that guide personal expectations and actions. For centuries, Moroccans have gathered around storytellers in the lively marketplace of Marrakech, the J'maa el F'na, to hear tales of life and love, of tragic plights and comic relief, of human foibles and heroism. The stories are often dramatically acted out in costume and mime, with the perils and triumphs accentuated by Berber drumming. Like storytelling and theater in cultures the world over, they convey personal mores, family values, and adaptive strategies for mastering life's challenges.

Cultural changes, disrupting traditional modes of understanding the self and others, generate heightened concern for coherence and integrity in life stories (Geertz, 1986). With today's technological advances, images and stories of marriage and family life are transmitted globally. They powerfully shape and reflect values and concerns, what it means to be a good husband or wife, father or mother, son or daughter; to be successful in life or to fail. These portrayals via satellite and the Internet are often strangely incongruent with local life. Not surprisingly, cultural anthropologists find multiple, conflicting identities in the life narratives of young people who are challenged by shifting norms and their own uncertain place in our rapidly changing world.

The multigenerational family transmission of stories and rituals conveys enduring values and traditions for stability and continuity amid rapid change. Those that preserve links to a family's cultural heritage are especially valuable for immigrant families, whose members can too easily lose their sense of identity, community, and pride amid pressures for assimilation to the dominant culture (Falicov, 2012, 2013). For transnational families living "between two worlds" and often feeling they belong to neither, Falicov encourages them to live with "two hearts" instead of a broken heart. It's important to ask about their families' migration experiences, attending to the traumas and losses they suffered and to the sources of resilience that enabled them to survive, regenerate, and make their way in a new world. Recovering such stories can restore a vital sense of connection and meaning, transforming their experience as they weave together the separate strands of their lives into a larger whole (see Chapters 11 and 14). Researcher Elizabeth Stone found that family stories told by new immigrants in the United States and their American-born children help retain affiliation with their country of origin, reinforcing a dual identity and affiliation (Stone, Gomez, Hotzoglou, & Lipnitsky, 2005). Stone views family stories as the DNA of family life.

In sharing stories we come to know our personal and collective histories and ourselves, building coherent identities to make sense of the larger social context and our place in it. Griffin (1993) asserts that we all have a deep need to be connected to the larger society and to our own history. She contends that all history is a part of us, so that when stories are told and secrets revealed—whether about our own family members or about tragic events or heroic deeds long ago or far away—our lives are made clearer to us.

Stories have particular significance in our response to major life challenges. Adversity and the accompanying distress become tensions and organizing principles for coherent life stories and belief systems (Bruner, 1986). Whether a widespread catastrophe, a personal tragedy, or persistent hardship, adversity generates a crisis of meaning and a potential disruption of personal integration. This tension prompts the construction or reorganization of our life story and beliefs. Over time, we revise our stories of adversity and resilience to gain narrative coherence and integrity (Cohler, 1991). A major therapeutic task involves the effort to reorganize a life story that presents past or ongoing misfortune as an impediment to the ability to move forward.

All helping professionals can offer a healing context for dialogue and storytelling. Kleinman (1988) found that most family members who have experienced serious illnesses benefit greatly from the opportunity to tell their stories of suffering. Yet professionals need to be attuned to cultural differences. For instance, counselors for Cambodian refugees who fled widespread massacres in the 1970s found that many families told their stories of the terror and torture just once, and then preferred to go on with their lives and speak of it no more (Mollica, 2006). Community-based, resilience-oriented approaches elicit stories of courage, perseverance, and mastery alongside suffering with those who have experienced extreme trauma (see Chapters 8 and 11).

Therapists can help clients to recover important stories from the past that have become fragmented or lost, often in family processes of secrecy, denial, distortion, and relational cutoff (Byng-Hall, 2004; Imber-Black, 1998). Such stories may concern stigmatizing situations, such as gender-nonconforming relationships, or recount blame-, shame-, or guilt-laden incidents involving substance abuse; violence or sexual abuse; suicide; or accusations of unethical, scandalous, or illegal conduct. In narrative therapy approaches (Freedman & Combs, 1996; White & Epston, 1990), the therapist and family collaborate in developing alternative meanings and new, more hopeful, affirming stories in place of problem-saturated narratives.

Important beliefs for family resilience can be organized into three key processes, as outlined in Table 3.1: making meaning of adversity, a positive outlook, and transcendent or spiritual pathways for rising above adversity.

MAKING MEANING OF ADVERSITY

How families make sense of a crisis situation and endow it with meaning is crucial for resilience (Antonovsky, 1998; Patterson & Garwick, 1994). For instance, Kagan (1984) found that families can have a positive mediating

TABLE 3.1. Key Processes in Family Resilience: Belief Systems

Making meaning of adversity

- Relational view of resilience—versus "rugged individual."
- Normalize, contextualize distress: common, understandable in adverse situations.
- Sense of coherence: view crisis as a shared challenge; meaningful, comprehensible, manageable.
- Facilitative appraisal: explanatory attributions, future expectations.

Positive outlook

- Hope, optimistic bias; confidence in overcoming challenges.
- Encouragement: affirm strengths and build on potential.
- Active initiative and perseverance (can-do spirit).
- Master the possible; accept what can't be changed; tolerate uncertainty.

Transcendence and spirituality

- Larger values, purpose.
- Spirituality: faith, contemplative practices, community; connection with nature.
- Inspiration: envisioning new possibilities, aspirations; creative expression; social action.
- Transformation: learning, change, and positive growth from adversity.

influence in children's adjustment to an emotionally stressful experience, such as a father's prolonged absence or parental divorce, by sharing helpful perceptions and an understanding of what is happening and what will happen to them. The ability to clarify and give meaning to a precarious situation makes it easier to bear.

As Reiss (1981) observed, a family's shared world view influences how members approach a stressful new situation and the meanings they attach to life challenges. A critical event or disruptive transition can catalyze a major shift in a family belief system, with reverberations for immediate reorganization and long-term adaptation.

Relational View of Resilience

The protest song "We Shall Overcome" became the anthem of the 1960s Civil Rights movement and has inspired hope and creative action in many parts of the world. This simple yet profound phrase expresses the core conviction in relational resilience: in joining together, we strengthen our ability to overcome adversity.

The individualistic ethos underlying the myth of the rugged individual denies the crucial importance of the interpersonal and the communal. At

the core of strong families is the value of kinship and pride in family identity (Beavers & Hampson, 2003). Genuine caring is effective even in families where parenting skills are more modest. An expectation of satisfaction
from relationships, in turn, reinforces involvement and mutual investment.

Meaningful kin and community connections are vital lifelines in
times of distress. As we will see in Chapters 4 and 5, a relational view is
expressed in a family's organizational processes and in communication
and problem-solving processes. For instance, a shared commitment to the
marital vow "in sickness and in health" sustains bonds through serious illness or disability and can bolster collaborative actions to support optimal
recovery (see Chapter 12). When families view a crisis as a shared challenge to be tackled together, their resilience is strengthened.

Trust is essential. When families hold a positive world view of human
nature as essentially good, or at least as not malign in intent, it enables them
to relate with trust (Beavers & Hampson, 2003). However, the ability to be
trustful and to view others as caring can be impaired by repeated experiences of betrayal, exploitation, abuse, or discrimination. Yet family members
must at least be able to assume benign intentions in their own significant
relationships rather than believe that others' actions are hostile or destructive
in intent. Confidence in one another's basic goodwill is essential to achieve
closeness and collaboration, and to support trust, joy, and comfort in relating.

Families are better able to weather adversity when members have an
abiding loyalty and faith in each other, rooted in a strong sense of trust.
They share confidence that home is a safe and welcoming place and that
they can count on one another. Here again, beliefs and actions are intertwined. When members are trustworthy they stand by their word and stand
by each other. Relationships are strengthened by actions that show trustworthiness, and that are based on consideration of one another's welfare.
Trust fosters open communication, mutual understanding, and problem
solving, as pioneer family therapists observed. Boszormenyi-Nagy (1987)
emphasized this ethical dimension of family relationships in his concept of
"merited trust," involving multigenerational legacies of parental accountability and filial loyalty, which sustains a strong relational foundation and
buffers periods of stress and disorganization.

Normalizing and Contextualizing Adverse Experience and Distress

In facing a crisis or multi-stress conditions, people commonly feel overwhelmed and unable to control events impinging on their lives. Families

gain valuable perspective when they can view their problems in context. We can foster their resilience by *normalizing* and *contextualizing* distress, so that family members can enlarge their understanding to see their reactions and difficulties as understandable in light of their adverse situation, such as a painful loss or daunting obstacles. The tendency for blame, shame, and pathologizing is reduced in viewing their complicated feelings and dilemmas as "normal," in other words, common and expectable among families in similar predicaments or environmental contexts.

Viewing adversity in a developmental context also facilitates resilience (see Chapter 9). Positive adaptation is fostered through acceptance of the passage of time and the need for change with new developmental challenges. Life cycle transitions or other disruptive events can also be seen as milestones that may spark reevaluation of assumptions about one's place in the world. In this way, painful transitions can catalyze growth and transformation.

Sense of Coherence

The concept of *sense of coherence* was developed by Antonovsky (1998) as a model for understanding the emergence of health—a "salutogenic" orientation in contrast to the dominant "pathogenic" paradigm in biomedical research and practice. Antonovsky remarked that, given the stress-producing nature of the human condition, the miracle and mystery are that any organism ever survived for any length of time. The important question then is, what resources promote stability and health in the face of disruption and change?

Sense of coherence (SOC) is defined as a global orientation to life as comprehensible, manageable, and meaningful. A strong sense of coherence involves confidence in the ability to clarify the nature of problems: to understand and make sense of an adverse situation. Demands are believed to be manageable by mobilizing useful resources, including relational supports. Stressors are viewed as meaningful challenges that matter, that we are motivated to deal with successfully, and that enhance feelings of social integration and purpose in life. A sense of coherence has been found to contribute significantly to health, mental well-being, and quality of life in at-risk groups, and to be more influential than such individual traits as temperament or intelligence (Cederblad & Hansson, 1996). It taps into important elements missing in such concepts as *locus of control* and *mastery*, which focus more narrowly on self-reliance and specific coping strategies. The SOC concept cuts across such influences as culture, class, and gender, emphasizing flexibility in selecting varied strategies that are useful and preferred in dealing with diverse challenges.

Antonovsky and Sourani (1988) assessed *family sense of coherence* in families coping with a particular crisis. They studied working-class couples faced with the husband's disability and subsequent pileup of stresses. A high sense of family coherence predicted better coping and adaptation, with greater satisfaction within the family and in its fit with the community.

Appraisal of Adverse Situation and Future Course

Our appraisal of stress events and our resources to deal with them strongly influence our response (Lazarus & Folkman, 1984). The same event may be perceived as burdensome, threatening, harmful, benign, or irrelevant. Stressful life events are most distressing when we feel little control over them or when they pose a major threat to our lives, our loved ones, and our understanding of ourselves and the meaning of life (Cohler, 1991). The meanings attributed to problems and the ways distress is handled vary with different family and cultural norms. Epidemiologists report that at any given time, 75% of all Americans are "symptomatic," experiencing physical or psychological distress. Yet most don't seek treatment, instead defining their distress as part of normal life (Kleinman, 1988). Distressed families may attempt to deal with problems in various ways. Studies have found that highly resilient people do reach out for help when needed, turning to kin, social, and religious support systems—most often before going to professionals.

Causal and Explanatory Beliefs

When adversity strikes, we attempt to make sense of how things have happened through causal and explanatory attributions. Some blame others, or view themselves as victims in a dangerous and hostile world beyond their control. Many believe that adversity is simply a matter of bad luck. Some hold strong religious beliefs that misfortune is a sign that they have sinned and deserve to suffer or be punished. It's important to explore the family, cultural, and religious roots of such beliefs and their implications.

Western culture emphasizes personal responsibility, with the belief that we are masters of our fate. In U.S. society, we hold a curious split of individual and family responsibility: we tend to credit individuals for their success but blame their families for any problems. A Moroccan Muslim friend once told me of his father's drinking and abandonment of the family, and of his mother's retreat into her own sorrows. When, from my American perspective, I was puzzled that he harbored no anger or blame toward them for his own life difficulties, he replied, "But you don't understand. I'll always be grateful to them: my parents gave me life."

In many cultures and faith traditions, adversity is ascribed to fate, destiny, or God's will, and may be regarded as beyond human comprehension. Hindus believe that misfortune may be the result of bad karma, due to one's conduct or circumstances in a previous life. In many indigenous traditions, when things go wrong in a family, people externalize blame, believing that others who are envious, spiteful, or wish them harm may have brought about their plight; they turn to highly respected shamans or faith healers to restore health or good fortune (Falicov, 2013; Wright & Bell, 2009).

High-functioning families in mainstream U.S. culture tend to view problems as resulting from many contributing variables rather than from one cause—essentially holding a systemic orientation, although they never heard of systems theory (Beavers & Hampson, 2003). Their responses vary pragmatically with the situation. For example, parents see that attempts at autocratic control of children can trigger reactions of angry defiance, just as uncooperative defiance invites tyrannical control. Aware of mutual influences, family members avoid blaming or typecasting others as villains or victims. In contrast, poorly functioning families tend to adhere rigidly to one explanation, get locked into a belief in a single cause or personal failing, and are prone to blaming and scapegoating. Families whose members repeatedly blame one another tend to have more conflict and less solidarity than families who unite by attributing blame beyond their borders (Wright & Bell, 2009). A united front mobilized by the belief "Us against the world" may be a survival strategy in highly challenging contexts, yet can have a cost in social isolation, alienation, and mistrust.

How family members define and frame a problem situation will influence how they attempt to deal with it. A family's general world view may not fit well with a particular challenge. For instance, a family that believes no effort should be spared until a solution is found may have difficulty accepting and living with a problem that can't be solved or an illness that cannot be cured.

In all family assessments, it is useful to explore patterns of problem explanation and attribution. Preoccupation with causal questions and accusations—"Who is at fault?"—is natural in situations of tragedy that go unexplained, such as the disappearance of an airliner. In families, parents (especially mothers) are particularly vulnerable to blame and guilt when something happens to a child, due to expectations of responsibility for their children's well-being. When adversity strikes, issues of blame, shame, and guilt can become problematic, tearing family members apart.

One couple, Jean and Jerry, were on the brink of divorce several months after their 3-year-old son had drowned in the lake behind their vacation cabin. Each blamed the other for not watching the boy, who waded into water to retrieve a ball and dropped from sight. They fought bitterly, faulting each other for negligence. It was crucial to explore and acknowledge each parent's painful self-doubts and self-blame under the surface of their mutual attacks. Eventually, they both owned partial responsibility for the ambiguity in their communication about who was "on duty" at the time of the accident. Other contributing factors were also acknowledged, such as the rocky shoreline, which increased the risk of a fall. In shifting from blame to a fuller appreciation of the many variables, Jean and Jerry became better able to share their sorrow, to consider what might be learned from the tragedy, and to begin a healing process together.

When people are locked into a particular explanation of their experience and we invite them to reflect on their beliefs, they become freer to consider other possibilities. The following questions can be useful to guide inquiry with families in crisis: How do family members try to make sense of the situation? How do they think it occurred? What additional factors may have been involved? Do they fault themselves? Anyone else? Do they believe it was accidental or intentional? Are family members overly preoccupied with blame, shame, or guilt? How do they agree or disagree in their views? What connections do they make to other adversities that have occurred in their lives and in their family's past history? How do cultural beliefs influence their views? Often this is the first time members have shared their private beliefs with one another. They may be surprised to learn that, deep down, each person blames himself or herself in some way, or that they've been fighting over assignment of blame in order to deflect unbearable pain, which can be eased through more empathic interaction.

Future Expectations and Catastrophic Fears

In troubled and uncertain times, we look to the future with anticipation or dread. We worry about what will happen to us and what can be done to improve our situation? Our expectations, both conscious and out of awareness, are validated or disconfirmed in our daily lives and transactions. Assumptions that we will succeed or fail may lead us to take actions that fulfill our prophecies. Beck (Beck, Rush, Shaw, & Emory, 1979) identified three self-defeating cognitive distortions, or types of faulty thinking, that increase human vulnerability: (1) minimizing or underestimating strengths; (2) magnifying or exaggerating the seriousness of each problem or mistake; and (3) "catastrophizing," or expecting the worst. These beliefs can be a major source of depression.

Catastrophic fears are paralyzing assumptions that block constructive action and fuel self-defeating behavior. For instance, heightened fears of loss, rooted in parental rejection or multiple foster care placements, can lead a child to misbehave in ways that bring about another loss. Fear of abandonment may propel a partner to leave a relationship before being left. James, remarried after the death of his first wife from breast cancer, left his second wife abruptly within weeks of her diagnosis of breast cancer. She recovered; their relationship did not.

Perceptions of a current event intersect with legacies of previous multigenerational family experiences in making meaning of life challenges (McGoldrick, Garcia Preto, & Carter, 2016). Traumatic past experiences—especially at the same nodal point in the life cycle as in a previous generation—load apprehension onto the present situation, particularly in a similar situation (Walsh, 1983). Yet if a family showed courage and experienced success in mastering the past ordeal, its members will tend to approach the new situation with greater confidence. It is important to search for such stories in dealing with past adversity—they offer positive models that can be transposed to new challenges.

In our mastery-oriented culture, parents need to encourage their children to perceive success as largely due to their efforts, resources, and abilities. Families help them to assume realistic ownership for their achievements and possess a sense of some personal control over what happens in their lives, which enhances self-esteem. In contrast, children with low resilience more often believe that success and failure are matters of chance or luck, forces beyond their control. Such perceptions lower their confidence of future success. When mistakes or failure occur, highly resilient children view them as experiences from which to learn, rather than as occasions of defeat. They are more likely to attribute mistakes to factors they can change, such as insufficient effort or an unrealistic goal. In contrast, children with low resilience and self-esteem are prone to believe that their mistakes are due to their own deficits (e.g., "I'm just stupid"), which can't be modified. The sense of competence and control are intertwined.

Severe and persistent adverse conditions that involve forces largely beyond personal control, such as chronic poverty, breed helplessness and hopelessness. For poor minority youth, both self-esteem and resilience erode when job opportunities and encouragement to succeed are lacking. Future success becomes less likely as individuals and their families expect to fail and retreat from demands, or resort to self-defeating coping strategies that worsen their situation.

High-functioning families recognize that success in human endeavors depends, in part, on variables beyond their control; yet they share the conviction that with goals and purpose, they can make a difference in their lives (Beavers & Hampson, 2003). They accept human limitations, believing that no one is completely helpless or all powerful in any situation. And they foster self-esteem by achieving relative competence in dealing with a challenging situation. It's important for clinicians to explore beliefs about personal agency, power, and control. Who and what could be helpful in making things better? Can their efforts make a difference? We can help families find ways for all members, even small children, to contribute in some valuable way.

POSITIVE OUTLOOK IN OVERCOMING ADVERSITY

Abundant research finds that a positive outlook is vitally important for resilience. Key elements involve hope and optimism; a focus on strengths and potential; initiative and perseverance; and "mastering the art of the possible."

Hope: "Oxygen for the Spirit"

"What oxygen is to the lungs, such is hope to the meaning of life" (Brunner, 1984, p. 9). Sustaining hope in the face of hardship or overwhelming odds enables us to carry on our best efforts. The word *hope*, originating in Old English, has a similar connotation in many languages: "to leap with expectation." Hope combines an internal decision—a leap of faith—with an external event we strongly desire to happen.

Hope is a future-oriented belief; no matter how bleak the present, we can envision the possibility of a better future. Hope for a better life for their children keeps beleaguered parents in impoverished communities from being defeated by their immediate circumstances. As the Reverend Martin Luther King Jr. avowed: "We must accept finite disappointment but we must never lose infinite hope."

Hope is essential in repairing troubled relationships. Too often, partners give up on a marriage when they have lost hope that change can occur. Research-based couple interventions find that in many seemingly hopeless relationships, "reservoirs of hope" can be found and strengthened (Markman, Stanley, & Blumberg, 2010). In the wake of devastating loss or trauma, we need to help families reorient hope to invest in rebuilding their lives and revise dashed hopes and dreams.

In truly dire situations, Weingarten (2004) cautions us to hold *reasonable* hope, with acknowledgment of the complexities and contradictions of our lives and an accommodation for doubt and despair. In contrast to denial or blind optimism, the challenge is to fully grasp the messiness and uncertainties in our situation without losing hope. She views hope as something we actively do with others. Because its effects on body and soul are so significant, hope must be the responsibility of the community.

Optimistic Orientation

Although the "power of positive thinking" has become a cliché, considerable research documents the strong effects of an optimistic orientation in dealing with stress and overcoming adversity. High-functioning families tend to hold a more optimistic view of life (Beavers & Hampson, 2003).

In the field of positive psychology, the concept of *learned optimism*, introduced by Seligman (1990), has relevance for fostering resilience. Seligman's earlier studies on "learned helplessness" found that individuals can be conditioned to become passive and helpless and give up on trying to initiate action or solve problems when rewards and punishments are unpredictable or random and their efforts are futile. Generalizations of permanence, pervasiveness, and personalization contribute to learned helplessness in such beliefs as "Nothing ever works out." Depression and pessimism are mutually reinforcing and can deplete the immune system, impair physical health, and even hasten death.

In an encounter with Jonas Salk, at a conference on psychoneuroimmunology, Salk said that if he were a young scientist today, he would focus on *psychological* immunization. Seligman proposed that if helplessness can be learned, then it can be unlearned by experiences of mastery when people experience success and come to believe that their efforts and actions can work. His research team worked with youth at risk for depression, their parents, and teachers, using cognitive-behavioral techniques. He found that children who learn such skills as challenging their negative thoughts and negotiating with peers showed less depression than control youth, with effects increasing over time. Such findings point to the importance of strengthening family communication skills for active agency, problem solving, and success (see Chapter 5).

Yet a cheerful mindset is not sufficient (Ehrenreich, 2009): Successful experiences and a nurturing context are needed to reinforce a positive outlook. Another caution is required: in warfare or conditions of extreme atrocity, promoting a positive mindset can be harmful and can heighten posttraumatic stress and moral injury (Litz et al., 2009; see Chapter 11).

In epidemiological research, Shelley Taylor (1989) found that people who hold selective positive biases about their chances of overcoming highly stressful situations tend to do better than those who accurately grasp "bad news," such as a poor prognosis in a life-threatening illness (see Chapter 12). These "positive illusions" sustain hope, enabling them to carry on their best efforts to overcome the odds. Taylor distinguished positive illusions from defensive denial or repression of distress, as incorporating information about the stressful situation and absorbing its implications (Taylor, Kemeny, Reed, Bower, & Gruenwald, 2000). They function as a buffer against stress and are associated with a variety of indices of adaptive coping, such as persistence at tasks, willingness to help others, and high functioning.

Such positive illusions are also common in couple and family relationships. Despite high divorce rates, few people believe that they will be among the divorce statistics (Fowers, Lyons, & Montel, 1996). Looking more closely at "marital illusions"—fantasies and unrealistic ideas people hold about marriage in general and their own relationship in particular—Fowers found that happy couples tended to hold rosy images of their relationships. They idealized their spouses, attributing more positive qualities to them and crediting them for the positive aspects of their marriage. However, extremely unrealistic expectations that a partner could meet all needs placed an undue burden on the relationship.

It is important to underscore that resilience is not fostered by simply looking at "the bright side" without acknowledging painful realities or contextual constraints and giving voice to concerns (Ehrenreich, 2009). Each family's suffering is unique, and attempts to have members "cheer up" or "count their blessings" can unintentionally trivialize their experience. Reassuring platitudes such as "It'll all work out" or "Life could be worse," though meant to offer comfort and solace, are usually not felt to be empathic or helpful when the pain and heartache experienced are not heard and validated.

Shared Confidence in Overcoming Challenges

When Norman Cousins (1979/2001) was told he had an incurable collagen disease and had only months to live, deep down he believed he had a good chance to survive for much longer and strove to beat the odds. Fully mindful of the seriousness of his condition, he observed, "I have learned never to underestimate the capacity of the human mind and body to regenerate—even when the prospects seem most wretched." With the conviction that his own total involvement was necessary in achieving his aim, he didn't do it alone: he selected a physician with whom he could collaborate to fully mobilize all his resources.

In resilient families, members encourage each other's steadfast confidence through an ordeal: "We always believed we would find a way out." This conviction, a shared "can-do" spirit, and the relentless search for solutions fuel optimism and make family members active participants in the problem-solving process. Confidence that they will all do their best builds relational resilience as it sustains individual efforts.

Encouragement: Affirming Strengths, Building on Potential

The word *courage* is embedded in the word *encouragement*. Personal courage is strengthened by the encouragement of family, friends, and community. One woman, abandoned by her husband, dreaded her divorce hearing and the difficulties that lay ahead. Her brother accompanied her to the hearing, saying simply, "I came to sit at your side to give you courage."

The courage shown in the everyday life of ordinary families often goes unnoticed. In inner-city neighborhoods in Chicago, children face daily threats of gun violence on their way to and from school; parents' return home from a late-night shift is always hazardous. Mothers show enormous courage in steeling themselves each morning to get their families through another harrowing day, and encourage their children to strive for a better life.

When families are dealing with a major crisis or pileup of stresses, they can easily lose sight of their strengths and resources. Therapy, like family life, can become problem-saturated, attending to all that has gone wrong, becoming stuck in blaming and scapegoating, or sinking into despair with recurrent crises. By noticing, affirming, and commending family members for their strengths and potential in the midst of difficulties we help them to counter a sense of helplessness, failure, or blame (see Chapter 7). When we see potential in everyone, it reinforces a sense of pride and confidence and a "can-do" spirit.

Active Initiative and Perseverance

For resilience, a positive outlook must be acted upon by taking initiative, rather than waiting passively for things to work out. We can help families to see and seize opportunities. The belief that their efforts and actions can make a difference can fuel this initiative.

Perseverance—the ability to "struggle well" and persist in the face of overwhelming adversity—is a core element in resilience. What some might call stubbornness may also be seen as tenacity, a strong determination to overcome obstacles. It requires us to rebound from setbacks and try again—or try a new way—until we succeed. As one mother put it, "We fall down seven times but we get up eight." The father added, "When any of us is down, the others pull us back up."

At times, all that can be done is to make the best of a grim situation and stand firm with resolve. The endurance and survival of harrowing life experiences can themselves be a source of pride, as in the resilience of families who have survived over generations of slavery, racial discrimination, and poverty (Pinderhughes, 2004). Elie Wiesel (1995), in describing the dehumanizing effects of the Nazi concentration camps, said that to survive while remaining a human being was itself heroic.

In Memory's Kitchen (DeSilva, 1996) is a remarkable collection of recipes, poems, and stories written by the women starving in a Nazi concentration camp at Terezin, Czechoslovakia. In an effort to endure the hunger, cold, and terror at the camp, the women met secretly to share memories of the family life to which they might never return. They believed that they needed imagination and a link to their traditions to survive and preserve their identity and heritage. Their way of coping was to think of wonderful food—to transport themselves back into their kitchens and dining rooms, filled with joyous gatherings, loving families, and lively children. The recipes evoked memories of feasts and celebrations, such as "Mrs. Pachter's *Gesundheit* Kuchen," "good health" cakes traditionally taken to the mothers of newborn babies. Their positive remembrances were written on scraps of paper, stitched together by hand, and hidden to be retrieved after the war as a legacy of their lives. Although the women did not survive the camp, their endurance and their collected memories attest to the survival of the spirit.

Mastering the Art of the Possible

In Higgins's (1994) study, resilient adults reported that they had overcome childhood adversity by channeling their energy and efforts to master what they could control and accepting what couldn't be changed. Higgins aptly called them "masters of the art of the possible." They believed that it was a waste of energy to be preoccupied with regret, retribution, or old wounds. Rather, they took stock of their situation—their challenges, constraints, and resources—and then focused on making the most of their options. Both active mastery and acceptance—akin to the Serenity Prayer in addiction recovery movements—are required.

In the experience of immigration, posing the dual challenges of loss and adaptation, strengths are forged through interweaving the old and the new for continuity and change (Falicov, 2012). Immigrant women have often found cooking to be both a source of livelihood in the new land and a cherished link to the families and homelands left behind. My great-grandmother Frimid and her husband came to Milwaukee from Budapest, fleeing pogroms against the Jews in the 1880s. With her admired cooking skills, she launched a catering business while her husband found work in a brewery. The story was told that one year, the strange weather reminded her of a certain season in Hungary when all the onion crops had failed. With her husband's encouragement, she withdrew all their savings from the bank and invested in onions. Sure enough, the crop failed, and, having cornered the market, they did quite well. Her picture on the front page of the local newspaper was captioned, "Frimid: The Onion Queen." Family stories of her bold resilience have been a source of inspiration for me, as her namesake. (However, I have yet to realize any financial windfall!)

Beliefs concerning mastery and acceptance need to be counterbalanced as we recognize both our possibilities and the realistic limits of our power. A philosophical acceptance is more common among older people, and is an important source of wisdom that comes with aging (Walsh, 2013). Traditional Eastern and Native American teachings are less focused on mastery and more attuned to living in harmony with nature. Those of us with a Euro-American mindset are often uncomfortable in situations beyond our control. Striving to "beat the odds" fits our competitive culture. Western medicine has emphasized control over life and death. But each time a patient dies, or "fails" to recover, doctors—and family members—must confront the reality we live in an uncertain universe and can't "master" death. Still, we do have the ability to heal and to grow psychosocially and spiritually from an illness or traumatic experience that we can't control or reverse.

Although family members may not be able to control the *outcome* of events, they can make choices and find meaningful ways to participate actively in the *process* of dealing with unfolding events, influencing the quality of their lives and relationships. In situations beyond their control, or those with high uncertainty, they can be encouraged to carve out aspects they can influence. For instance, when an illness is terminal and no treatment options remain, family members can actively choose ways to participate in caregiving, the relief of suffering, and preparation for death (see Chapter 12). In such ways, they make the most of the time they have together, focus on their priorities, and find comfort in loving one another well in the face of loss (Gawande, 2014).

TRANSCENDENCE AND SPIRITUALITY

Transcendent beliefs and experiences provide meaning, purpose, and connection beyond our selves, our families, and our immediate plight. They provide continuity with the past and into the future, with generations before us and those to come. They offer clarity about our lives and solace in distress; they render unexpected events less threatening and foster acceptance of situations beyond our control. Most commonly, transcendent beliefs are anchored in spiritual faith and cultural heritage. They may also be expressed through secular humanist values and deep philosophical, ideological, or political convictions.

Values and Purpose: A Moral Compass

A transcendent value system, whether conventional or not, enables us to define our lives and our relationships with others as meaningful. Just as individuals prosper within significant relationships, couples and families thrive when connected to larger communities and value systems (Beavers & Hampson, 2003; Doherty, 2013; Walsh, 2009d). To accept the inevitable risks and losses in loving and being close, families need a value system that transcends the limits of their experience and knowledge. It enables members to view their particular reality, which may be painful, uncertain, and frightening, from a perspective that makes some sense of events and allows for hope. Without this larger view, or moral compass, we are more vulnerable to hopelessness, alienation, and despair.

In surveys, most Americans have ranked "family ties, loyalty, and traditions," and secondly, "moral and spiritual values," as the main factors thought to strengthen the family (Walsh, 2009d). In clinical practice, it's important to explore each family's core values and how they may have been strengthened or shaken by crisis events. Persistent adversity may prevent families from fully living out their values. Family members can be encouraged to get in touch with their deepest values and to commit themselves to live in ways that support their best aspirations.

Spirituality

It is important to clarify our understanding of the terms *religion* and *spirituality* (see Walsh, 2009d, 2012d, 2013). *Religion* refers to an organized, institutionalized faith system with shared traditions, doctrine, moral values, and practices, a community of followers, and belief in God or a higher power. Through sacred scriptures, teachings, rituals, and ceremonies, religions provide standards for individual virtue, relational conduct, and family life as they connect individuals with their shared community, its history, and its survival over adversity. Congregational affiliation provides clergy guidance and a community of shared faith for support in times of need. All faith traditions counsel compassion and forgiveness in healing and resilience (Hargrave, Froeschle, & Castillo, 2009; see Chapters 11 and 14).

Spirituality, a broad, overarching construct, refers to transcendent beliefs and practices lived out in daily life and relationships. It is the heart and soul of religion (Pargament, 2007) and can also be experienced outside religious structures and by people who are not religious. Spirituality involves an active investment in internalized beliefs that bring a sense of meaning, wholeness, and connection with others. It may involve belief in an ultimate human condition or set of values toward which we strive; belief in a supreme power or an inner light; or belief in a holistic oneness with the human community, nature, and the universe. Spirituality invites an expansion of awareness, with personal responsibility for and beyond oneself, from local to global concerns. In sum, spirituality is relational: it involves a deep connection within oneself and with all others.

Spirituality can best be seen as a dimension of human experience. As such, it requires an expansion of systems theory to encompass biopsychosocial–spiritual influences and their interplay in personal and relational well-being and in suffering, healing, and resilience. Like culture or ethnicity, spirituality involves streams of experience that flow through all aspects of life, from multigenerational heritage to shared belief systems and their expression in ongoing transactions, spiritual practices, and response to adversity. Spiritual beliefs and practices come to the fore in situations of adversity. It is important to explore their importance in family life; ways that they may contribute to distress; and ways that spiritual resources, fitting a family's orientation and preferences, may be drawn on for resilience (see Chapters 6 and 7; Appendix 3).

Exploring Spiritual Sources of Distress

Suffering invites us into the spiritual domain (Wright, 2009). Yet spiritual distress can impede coping, mastery, and ability to invest life with meaning. Religious beliefs may become harmful if held too narrowly, rigidly, or punitively, or if used to rationalize the abuse of women or children. Deeply held religious beliefs are common sources of meaning when tragedy occurs. One husband attributed the couple's infertility to God's punishment for his past infidelity. In some cases, a crisis may precipitate a questioning of long-held spiritual beliefs—a father who turns away from God and his church after the death of his child, wailing, "How could a loving God take the life of an innocent child?" In other cases, it may launch a quest for a new approach to faith that can be sustaining, as when gay, lesbian, or transgender persons have been condemned by their family's religion.

Drawing on Spiritual Resources for Resilience

Numerous studies reveal the significant influence of spirituality in resilience (see Walsh, 2009c) and in posttraumatic growth (Tedeschi & Calhoun, 2004). Spiritual beliefs and practices offer meaning, support, and comfort in the face of adversity, especially in situations beyond comprehension, clarity, or control. Strong faith supports efforts to endure hardships, overcome challenges, and turn lives around (Werner & Smith, 2001).

For immigrant families and African Americans, religion has been a wellspring for resilience, countering discrimination and despair (Boyd-Franklin, 2004; Falicov, 2013). The Reverend Martin Luther King Jr., a guiding spirit to many oppressed people, held abiding faith that social justice would prevail. Yet rather than waiting for God's deliverance, he urged collective action to bring about change, emphasizing personal responsibility and shared initiative.

Mounting neurobiological evidence reveals that strong faith and contemplative practices, as in prayer or meditation, can promote health and healing, reduce stress, and strengthen the neurological, immune, and cardiovascular systems (Kabat-Zinn, 2003; Koenig, 2012). Although congregational affiliation has been declining, what matters most is drawing on the power of personal faith to give meaning to a precarious situation and find hope, comfort, and solace.

Couple and family research finds that shared spiritual beliefs and practices strengthen relationships and the ability to transcend troubled times (Beavers & Hampson, 2003; Mahoney, 2010; Marks, 2006; Stinnett & DeFrain, 1985; also see Walsh, 2009d, 2012d). When values are lived out in family life and meaningful shared practices—and when parents practice what they preach—at-risk youth find them a resource in resisting harmful influences and in dealing successfully with challenging social environments.

Spiritual connectedness and renewal can be found in communion with nature, as in the powerful beliefs and practices of indigenous peoples from earliest times. Native Americans and others who have suffered cultural genocide and the decimation of their land, water, forests, animals, and people, continue to espouse their kinship with all living things (Robbins, 2013). In modern life, we may experience this deep connection in varied ways, from bonding with companion animals, tending a garden, or hiking through the woods, to feeling in harmony with the rhythm of waves on the shore. Many are drawn to places with high spiritual energy, such healing waters, or make pilgrimages to sacred sites.

The expressive arts, in many forms, can be a powerful spiritual resource with healing effects. Through art, music, literature, and drama, we can communicate profound suffering, our common humanity, and the triumph of the human spirit. Music offers a powerful transcendent experience in every culture. African American gospel singing, blues, and jazz arose out of the cauldron of slavery and oppression, soaring to creative new heights. As the Hopi Indians say, "To watch us dance is to hear our hearts speak."

For me, music has a deep spiritual resonance and a connection with my mother and my daughter. My mother, a gifted musician, was the piano teacher in our town and, with an ecumenical command of the great hymns, she also served as organist for the Jewish temple and, on holidays, for various Christian congregations. Music, whether sacred or secular, released the weariness and sorrow she carried from the hardships and losses in her life; I could see, as she played Chopin or Schumann, she was transported to another realm. (See her story in Chapter 14.) Music has also been a spiritual wellspring for me and for my daughter, especially through difficult times. Although I don't share her love of hip-hop, and I prefer yoga to her Zumba, we share a deep appreciation of world music and dance.

Resilience, faith, and intimacy are linked (Higgins, 1994). Faith is inherently relational from early in life, when fundamental convictions are shaped and nourished within caregiving bonds. Loving relationships with partners, family members, and close friends—soul mates and kindred spirits—infuse our lives with meaning. Viktor Frankl (1946/1984) recounted how in Nazi prison camps he was sustained by his deep spiritual connection with his wife, visualizing her image: "I didn't even know if she were still alive. I knew only one thing—which I have learned well by now: Love goes very far beyond the physical person of the beloved. It finds its deepest meaning in the spiritual being, the inner self" (pp. 59–60).

Inspiration: Innovation, Creative Expression, Social Action

Creativity is often born of adversity. The struggle to overcome life challenges can bring new vision to our lives. Our imaginations can transport us beyond our immediate troubles to illuminate pathways out of our dilemmas and into a better life ahead. Resilient persons—and communities—often draw something positive out of a tragic situation.

Families must also be inventive to weather and rebound from adversity. A well-functioning family draws on a wide variety of inspirations to solve its problems, including past experience, family stories, creative fantasy, and new and untried solutions. Madsen (2009, 2011) sees the need for an attitude of disciplined improvisation, aiming toward a preferred life vision. With societal transformations worldwide, we are all called upon to envision viable models of human connection, meaning, and fulfillment.

Role Models and Heroes

We can be inspired to transcend the constraints of our own situations through the positive examples of others who demonstrate resilience. Beyond the borders of our everyday world, we are drawn to the life stories of men and women of high attainment who have overcome adversity. Sports heroes often inspire youth, especially those in highly challenging social environments. In Chicago, we were all fans of Michael Jordan, the basketball giant who embodied many of the qualities of resilience throughout his career. Not resting on the laurels of his extraordinary talents, he worked out tirelessly—honing his skills, pushing his limits, always striving for excellence, and developing new ways to compensate for injuries and aging. He maintained a tenacious will to win, to persevere, and to rebound from failure and loss, which he viewed as challenges sparking him to try even harder. Although Jordan was seen as innately gifted, his many qualities of resilience were relationally honed in his strong family upbringing. He once noted his most important skill: "to focus, focus, focus." In his mother's memoir of their family life (Jordan, 1996), she recalled, "I always taught my children to focus, focus, focus!" Jordan's own heroes were his parents—his nurturing and spiritually devout mother, who instilled strong values, and his father, who was his mainstay and closest companion. Yet despite his success and fame, he was not spared tragedy when his father was brutally murdered in a roadside robbery. In shock and grief, he left basketball, losing passion for the sport with the loss of his father. After turning to baseball (a childhood connection with his father), he returned to basketball to lead a remarkable Chicago Bulls team in winning a fourth NBA title—on Father's Day. Hugging the trophy, he wept openly, dedicating the victory to the memory of his father.

The life story of Supreme Court justice Sonia Sotomayor (2013) is a remarkable account of resilience, nurtured by her grandmother and by deep Puerto Rican cultural roots. She grew up poor in a Bronx housing project at a time when the neighborhood was plagued by gangs, drugs, and violence. She learned she had juvenile diabetes at age 7. A couple of years later, she lost her father, an alcoholic whose unpredictable behavior had cast a shadow over her family life. Her best friend in childhood was her cousin Nelson. She relates that they were inseparable and virtually identical—except that he was smarter and had the father she wished for. Yet Nelson became a heroin addict and died of AIDS before his 30th birthday. Why, Justice Sotomayor wondered, did she manage to survive when Nelson failed, consumed by the same dangers that had surrounded her? The culture of machismo played a role, she writes, pushing boys out onto the streets while protecting girls. Her own force of will was crucial too, with a sense of discipline and perseverance honed from her determination to manage her diabetes. It was the love and protection of her grandmother, Abuelita, that gave her "a refuge from the chaos at home" and allowed her "to imagine the most improbable of possibilities for my life." Her first dream was of growing up to become a detective like her favorite heroine, Nancy Drew, because she thought her mind worked in similar ways. She then became fascinated with the idea of becoming a lawyer or judge from watching law dramas on television.

Reading and absorbing life stories can open up the world, enabling us to envision and reach for possibilities beyond our limited circumstances. Parents can open windows to many realms by reading with their children from early childhood. I grew up in a poor, working-class neighborhood where most of my classmates married and got factory jobs after high school. My own aspirations were enlarged through reading: my library card was my ticket to an expanded world view. Some stories were constraining: such classic fables as "Cinderella" and "Snow White" were stifling in their gendered expectations that if I was sweet, compliant, and uncomplaining, I would be rescued by a prince to live happily ever after. Fortunately, I found inspiration in such biographies as those of Jane Addams, a social work pioneer who founded Hull House, and the scientist Marie Curie. Although I didn't plan to follow those particular pathways, curiously enough, I later found myself drawn to social change and research. The book I recall most vividly from early childhood was *The Little Engine That Could*, about a small blue train engine that couldn't keep up with the big engines, but through strong determination ("I think I can; I think I can; I know I can!") was able to get over the mountain. When tempted to think of my own resilience as self-made, I need only recall that it was my parents who read that story to me at so many bedtimes.

We often fail to see the many examples of resilience in our own families and communities. We attribute neglect to single mothers working out of the home when we need to appreciate their heroic feat in managing job, parenting, and household demands. Stories of uncommon courage and triumph over tragic events are valuable, but so too are stories of the remarkable strengths and vitality of ordinary families in weathering the storms of life. In *Hope Dies Last*, Studs Terkel (2003) documents the courage and comebacks everyday people make every day—the heroic feats that don't get media fanfare. For helping professionals, seeing the ways ordinary families draw on the capacity for resilience can inspire us to see and affirm the unrecognized strengths in every family we work with.

Compassionate Outreach

Suffering and struggle can also open hearts to greater compassion for the plight of others and efforts on behalf of those endangered—from at-risk individuals, families, and larger communities to all life on our shared planet. Giving love (concern, assistance, support, empathy) when one is facing adversity oneself is an act of power that redefines the context of the interaction/situation and thereby creates new meaning. We change our position in any adverse interaction by defining ourselves as givers of love rather than victims (Mollica, 2006). As studies of resilience and positive growth document, resilient individuals and families commonly emerge from shattering crises with a heightened moral compass and sense of purpose in their lives. In an altruism born of suffering (Staub, 2013), they gain compassion from their experience and strong motivation to prevent or ameliorate the suffering of others. Sonia Sotomayor's (2013) early family and community experience, including a keen awareness that the poor and minorities are disproportionately victims of crime, infused her legal career with an abiding commitment to fairness and to fixing broken systems.

Families commonly develop increased compassion for others as a result of their own experiences with adversity. Resilient families often desire to give back to their communities and seek to help others to prevent or alleviate similar suffering (Lietz, 2007; Patterson, 2002). This often sparks commitment to local community action or a nationwide campaign, such as that started by the bereaved parents who organized Mothers Against Drunk Driving (MADD) so that other families could be spared their tragedy. Many express their spirituality through working passionately for social justice or environmental causes, as in the Jewish tradition of *tikkun olam*, or efforts to repair the world (Perry & Rolland, 2009). Lietz (2011) found that in many ways "empathic action," in turn, increased families' own healing and resilience.

Transformation: Learning, Change, and Positive Growth

Hardship, tragedy, or failure can be instructive and can serve as an impetus for personal and relational change and growth. Resilience is gained when family members survey their experience and attempt to draw lessons from it that can be valuable in guiding their future course. In accepting what has happened and any persisting scars, they try to incorporate what they have learned into efforts toward living better lives.

In such ways families forge new meaning and growth out of the cauldron of adversity. Resilient families believe that their trials have made them more than what they might have been otherwise. One couple nearly lost a son in a freak accident that shook the very foundation of the family. They experienced this crisis as an epiphany, crystallizing a deeper appreciation of their family bonds, a stronger sense of purpose in life, and a dedication to practice their values more fully. In the uncertainty and pain wrought by a life crisis, core beliefs come to the fore. As events are assimilated, they may come to be seen as a gift that opens a new life phase and more meaningful pursuits (see Tedeschi & Calhoun, 2005).

The paradox of resilience is that the worst of times can bring out our best. A crisis can yield transformation and growth in unforeseen directions. It can awaken family members to the importance of loved ones or jolt them into healing old wounds and reordering life priorities. Families in problem-saturated situations need to envision a better future through their efforts. When their hopes and dreams have been shattered, they need to imagine and invent new possibilities that can yield transformation and positive growth.

CHAPTER 4

Organizational Processes

Relational and Structural Supports

A tree, deeply rooted, nourished, and sheltered, bends in
the storm but does not break.
—An image of resilience by a Japanese colleague

Families, with varied forms and relational networks, must provide
structure to support the integration and adaptation of the family unit and
its members (Minuchin, 1974). Family organizational patterns are maintained by external and internal norms, influenced by cultural and family
belief systems. Patterns are also based on mutual expectations in particular
families and persist out of habit, personal preferences, mutual accommodation, or functional effectiveness. To deal effectively with crises or persistent adversity, families must mobilize and organize their resources, buffer
stresses, and reorganize to fit changing conditions. This chapter identifies
the organizational elements in effective family functioning, highlighting
key processes for relational resilience: flexibility, connectedness, and social
and economic resources (see Table 4.1).

FLEXIBILITY

Families need to develop a flexible structure for optimal functioning in the
face of adversity. Like all human systems, families tend to resist change
beyond a certain familiar or acceptable range. Yet change is an inevitable
part of the human condition. Families must be able to adapt to changing

TABLE 4.1. Key Organizational Processes in Family Resilience

Flexibility

- Rebound, adaptive change to meet new challenges.
- Reorganize, regain stability with disruption: continuity, dependability, predictability.
- Strong authoritative leadership: nurture, guide, protect.
- Varied family forms: cooperative parenting/caregiving teams, households.
- Couple/coparent relationship: mutual respect; equal partners.

Connectedness

- Mutual support, collaboration, and commitment.
- Respect individual needs, differences.
- Seek reconnection, repair relational grievances.

Mobilize social and economic resources

- Recruit extended kin, social and community supports, models and mentors.
- Build financial security; navigate stressful work–family challenges.
- Transactions with larger systems: enlist institutional, structural supports.

developmental and environmental demands—both normative (expectable, predictable) and nonnormative (uncommon, untimely, or unexpected). Flexibility, a dynamic balance between stability (*homeostasis*) and change (*morphogenesis*), enables a family to maintain structure while also adapting to meet life challenges (Olson & Gorall, 2003).

Adaptive Change: "Bouncing Forward"

The capacity for adaptive change is essential for high functioning in couples and families, especially under stress. Virginia Satir (1988) observed that in healthy families the rules for members are flexible, appropriate to situations, and alterable. Similarly, couples studies find that the capacity for adaptability, flexibility, and change predict the long-term success of the relationship. Partners must be able to evolve together and cope with the multitude of internal challenges and external forces in their lives. When people hold a rigid conception of marriage as an institution with unalterable rules and roles, they are more wary of long-term commitment. As the fabled Hollywood film star Mae West once put it, "It's not that I'm opposed to the institution of marriage; I'm just not ready for an institution." Today, couples and families are constructing relationships with a flexible structure that they can mold and reshape to fit their emerging priorities and challenges over time (see Chapter 9).

Resilience is commonly thought of as "bouncing back," like a spring, to a precrisis shape or norm. It is more apt to think of "bouncing forward," rebounding and reorganizing adaptively to meet new challenges or changed conditions (Walsh, 2002b). With a highly disruptive crisis, it may not be possible to go back to the way things were. With major losses, such as a loved one's death or a divorce, we must forge new pathways. When events of great magnitude occur, such as a major disaster, families may not be able to return to "normal" life as they knew it. Residents of New Orleans speak of "life before" and "life after" Hurricane Katrina. We may be forced to question old assumptions and grapple with a fundamentally altered conception of ourselves in relation to others in our shared world (see Chapter 11). In rebuilding lives, we recalibrate "normal" settings to meet unanticipated challenges, constructing a new normal.

Restabilizing with Disruption

In the upheaval of a crisis, disruptive transition, or pileup of stressors, family members yearn for calm and order. Families commonly lose structure, daily routines fall by the wayside, birthdays are forgotten, and established patterns of living can become disorganized. We can foster resilience by helping members sustain important functioning in the midst of turmoil and regain stability in the aftermath, restoring predictable, consistent rules, roles, and patterns of interaction. Family members—especially children— need to know what they can expect of each other. Reliability is crucial: they need assurance that they can depend on one another to follow through with commitments.

Family rituals and routines maintain a sense of continuity through disruption, linking past, present, and future through shared traditions and expectations (Imber-Black, 2012). Families and communities gather in the celebration of holidays, traditions (such as anniversaries and reunions), and rites of passage (such as weddings, bar/bat mitzvahs, graduations, and funerals) (Harvey & Hill, 2004). Rituals can also facilitate difficult transitions, such as remarriage and stepfamily integration. They mark important milestones, restore continuities with a family's heritage, create new patterns, and foster healing from trauma and loss.

Routines of everyday life, such as family dinnertime or Sunday brunch with Dad, provide regular contact and a sense of connection (Fiese, 2006). In family assessment, we can learn about structure by asking about a typical day and week, and how family life has changed with a crisis or major transition. Some families become too overloaded and fragmented for

nightly dinner together. Seemingly small routines can make a big difference. Often children with school or behavior problems have no set bedtime,
or it is a nightly hassle, with overtired children becoming more wound up
and exhausted parents' tempers likely to flare. Everyone benefits from setting a reasonable bedtime routine with pleasurable contact, such as reading
together or a bedside chat. Older children can be enlisted to assist with
younger ones, building their competencies and sibling connections, and
allowing adults much-needed time for respite.

   In times of crisis and major transitions, disruption in family structure
and daily routines compounds upset and confusion, especially for children.
One resilient family rallied when a parent's illness required several hospitalizations at a distance. Extended family members took turns moving in
to stay with the children. This enabled them to sleep in their own beds,
have their belongings at hand, and keep up daily routines and friendships,
rather than experience further dislocation by shuttling to stay with various
relatives each time. When family life is reorganized, as with divorce, it is
important for families to create new routines that provide the continuity
of significant bonds, such as Friday-night pizza with Dad. After a divorce,
the predictability and reliability of contact with a nonresidential parent are
crucial for children's adjustment (Hetherington & Kelly, 2002; see Chapter
9). Children are more likely to feel abandoned or unloved when a parent
drops in and out of their lives without clear expectations about contact and
support, or when promises are vague and plans repeatedly fall through.

Strong Leadership: Nurture, Guide, and Protect

Parents and their elders are the architects of a family, laying the foundation
for healthy family life in the structural arrangements, roles, and rules they
construct. With adversity, strong leadership is crucial to nurture, guide, and
protect children, and to care for elders and members with special needs.
Leadership is also needed to provide basic resources (e.g., money, food,
clothing, health care, and shelter) and to manage the many pressures and
demands of family life (Ryan, Epstein, Keitner, Miller, & Bishop, 2005).

   Research by Olson and colleagues (Olson & Gorell, 2003) has shown
that strong, clear leadership is important for adaptability. Adults in charge
uphold their authority and responsibilities, yet they are careful not to abuse
their power. Children's choices and responsibilities increase with developing maturity. Frustrating power struggles occur infrequently. Families with
moderately structured relationships have somewhat democratic leadership, with some negotiations including the children. Roles are stable, with
some role sharing. Rules are firmly enforced with few changes. Those with

moderately flexible relationships have more egalitarian leadership, with a democratic approach to decision making. Negotiations are open and actively include the children. Roles may be shared, and change is fluid when necessary. Rules are age-appropriate and can be modified over time.

Families are also critical social learning contexts. They function best when they exchange benefits far more frequently than punishments or coercion (Sexton, 2011). Parents encourage children's success and reward adaptive behavior through attention, acknowledgment, and approval. They try not to reinforce maladaptive behavior. In less functional families, parents use more coercion and focus on misbehavior, failure, control, and punishment. Positive efforts and successes go unnoticed and unrewarded. Therapists can serve as models, helping families to affirm positive intentions, efforts, and behaviors and to encourage interests and talents. We can help distressed families find opportunities for rewarding exchanges that enhance their relationships, along with individual competence and self-esteem.

Families need effective methods of monitoring and control to keep children's behavior within bounds and neither dangerous nor destructive. Authoritative yet flexible rules and behavior control are most effective (Olson & Gorell, 2003; Steinberg, Blatt-Eisengart, & Cauffman, 2006). Standards are reasonable, with opportunity for negotiation and change. Parents/caregivers are in accord when setting and enforcing rules. They are clear about what behavior is unacceptable and intervene consistently when infractions occur. They make allowances when a situation calls for it, yet still maintain consistent expectations. In highly disruptive crisis situations, very strong leadership is essential to maintain or restore order and reduce chaos or overwhelming stress. More authoritarian leadership may be needed in families living in high-risk social contexts where community structures have broken down. Above all, caring discipline with firmness *and* warmth is most effective.

The resilience literature underscores the vital importance of *mentoring*: guiding and inspiring children in positive directions, especially at-risk youth in impoverished environments. In clinical and juvenile justice fields, there has been an overfocus on behavior control with insufficient attention to the ways that parents, older siblings, extended family members, and community elders can all play a part in providing values, motivation, modeling, and active mentoring (Ungar, 2004; see Chapters 8 and 13). Rather than lecture youth about what they should and shouldn't do, a mentoring relationship actively invests in each child's interests and talents and nourishes hopes and dreams. In our practice, we can usefully approach this dimension by identifying and encouraging mentoring opportunities within the family network, supplemented by community resources.

Varied Family Forms: Cooperative Teams

In today's diverse family structures, leadership patterns are varied, from an intact two-parent family to single-parent and binuclear households, stepfamilies, and extended kinship care (Walsh, 2012c). Families function best and children thrive when parents and other involved kin work collaboratively with mutual respect and accommodation within and across households. Clarity and consistency in expectations and consequences for children are crucial. Parenting arrangements that involve a grandparent or nonresidential parent and separate households can work well as long as lines of authority and responsibility are clearly drawn.

Couple and Coparental Relationships: Mutual Respect, Equal Partners

Couple and coparental relationships function best when partners value and support each other's contributions in a mutual, equitable way, with role flexibility and overall balance. Mutual respect and consideration are important. Children are affected by how parents treat each other, not only how each parent relates to the child (Ryan et al., 2005). In well-functioning families, partners' contributions may vary, but neither carries disproportionate burden or privilege. Most men today are more involved than their fathers were on the home front yet still carry far less household responsibility than their wives. When both partners hold jobs and share childcare and housework, a division of labor needs to be worked out for their particular situation, with demands, skills, preferences, and fairness taken into account. Bombarded by multiple, conflicting job and family pressures and by changes in role expectations, dual earners need to establish a very clear structure and yet to be highly flexible so they can shift gears and cover for each other as needs arise.

Gender-based disparities in power and privilege still commonly occur in family role expectations, relational styles, and constraints, reinforced by cultural norms and institutional policies. Women and men increasingly challenge gender-linked role constraints and seek more equitable partnerships in work and family life, yet, as discussed in Chapter 2, this is still a work in progress (Knudsen-Martin, 2012).

The balance of power is a fundamental issue in all couple relationships, contributing to relationship success, intimacy, stability, and satisfaction (Driver, Tabares, Shapiro, & Gottman, 2012). In high-functioning families, partners strive to share strong egalitarian leadership and authority (Beavers & Hampson, 2003). They experience power through close, loving bonds, not through coercion or control over one another. The greater the power imbalance, the greater is the risk for conflict and dissolution.

Reciprocity over time is essential for a fair and equal partnership. A good relationship requires continuous balancing in terms of partners' priorities and responsiveness so that each carries a fair share of responsibilities and enjoys equal privileges. This give-and-take is based on trustworthiness and follow-through—mutual assurance that each member's needs will be honored and that their exchange will balance out over time. We can help partners negotiate to rebalance power and entitlement, to share burdens more equitably, and to appreciate each other's contributions (Knudsen-Martin, 2012).

Family therapists have become aware that a therapeutic stance of neutrality tacitly reinforces cultural biases and ignores harmful power skews in families and society. Ethically, we must foster equal respect and challenge beliefs and practices—in families and larger systems—that perpetuate abuses of power, particularly in demeaning treatment and in violence or sexual assault. Change is also needed in societal, institutional, and workplace structures for equal opportunities, status, and pay and for more flexible work and child care arrangements. Relational resilience is strengthened when men and women can share fully and equally in the responsibilities and joys of family and work life.

Navigating Stressful Life Challenges: Counterbalancing Stability and Change

Family resilience requires the ability to counterbalance stability and change as family members deal with adversity. Skiing offers a useful metaphor for visualizing the dynamic balance needed to navigate life challenges. Going down the mountainside, good skiers maintain stability while shifting position fluidly to meet the changing demands of the terrain. When a skier stiffens up out of fear of losing control, the rigid stance heightens the risk of falling and of serious injury.

My personal experience with skiing held valuable lessons for my practice as a therapist. As a novice, with a catastrophic fear of speeding out of control and tumbling all the way to the bottom of the mountain, I sat down on the slope and refused to budge from terra firma. Lessons with a pro enabled me to overcome my fear and enjoy skiing and supplied useful clinical insights. A good ski instructor first teaches novices how to stop (control over runaway processes) and how to fall and minimize injury. Next, skiers learn how to sustain that dynamic balance of steadiness and flexibility, which requires repeated adjustments, as they shift positions while moving forward through changing conditions. Although my internal cues signaling fear (e.g., pounding heart) protested that I wasn't ready, my instructor calmly yet firmly encouraged me to take a few breaths and try a short run on a gentle slope (behavior change facilitating internal change). He provided a secure mentoring relationship by demonstrating skills and going just ahead of me, guiding my way and assuring me that he would catch me (quite literally a "holding environment") if I went too fast and lost control. Each small success, along with his praise and encouragement to do more, increased my competence and confidence.

Applying this analogy to work with families helps me understand much of what is commonly labeled as "resistance" to change and how to work with it. Change is frightening largely because family members fear losing control of their lives in a runaway process that might leave them even worse off than their present predicament. Fear of the unknown can outweigh current distress, which is painful yet familiar. Those who have been in crisis and have experienced terror or overwhelming chaos quite understandably hold catastrophic expectations about change; they may feel an acute sense of helplessness and fear that their lives will spiral out of control yet again. This apprehension is especially intense after major traumatic events (see Chapters 11 and 13) and for multi-stressed families (see Chapter 13). Therapy may seem particularly threatening when its objective and methods promote change. Therapists, indeed, are often thought of as change agents.

Helping professionals need to respect clients' hesitation to engage in a change process when they are already in crisis or in a precarious situation, or when they are struggling with an overwhelming pileup of stressors. We need to better appreciate their yearnings for less change and more stability, and strive to achieve a flexible balance. Like the ski instructor, we can encourage a collaborative process in which we actively structure the therapy and contribute our expertise and support, yet help clients to feel in control of the therapy process and more in charge of their lives. Families in crisis commonly experience an immediate period of rapid disorganization, which is disorienting and chaotic. It can be reassuring to normalize this experience, to slow down change processes, and to provide a strong structure to contain reactions and support the ability to tolerate uncertainty as families gradually attain a new, more functional equilibrium. An initial priority is to help them learn how to prevent runaway change by building skills and confidence in small, manageable increments. Tasks and directives can be helpful in learning how to fail (fall) safely, try again, and succeed.

We can also help them maintain continuities and build new structures as they undergo disruptive transitions and must reorganize (e.g., after the loss of a parent). In exploring what clients need and value—what family members *don't* want to change or lose—we can then help them find ways to conserve those elements, or to transform or replace them.

Crisis events often require a family to reorganize. With a major transition, such as stepfamily formation, a basic shift of rules and roles may be needed. Significant losses stress the family even further and require major adaptational shifts of family rules to ensure both the transformation and continuity of family life.

CONNECTEDNESS

A second key process in family organization involves *connectedness*, or *cohesion*, the emotional and structural bonding among family members (Beavers & Hampson, 2003; Olson & Gorall, 2003). In highly connected families, members enjoy time together, and share involvements in and outside the home, including fun activities and chores. Families tend to do best when they balance closeness, mutual support, and commitment with respect for separateness and individual needs and differences.

Mutual Support, Commitment, and Teamwork

In dealing with serious life challenges, family members need to be able to turn to one another for support. A well-functioning family provides a safe harbor in storms for its members, with assurance of secure attachment, trust, and commitment (Bowlby, 1988; Byng-Hall, 1995). Family members take an active interest in what is important to each other, even when interests vary, and can respond empathically to others' distress. The comfort and security provided by warm, caring relationships is especially critical in times of crisis, when anxieties and intense upset can precipitate conflict and cutoffs.

In facing adversity, families function best when members rally together and know they can count on each other. Pulling together is one of the most important processes in weathering crises (Stinnett & DeFrain, 1985). Every member can have a part to play in easing family burdens or offering support, and each feels valued by being included in some way. For instance, if a family member is seriously ill, children tend to do better when they are involved in some helpful way, rather than feeling helpless on the sidelines. A small child might draw a picture or pick flowers to bring cheer or might make a card expressing love or appreciation.

In highly connected families, emotional closeness and loyalty are strong. Time spent together is highly valued, and many interests, activities, and friends are shared. When separated or living apart, it's important to sustain connections through regular contact, now facilitated by the Internet, as well as photos, stories, and keepsakes. Well-functioning families encourage members to be both differentiated and connected, valuing every individual's uniqueness and validating his or her efforts, sense of competence, and self-worth.

Although cultural norms and family organizational styles vary considerably, extreme patterns of *enmeshment* and *disengagement* tend to be dysfunctional under stressful conditions. When family members are enmeshed, diffuse boundaries, blurred differentiation, and strong pressure for togetherness can block competence. Individual differences may be seen as threats to group survival and sacrificed for the sake of unity and loyalty. Pressures for consensus can interfere with communication and problem solving. Even with a large network proffering support, in crisis family members can readily become overloaded and overreactive and have difficulty managing stress. When families are disengaged, unsupported family members drift off on their own or cut off emotionally and are left to fend for themselves.

A family's *organizational style* should not be equated with its *level of functioning*. Family and cultural norms vary widely in preferences for closeness and separateness. In ethnic groups that value solidarity and community, families expect individual needs to be deferred to the common good. In clinical practice, caution is required not to erroneously label as pathological "enmeshment" or "disengagement" patterns of high connectedness or separateness that may be typical and/or functional in different contexts. High cohesion may even be necessary to deal with a crisis, a pileup of stressors, or caregiving challenges (Green & Werner, 1996). In many ethnic groups, such as Latin American, Asian, and Middle Eastern families, high concern and involvement in each other's lives is normative. Adult children may be expected to subordinate their own pursuits to attend to family priorities, such as financial contributions to relatives in need (Falicov, 2013). The emphasis on independence and self-reliance in the dominant U.S. culture can lead to faulty assumptions of dysfunction and inappropriate therapeutic goals. Most other cultures prioritize interdependence and place family and community commitments above individual preferences.

Family boundaries—rules defining who participates how—clarify and reinforce roles and support family functioning (Minuchin, 1974). Boundaries need to be clear and firm, yet also be flexible enough for restructuring in response to stress. The *clarity* of boundaries and subsystems, particularly between adults and children, is important. Ambiguity in boundaries, roles, and membership can complicate adaptation (Boss, 1999). *Interpersonal boundaries* define family members, promoting individual identity and autonomous functioning. High-functioning families strive to maintain clear boundaries. Members take responsibility for their own thoughts, feelings, and actions. They respect the unique qualities and subjective views of others. When boundaries become blurred and confused, members intrude into other's personal space and may fuse their own identity with that of others. As one father said, explaining why he hits his son, "When I look at him, I see me; he's got all my bad habits, and I try to knock 'em out of him."

Generational boundaries maintain hierarchical organization in families. Established by parents or kin caregivers, they reinforce leadership and authority and differentiate rights and obligations. They guard a couple's relationship from intrusion and protect children from abuse by adults. When parents and grandparents are actively involved in family functioning, intergenerational tensions can arise around authority issues. A variety of arrangements can be workable if the social organization and generational hierarchy are clear and consistent. In a two-parent family, a strong parental alliance with clear generational boundaries is important.

In early family systems theory, parentification of a child was assumed to be dysfunctional. However, in multi-stressed and underresourced single-parent or large families, it may be necessary and functional for older children to take considerable responsibility to assist with housekeeping, child care, and financial demands. When a parent is absent or has a disabling illness, a child may be thrust into premature responsibilities, such as a caregiving role or a job to help out. Such role assignment is best delegated, with children assisting adults, who remain in charge. These responsibilities can foster early competence and are not necessarily harmful, as long as the burden is not excessive and other family members share tasks to the best of their ability. Boundary blurring becomes dysfunctional if adults abdicate leadership. It is most harmful if a child is exploited, emotionally embroiled in adult conflicts, or sexually abused (Scheinberg & Fraenkel, 2001).

Good teamwork facilitates resilience under stressful conditions. In well-functioning families, members form multiple and varied alliances around shared interests, concerns, and responsibilities. They avoid triangulation (Bowen, 1978; Minuchin, 1974), when two members (often a couple) draw in a third (typically a child) to deflect tension between them. Distress increases when members become embedded in multiple triangles, often involving extended families. For resilience, flexible alliances and teamwork are organized around varied strengths and resources to share and allocate tasks. Progress is tracked with members held accountable for their part. It is important that no one is overburdened, with others underfunctioning. Family members flexibly fill in for one another as needs arise. In practice, I find that families like the metaphor of a sports team in approaching their own effective team functioning.

SOCIAL AND ECONOMIC RESOURCES

Mobilizing Extended Kin, Social, and Community Resources

In Bali, as in many traditional cultures, all villagers participate in some way in the construction of every home. By contributing their efforts, they all support the firm foundation of the community. Similarly, in rural areas worldwide, neighboring farm families pitch in to help each other in harvesting crops. In strong communities, everyone rallies to assist families who have suffered losses in the wake of a major disaster. When families are open and generous in supporting others in crisis, they in turn can count on others in times of need. In our era of social fragmentation and self-reliance, we need to encourage families to build these vital networks for interdependence.

Family transactional processes with their social environment are crucial for family resilience. Well-functioning families are open systems with clear yet permeable boundaries, much like living cells with their dense network of connections, cohesive within their borders yet sustaining interchange with the outside world (Bateson, 1979). Members are actively involved in their environment, relate to it with optimism and hope, and bring varied interests and resources back into the family (Beavers & Hampson, 2013).

Relational lifelines with extended kin and social networks can provide practical assistance, emotional support, and vital community resources. In times of crisis or hardship, they offer information, concrete services, support, companionship, and respite. They also promote a sense of belonging, with security and solidarity. Community programs and religious congregations support individual and family well-being through regular participation in a wide array of functions, such as church suppers, choral singing, seniors' clubs, youth activities, and community service. Research suggests that there is something life-protective in belonging to a group and having regular social activity of any kind, especially to avoid isolation and alienation.

When my father was widowed with no family members nearby, he was initially quite lonely. Increasing involvement in his men's organization brought him meaningful activities and structured social gatherings for many years. Living modestly on his Social Security check, he devoted his full time and energies to volunteer work, going daily to the staff office to assist in fund-raising events on behalf of hospitals for children with disabilities. This involvement held special meaning for him, since my father had suffered disability himself as a child (see Chapter 14 for his story). As my esteem rose for my father, so too did my recognition of the value in such groups, which I had earlier derided as "men marching in parades in funny hats." When my father died, all his lodge brothers, in their hats and full regalia, turned out for his funeral and gave him a glorious send-off.

Linkages with the social world are vitally important for family resilience. Stinnett and colleagues (Stinnett & Defrain, 1985) found that strong families have the strength to admit they have difficulties and need help. When they can't solve problems on their own, they are more likely to turn to extended family, friends, neighbors, community services, and/or therapy or counseling. Conversely, family isolation and lack of social support contribute to dysfunction under stress. Research has documented that it is not simply the size of the network or the frequency of contacts that makes a difference; their helpfulness depends on the quality of the relationships. Some are better with practical assistance, others with emotional support; and some make matters worse. Therefore, a dense network can provide varied kinds of support without overburdening anyone. Since most people come for help when in crisis, our assessment of social networks should also identify conflicts or cutoffs that, if repaired, could be supportive. It's important to search for hidden resources and foster potential new connections. We also need to offer information about community resources and facilitate linkages.

Informal kin and chosen family members can be lifelines for resilience. These richly textured bonds have enabled struggling families to survive the ravages of poverty, racism, blighted communities, and inner-city violence (Boyd-Franklin, 2004). Such resources are particularly vital for underresourced single parents (Anderson, 2012). As one struggling mother said, "I have no family nearby, except my brother, and he's lost to drugs. I don't know what I'd do without my friends—I can always turn to them; they are really my 'next of kin.' "

For immigrants, migrant workers, and refugees, supportive kin and community ties may have frayed. Those in transition can become marginalized, on the edge of two social worlds, belonging to neither, and with tugs in incompatible directions. Our objective should be twofold: to support their adaptation and connection in their new social context and also to preserve valuable linkages with their kin, community, and cultural bonds (Falicov, 2012).

Multifamily groups serve as valuable networks for distressed families—for example, by linking undersupported single parents or families coping with the strains of a serious illness. The Internet has also become a increasingly vital source of information, social networking, and virtual communities.

It's important to pursue many kin and community options in seeking out models, mentors, and other inspirational figures, especially for at-risk youth. Mentoring relationships can be cultivated in the extended kin and community network. Isolated elder persons can play a mutually beneficial role in tutoring children. Programs such as Big Brothers/Big Sisters have demonstrated powerful effects in preventive efforts with at-risk urban children: involved youth are less likely to join gangs or use alcohol or drugs, and they show higher school performance. The key in such a relationship is spending time together engaging in chores and productive responsibilities, as well as fun activities, with a caring, positive role model, someone to look up to, learn from, and be inspired by. We also need to expand the narrow dyadic view of the relational base of resilience, and not expect one caregiver or mentor to meet all needs. When children are raised in a thick network of caring relations in family and community, the possibilities for nurturance and mentoring are many and varied. The African adage "It takes a village to raise a child" holds true today more than ever.

Financial Security and Family–Work Balance

To strengthen family functioning, clinicians need to take financial resources into account and examine the structural supports and balances linking family and work systems (Bianchi & Milkie, 2010). In today's highly stressful life, two-earner and single-parent households experience tremendous role strain with the pressures of multiple, conflicting job and child care demands and inadequate supports. One dual-earner mother and father described their lives as being "like two speeding commuter trains meeting briefly at the station and racing on." Surveys repeatedly find the leading issues of concern to working parents are the constant difficulty of balancing job and family obligations and the lack of affordable, high-quality child care. Many overburdened parents manage to keep their families and children functional only at a high cost to their own well-being; too many overloaded families break down as strains leave them more vulnerable to conflict and dissolution. If families are to thrive, the workplace must be restructured to help all workers achieve a better balance in their lives.

We can look to other nations' examples in developing new models to sustain family resilience. Although all industrialized countries have experienced social and economic upheaval, disruptions elsewhere are cushioned by social policies that safeguard family well-being, child and elder care, and expanding roles for men and women. Throughout Europe, family policy is part of general economic policy, and governments provide a range of supports for families across income groups and without stigma attached. In

Scandinavian countries, family life and child welfare are considered crucial to the well-being of society. Public policies actively encourage a balance between family life and paid work based on two assumptions: (1) that men and women are equally responsible for the financial support, daily care, and well-being of their children, and (2) that involvement in parenthood should not disadvantage people in job security, earnings, or advancement. Parental leave and a variety of child care arrangements are guaranteed *child* entitlements (Cooke & Baxter, 2010).

We must counter the myth of family self-reliance that has grown out of society's individualistic strain. Many problems of families today largely reflect difficulties in adaptation to the social and economic upheavals of recent decades and the unresponsiveness of larger community and societal institutions. These structural problems make it difficult for families to sustain mutual support and control over their lives.

With mothers, fathers, and other caregivers in the workforce today, and with diversity in family structures and resources, families require a national commitment to affordable, high-quality child and elder care, universal health care, and more flexible job structures and schedules in order to support healthy family functioning and the well-being of all members. Employers need to develop innovative options—including job sharing, a shorter work week, and home-based employment—to meet the child-rearing needs of both fathers and mothers, and to fit the abilities and constraints of older people who want or need to keep working through their later years. Some countries have advanced legislation that recognizes family diversity and ensures that parental responsibility for a child's well-being always outweighs parental rights over a child. We also need to grapple with economic disparity and the impact of poverty and disempowerment on families and their members—particularly on women, children, the elderly, and people of color.

In clinical work, family assessment and interventions must not be limited to the interior of the family. We must also attend to the family's transactions with other systems and resources: how they can effectively navigate and negotiate to overcome obstacles and support their resilience (Ungar, 2011). It's important to inquire about income, financial situation, and major shifts in employment. A parent may benefit from coaching to negotiate a pay raise or a change in job schedule. Children may exhibit symptoms that reflect family concerns; for example, a son's school failure often coincides with his father's job loss.

In one family assessment interview, Mario and Alicia presented a tirade of complaints about their son's recent failing grades and stealing of Alicia's savings from under their mattress. In exploring recent stresses in the family, we learned that Mario had recently lost his second job, severely straining the family's finances, jeopardizing their home ownership, and fueling marital tensions. Feeling deficient as a provider, Mario felt like a total failure to be a "good" husband and father. We examined expectations about what a "good father" meant for family members and noted how their Italian American cultural beliefs equated "good father" with "successful breadwinner." We explored qualities other than a paycheck for which family members valued the father. Mario hadn't realized before how much he meant to them and how many ways he could contribute to raising his children well. Couple sessions focused on ways to support each other's efforts, budget their expenses, find ways they could both contribute to strengthening the family's financial security, and tap kin support until they regained solid footing.

With major shifts in the economy, companies have displaced workers at all income levels and life stages. Those with the least education and skills are hardest hit, and their families are seriously affected. Rates of alcohol and drug use increase, along with couple and family conflict. Family support is crucial for displaced workers to regain confidence and build new areas of competence. (See Chapter 8 for a model family resilience program.)

For many families this crisis is worsened by inadequate structural supports in the larger society (Bogenschneider & Corbett, 2010). Scarce resources, institutional barriers, and a pileup of employment, health care, and social problems burden too many families, especially those living in conditions of poverty and urban decay. Harry Aponte (1994) stresses that societal fragmentation, with its climate of stress, isolation, and distrust, has increased vulnerability, violence, and despair. The poor "have all the personal and family problems everyone else has, along with the complications of a personal, family, and community ecosystem weakened by chronic social and economic problems" (p. 9). They are at highest risk of early, unwed pregnancy, single-parent families, divorce, substance abuse, and violence. Aponte sees the poor as our "canary in the mines," warning us of our unsafe environment. Because the same conditions are also affecting everyone else, addressing larger structural problems may also heal and strengthen our whole society.

FAMILY SHOCK ABSORBERS

No family form or style is inherently healthy or dysfunctional. Each family, influenced by its cultural values, resources, and social context, develops its structure and preferences for certain transactional patterns. Whether those organizational processes are functional depends largely on their *fit* with family challenges. We need to extend our focus beyond the household to significant relational networks: All individuals are members of kinship groups, whether formal or informal, living under the same roof, within a community, or scattered at a great distance. The myth of the isolated nuclear family, intact and self-sufficient, should not blind us to the intimate and powerful connections among kin living apart. We need to recognize the significance of these relational lifelines for resilience, and to do all we can to strengthen them.

Leading clinicians, as well as researchers, have noted the importance of core organizational patterns for healthy family functioning. Above all, Minuchin (1974) urged us to view the family as a social system in transformation. With this orientation, many more families in distress can be seen and treated as average families in transitional situations, suffering the pains of accommodation to new circumstances.

Family and social networks are natural "shock absorbers" in times of crisis. Family therapy pioneer Carl Whitaker once presented a videotape of an interview with a "healthy family" at a meeting of the American Psychiatric Association. Many attendees challenged him, pointing out a host of pathologies they detected. Labeling the father an "obsessive–compulsive personality," they saw him as rigid and absorbed in his work. Whitaker rose to their challenge: He met with the family annually over the next 5 years and then returned to the conference to present his findings. All family members were still functioning well. Most remarkable, for Whitaker, was their flexibility during crises that had occurred, as is inevitable in all families. When the maternal grandmother became critically ill, the mother turned her attention to providing the needed care, while the father made more time for the family. Rallying in response to the crisis, he showed unexpected role flexibility in taking over most household and child care responsibilities during those difficult months, and was able to comfort and support his wife and children through the illness and death of the beloved grandmother. As Whitaker noted, this family summoned its resources and showed its greatest strengths when challenged by crisis. We need to share Whitaker's conviction that in all families, such resources can be brought forth to strengthen family resilience.

CHAPTER 5

Communication Processes

Facilitating Meaning Making,
Mutual Support, and Problem Solving

Our greatest glory is not in never falling, but in rising
every time we fall.

—CONFUCIUS

Good communication facilitates all aspects of family functioning
and resilience. The complex challenges in contemporary family life make
it all the more important. In times of crisis, disruptive transitions, or prolonged stress, communication is more likely to break down—at the very
times when it is most essential.

Communication involves the transmission of beliefs, information
exchange, emotional expression, and problem-solving processes (Ryan et
al., 2005). Every communication has a "content" aspect, conveying facts,
opinions, or feelings, and a "relationship" aspect, defining, affirming,
or challenging the nature of relationships. For instance, the statement
"Take your medicine" is a command with the expectation of compliance.
All verbal and nonverbal behavior conveys messages, including silence,
withdrawal—or spitting out the medicine, which might mean "I don't
like it!" (feelings); "It won't help!" (belief/opinion); or "I won't obey you!"
(relationship statement).

A large body of research on couple and family interaction has focused
on key elements in good communication. Olson's Circumplex Model and
FACES-IV instrument (Olson & Gorall, 2003) target specific skills, such

82

as speaking and listening, self-disclosure, clarity, continuity tracking, respect, and regard. Speaking skills involve speaking for oneself and not for others. Listening skills include attentive focus and empathic response. Self-disclosure involves sharing information and feelings about oneself, significant experiences, and the relationship. Within families, parent–child differences are common: parental requests for open communication may be viewed by adolescents as prying and intrusive.

Cultural norms vary widely regarding what information or feelings are deemed appropriate or helpful to share in families, and how directly, with whom, and in what context they are shared. Midwestern Scandinavians have an adage about the man who loved his wife so much he almost told her! In Japan, children are taught to infer what others are trying to communicate from the context and the way in which something is conveyed, and to notice what is *not* said, in the belief that words cannot adequately capture meaning or emotions. Physicians may inform family members of a bad medical prognosis but not consider it advisable to tell the patient.

Intervention efforts with families dealing with adversity aim to increase their abilities to clarify their situation, to express and respond to each other's feelings, needs, and concerns, and to negotiate approaches to resolve problems and meet new demands. Clear information, open emotional expression, and collaborative problem solving are key processes for family resilience (see Table 5.1).

CLARITY

Numerous studies have found that communication clarity facilitates effective couple and family functioning (Beavers & Hampson, 2003; Olson & Gorall, 2003; Ryan et al., 2005; Satir, 1988).

Clear, Consistent Messages

Clear and consistent verbal and behavioral messages yield shared understanding. In well-functioning families, even with interruptions, members can effectively resume discussions and follow through behaviorally. Contextual clarity enables members to distinguish reality from fantasy, facts from opinions, and serious intent from humor.

Clear and consistent family rules organize interaction, set behavioral expectations, and define relationships (Minuchin, 1974). Unclarity can be problematic. For instance, what does it mean when a single mother calls the oldest son the "man of the house"? When communication is vague,

TABLE 5.1. Key Communication Processes in Family Resilience

Clarity

- Clear, consistent messages (words and actions).
- Clarify ambiguous information; truth seeking.

Open emotional expression

- Share painful feelings (sadness, suffering, anger, fear, disappointment, remorse).
- Share positive feelings and interactions (appreciation, affection, fun, humor, respite).

Collaborative problem solving

- Practice creative brainstorming, resourcefulness.
- Share decision making; repair conflicts; negotiate; show fairness, reciprocity.
- Focus on goals; take concrete steps; build on success; learn from setbacks.
- Shift from reactive to proactive stance: prepare for future challenges.

distorted, or left unresolved, it breeds anxiety, confusion, and misunderstanding. Members may operate on faulty assumptions or attempt mind reading. Heightened anxiety and communication confusion can also impede effective action and coordination during crisis events and in disaster response (see Chapter 11).

Clarifying an Adverse Situation and Options

As we've seen in Chapter 3, the ability to clarify and give meaning to a crisis or a precarious situation makes it easier to bear. Often family members glean different understandings of events and their implications, based on bits and pieces of information, rumors, or their own assumptions. Some fill in the blanks with their best hopes; others with their worst fears. The experience becomes more comprehensible and manageable when members share information and perceptions, discussing openly the meanings and the ramifications for their lives. They can then better appraise their options, deal constructively with their challenges, and avert future difficulties. When family members have limited or conflicting information, blocking their adaptation, therapists can encourage them to gather more facts and expand perspectives for a fuller picture.

Sharing Bad News

Family members commonly try to protect loved ones from painful or threatening information, particularly children, elders, or other vulnerable members. However, prolonged silence, secrecy, or distortion can create barriers to understanding, authentic relating, and informed decision making. When facts about a traumatic loss are hidden, this can greatly affect mutual trust and stability over time. Withholding information about a threatened or impending event can rob loved ones of time to anticipate and prepare for it. In one case, Mark, a man in his 40s, didn't tell his parents he was terminally ill with melanoma until a week before he died; as a result, his sudden, unexpected death was so shattering that it triggered a heart attack in his father.

Family members are often aware of unspoken issues and tensions, like having a proverbial elephant in the room that can't be talked about. Conversations tend to remain superficial and contact is avoided. When members block communication of knowledge, memories, expectations, or fears, the unspeakable may go underground, often becoming expressed in emotional or physical symptoms or surfacing in other relationships or life contexts.

Commonly, when parents are concerned about a serious issue, they try to spare their children and other vulnerable family members from worry by putting on a cheerful facade, as if all is "normal." However, children readily pick up underlying tensions, as do family pets (Walsh, 2009b). When parents don't explain the source of their distress (e.g., a precarious job situation), children may blame themselves for being bad or unlovable. Some act on their best behavior so as not to burden a parent further. When children's concerns are submerged and unvoiced, they can erupt in physical or behavioral symptoms. Yet the crisis of a child's problems can also jolt family members into the need to deal with unshared issues.

> One mother brought her 5-year-old son for an evaluation for sexual abuse, fearing he had been molested in his preschool because she often found him fondling himself. Carefully ruling out sexual abuse, the therapist referred the case to me. In a session with the mother (the father had refused to attend), I explored recent stressful events in the family. She reported that several months earlier, her husband had had exploratory surgery for "stomach pains." A cancerous tumor and most of his stomach were removed. At hospital discharge, he told his wife, "OK, they said they got it all; I just want to go back to normal life and not talk about it."
>
> To respect her husband's wishes, she told the children, "Daddy's fine" and no more was said. At a recent checkup, "something suspicious" was found and the future prognosis was now worrisome. The parents assumed their son wasn't upset because he hadn't asked any questions. The next week she noticed that when the family had said

grace before dinner, her son had added, "And please God, take care of Daddy's tummy." It was important to see the parents together to open their communication and share their concerns about the life-threatening development. They were encouraged to discuss it sensitively with their children. Instead of acting as if nothing had happened, they were helped to integrate the experience into their lives and to meet the challenges ahead with the life-threatening condition.

Sometimes parents postpone any discussion until all facts or a dreaded outcome are certain. When a situation is tenuous, such as a potential separation or divorce, children may become hypervigilant for cues, reading bad news into any conflict or hushed conversation between parents. It can be more reassuring when adults relate what information they can and acknowledge the uncertainties they are dealing with, helping the children absorb the evolving situation gradually. It's helpful for parents to encourage children to come to them if they have more questions or concerns. It's important for parents to assure them that they will fill them in as the situation becomes clearer. We can be helpful by coaching parents on ways to share potentially upsetting information with children—facts of an adoption, a parent's absence, or a death—in age-appropriate ways. In the aftermath of traumatic experiences, truth telling is a vital process in family and community recovery (see Chapters 11 and 14).

OPEN EMOTIONAL SHARING

In well-functioning families, transactions are notable for a warm, cheerfully optimistic tone, with joy and comfort in relating, grounded in trust (Beavers & Hampson, 2003). In dealing with adversity, resilience is facilitated by the ability of members to express and tolerate a wide range of feelings, both painful and positive—from negative feelings such as sadness, anger, regret, and fear, to pleasurable interactions expressing love, appreciation, gratitude, and joy, and offering respite.

Empathic Sharing of Painful Feelings

A climate of mutual trust (see Chapter 3) encourages and is reinforced by open, empathic sharing of emotions (Beavers & Hampson, 2003). Messages are conveyed in a considerate way to respect others' feelings and differences. With acceptance of uncertainty, ambivalence, and disagreement, members risk less in being open. They show interest in what others have to say and hold an expectation of being understood. Active listening may not be sufficient when changes are also needed. When a family member is upset or expresses unmet needs, others demonstrate empathic concern by responding in both word and deed. In one study, relational processes in the more resilient families facilitated ways to express painful emotions regarding a recent family crisis. In contrast, families with low resilience often described struggles in expressing their feelings (Cohen, Slonim, Finzi, & Leichtentritt, 2002).

Gender-based socialization can constrain full emotional sharing. Images of masculinity block many men from disclosing vulnerability and feelings that might imply weakness, fear, or sorrow. In emotionally laden interactions, men are more likely to become flooded or withdraw by stonewalling or distancing emotionally (Driver et al., 2012). Some sexualize emotional needs in affairs or submerge feelings by overwork or substance abuse. In strongly patriarchal cultures and families, girls and women may risk emotional or physical harm if they voice feelings that challenge male authority or are thought to dishonor the family. To speak truthfully, with mutual respect, family members must feel safe.

Owning Feelings, Respecting Differences

As families face hard times, loving tolerance and respect for differences are important. In a family system, members' emotional responses are likely to vary, owing to cultural or personal differences, the nature of relationships, and particular implications of the adverse situation. Members may be out of sync with each other in their reactions, emotional intensity, or the timing of feelings that surface. A teenager's delayed upset at the loss of a parent may erupt just when other family members are emotionally ready to move on with life. Individual members may express varied aspects of complex emotions in the family. For instance, in the wake of a tragedy, when a hard-hit family is forced to give up its home, one child may be profoundly sad, while another may express only anger, and another may suppress feelings to support a struggling parent or act like a clown to cheer up everyone.

In a crisis situation, individual members' own unacknowledged or mixed feelings can become split between partners, siblings, or branches of a family. For instance, members' highly emotional decision over whether to terminate life support for a loved one in critical condition can become increasingly polarized in intense, bitter conflict. Some families may try to suppress or deny negative feelings and behaviors, while playing up the positive ones, presenting a false united front. In more distraught families, negative or angry feelings may predominate, with rare expression of gratitude, praise, or affection. Family sessions can be valuable in all these situations, helping members to express a fuller range of emotions, and to hear and understand the various feelings of others.

Well-functioning families show strikingly little blame, personal attack, or scapegoating. Members take responsibility for their own feelings and actions and acknowledge their contribution to difficulties. In poorly functioning families, a climate of fear and mistrust is perpetuated through criticism, blame, and scapegoating. Emotional expression then becomes highly reactive, critical, defensive, or attacking (Bowen, 1978). Conflict can escalate out of control. A vicious cycle may ensue, for instance, when a parent overreacts to a son's misbehavior with threats to send him away, increasing his anxiety and provocative behavior, which then push the parent beyond tolerance and result in his expulsion.

Open communication is essential in dealing with a prolonged ordeal. One couple reflected on the importance of sharing their feelings through their son's cancer diagnosis, subsequent treatments, remission, and uncertain long-term prognosis. The husband said that his greatest lesson had been not to be afraid of fear; he had learned that bottling up his fears only intensified them, but that expressing them to his wife eased his mind and brought the couple closer.

Open communication does not mean constantly talking about problems, suffering, or fears. Over time, members also need respite from focus on their ordeal. What's crucial is that communication not be blocked so that members can feel free, as needs arise, to voice what is on their minds and in their hearts.

Positive Interactions

Sharing positive feelings and enjoyable interactions is vital through stressful times. Relationships can tolerate considerable conflict as long as it is offset by much more positive communication through expressions of love, appreciation, and respect, and pleasurable interaction (Driver et al., 2012; Markman et al., 2010).

Sharing Pleasure, Fun, Joy

With a shattering experience, family members may feel numbed; chronic stress may generate "battle fatigue" and a deadened sense in relationships. It can be helpful to revive pleasures that were once shared and to create new ways for satisfying connection. Families can be encouraged to plan activities together that give them an enjoyable shared focus, such as a movie or a sports event; that provide an opportunity for active collaboration, such as a family potluck or a picnic; or that offer a spiritually renewing experience to transcend their immediate distress and draw strength for coping.

Therapists need to aim beyond reduction of problems and negative interactions to active encouragement of positive shared experiences to revitalize families that have gone through hard times, as in the following case.

Therapy with Mrs. Lamm and her four children was stuck in their shared depression and passivity. They came for help after 12-year-old Jeffrey attempted suicide by drinking cleaning solvent. Family therapy focused on their sadness and anger at the father's "disappearance" 3 months earlier, leaving his family uncertain of his whereabouts or whether he would return. The father, who had a serious drinking problem, had drifted off several times in the past, but always showed up a few weeks later as if nothing had happened. This time they worried that he might never come back. The more family members talked about their helplessness and hopelessness, the more weighted down the therapy sessions became. The therapy, like the family, was in limbo, waiting for the return of the wayward father.

Invited in as a consultant, I asked the mother and children how things had changed with the father's absence. I noted that they seemed to have lost the life of the family when the father wasn't around. Although his possible return might be beyond their control, they could, if they pulled together, regain their liveliness. I asked what they had enjoyed doing together. Hearing that they had the most fun going fishing, I asked if they might plan to go fishing over the coming weekend. They nodded passively, seeming to be waiting for someone to make it happen, as the father had always taken charge. It was important not to put all responsibility on the mother, who was depleted by job and family demands. Encouraging a team approach, I asked each child what he or she might do to help make it happen. One child offered to clean the fishing poles in the basement and help his small brother dig for worms; the two others agreed to make sandwiches and pack a picnic lunch. The mother, brightening, offered to drive them to a favorite fishing spot on Saturday morning. She and the children became animated in discussing the plans and remembering past fun they had enjoyed.

To anticipate possible obstacles, I asked if they could imagine anything that might keep them from going (such as bad weather or a child's misbehavior) and suggested that they plan an alternative "rain date." Since the father's unpredictability in his comings and goings was so problematic, it was especially important for expectations and plans to be clearly communicated, and for all members to take responsibility for their own parts and to agree that they could count on each other to follow through. The family arrived at the next session energized, with spirits revived from their outing. After this "jump start," the Lamms were better able to actively take initiative in other steps toward coming to terms with the ambiguous loss of the father and, while not giving up all hope, moving forward with life.

Sharing Humor

When doctors told Norman Cousins (1979/2001) that he would die within months from a rare disease, he posited that if negative emotions can produce harmful chemical changes in the body, then positive emotions should have a therapeutic value. He checked out of his depressing hospital room and into a comfortable (and less expensive) hotel. He attributed much of his recovery to "laughter therapy"—watching old Marx Brothers films and TV comedy shows. Medical studies have documented that humor, indeed, can bolster our spirits and our immune systems in ways that encourage healing and recovery from serious illness.

Shared humor and laughter are especially needed in families facing adversity. In multi-stress conditions, humor may be lost altogether as members become overwhelmed and depleted. Humor helps families to cope with difficult situations, reduce tensions, and accept limitations (Wuerffel, DeFrain, & Stinnett, 1990). Finding humor in the midst of despair can detoxify threatening situations, lessen anxiety, and offer respite from unrelenting stresses. It can facilitate conversation, express feelings of warmth and affection, and restore a positive outlook. Humor can ease a direct confrontation, melt a defensive reaction, help a person to accept failure, and lighten heavy burdens. Humor can be particularly beneficial when it expresses the absurd aspects of a harrowing situation—the incongruous, bizarre, silly, or illogical things that happen.

In high-functioning families, members realize that while they can envision perfection, they are destined to flounder, make mistakes, get scared, and need reassurance. This encourages both a sense of humor and humility (Beavers & Hampson, 2003). Family therapy pioneers encouraged clinicians to appreciate both the grim and the absurd, humanizing therapy in providing a context for sharing laughter as well as tears. Whitaker stressed the importance of family humor and playfulness for creative fantasy and inventive process (Whitaker & Keith, 1981). However, humor can be destructive when used to demean a family member or to express anger, cruelty, or contempt through biting sarcasm. Encouraging shared humor—members laughing *with* one another—can revitalize families' spirits.

Respite from Cumulative Stresses and Burnout

Family members can become emotionally overloaded and depleted from efforts to deal with overwhelming stresses. Clinicians need to recognize family burnout and be careful not to pile more expectations on exhausted parents or caregivers, and instead encourage other family members to arrange respite time and space, covering the bases to make it happen. For instance, I might task children to give their mother an hour on the weekend for herself. Most often, an overstressed mother, offered time for herself, replies, "I just want to close the door and go to bed and tune out all the noise!" Recharging emotional batteries is essential. Likewise, a couple needs to recharge their relationship. I may ask parents when was the last time they went out on a date, and they laughingly admit they can't remember. I suggest that they take time out from their difficulties for an enjoyable date, with a pledge of "no problem-talk." I might also encourage them to designate their bedroom a "problem-free zone."

COLLABORATIVE PROBLEM SOLVING

Effective problem-solving processes are essential for families to deal with crises and persistent challenges. All relationships will have problems. What distinguishes relational resilience is the ability to manage conflict and address problems collaboratively. This requires tolerance for open disagreement and skills for solving problems in daily living and in troubled times.

The practical and emotional aspects of a crisis situation are intertwined. When family functioning is disrupted by basic instrumental problems, such as the loss of a job and income, the ability to deal with emotional needs is also strained. In turn, emotional distress impairs problem solving. A negative emotional tone between family members—anger, frustration, discouragement, or defeat—can block them from dealing successfully with serious or persistent problems. Members may be reluctant to share their opinions or avoid bringing up a sensitive issue or a difference of opinion if they fear hurting others' feelings or escalating conflict. Both the practical and emotional tasks must be addressed.

The McMaster group (Ryan et al., 2005) has identified several steps in effective problem-solving processes. Family members first need to recognize a problem and to communicate with those involved and those who might be potential resources. Collaborative brainstorming enables them to weigh and consider possible options, resources, and constraints, and to decide on a plan. They then need to initiate and carry out action, monitor efforts, and evaluate their success. Well-functioning families can efficiently manage, if not resolve, most problems in daily life. Their communication, decision making, and action flow reasonably smoothly. In reviewing results, they can fine-tune or revise their efforts as needed.

Identifying Problems and Related Stressors:
Creative Brainstorming

When help is sought for a presenting problem—a parent's depression, a husband's drinking, a child's misbehavior—it is important to explore other recent or ongoing stressors in family life that may be reverberating throughout the system. A child or adolescent's misbehavior is often a barometer of family tensions and may deflect concern from other family concerns that require attention.

It's important to involve family members in creative brainstorming of problematic situations. In well-functioning families, parents act as coordinators and coaches—bringing out others' ideas, voicing their own, and encouraging choice wherever possible. The contributions of members young and old are respected as valuable (Beavers & Hampson, 2003).

By identifying obstacles to problem solving, families can find ways to overcome them. We can encourage members to discuss both resources and constraints, and to consider various options, weighing the costs and benefits for the family and individual members. Openness to trying new solutions is a hallmark of adaptive families. Flexible and inventive approaches build resourcefulness in tackling future problems.

Shared Decision Making: Negotiation, Compromise, and Reciprocity

In research on resilient individuals, Higgins (1994) was struck by their ability to "love well" in long-term relationships. They showed a high degree of reciprocity and concern for one another and consistently tried to recognize others' needs. They made active efforts to withstand conflict, disappointment, anger, and frustration and negotiated difficulties successfully over time.

Studies across a broad diversity of families have found negotiation processes to be crucial for optimal couple and family functioning. In problem solving, a collaborative process of negotiation can be as important as the outcome, with family members' input sought on major decisions. It's crucial for therapists to note how important decisions are reached.

> Anna requested individual therapy for her recent depression, triggered by the decision to move to another part of the country so that her husband, Bob, could take a better job. I asked the couple to come in together initially, to explore the situation jointly and determine how to be most helpful. When I asked them how the decision to move was made, Bob replied, "I told her I had this great job offer that I told them

I'd probably take; what do you think about it?" Confronted with a decision all but made by Bob, Anna agreed because it was good for him, without considering her own feelings and needs. After they had made all arrangements, she became acutely depressed about leaving her job, family, friends, and community. Bob was angry at her for burdening him with her sadness and regrets after agreeing to the decision, wanting her to "pull her own weight" with the difficult practical demands of the transition. Although they both initially suggested that Anna needed individual counseling "to adjust to the move," I recommended combining individual and couple sessions.

The partners were strongly encouraged to review their decision-making process and to discuss the options, costs, and benefits more collaboratively. This process revealed that they both had mixed feelings about the move, but that Bob had expressed only the positive side, while Anna, passively accommodating, carried all the feelings of regret and loss. As their positions had polarized, their relationship became increasingly strained. Anna realized that she needed to participate more actively in the couple's decision making and to have her feelings acknowledged and her preferences weighed in the balance. Had she met with a therapist individually to "adjust" to the move, she would most likely have carried resentment along with her accommodation.

Negotiation involves airing and respecting differences while working toward shared goals. Striving for an equal partnership and working out the complex demands of dual-career family life put a premium on negotiation processes. Couples need to gain comfort and skill in open communication and conflict management. To be successful negotiators, family members need to be able to express their own feelings and preferences and to listen and respond empathically to others. It's crucial to interrupt negative cycles of criticism, blame, and withdrawal—the attacks and defensiveness that corrode relationships. Those who sustain strong relationships learn how to repair conversations that go badly and how to soothe each other when hurt or upset occurs (Driver et al., 2012). One person might say, "This isn't working; let's try talking about this again after a break" or "Let's both cool down and try to resolve our differences more calmly when we can hear each other." Such nurturing, monitoring, and support strengthen relationships as problems are tackled.

Negotiation and compromise can be hindered by struggles over power and control. Battles over the relationship aspect of communication keep substantive issues from being addressed. Accommodation may be viewed in terms of winning versus losing, or having power over others versus being controlled or "one-down." Positions become rigid and nonnegotiable when compromise is felt to be "giving in" to the other. When there is a skewed deference–dominance imbalance over time, resentments are stockpiled. A lack of trust in reciprocity breeds short-term "tit-for-tat" exchanges, or a withholding on one person's part until the other "evens the score" between them. Lack of nurturing and supportiveness contributes to resentment. Multiple stresses heighten tensions and conflict.

Traditional gender-based socialization and power dynamics influence negotiation processes and outcome. Men and women often enter into negotiation with different basic premises. Men reared for success in the workplace are more likely to argue their positions forcefully and convincingly, with the aim of winning—meeting their own needs as fully as possible. Women, reared to prioritize the needs of others, more often defer and accommodate. It can be helpful in therapy to contextualize this skew in terms of these differing premises, recognizing family of origin and sociocultural influences.

> As Anna and Bob addressed their situation, Anna observed, "Somehow I always seem to defer to him. Maybe it's just my problem." I contextualized their dilemma, noting that quite commonly men and women learn different rules about negotiation. We explored how this might be happening for them: "Let me see if I understand your positions. It seems that for you, Bob, good negotiation means making the strongest case on your own behalf and pushing to win your case. Is that so?" Bob grinned. "That's true—sure!" "And for you, Anna, good negotiation means consideration of Bob's needs and compromise of your own." Anna nodded, adding, "And since I never play by his rules and he never plays by mine, things always end up his way. But this decision to move is too important—I need my feelings to count, too."
>
> We explored how their childhood experiences contributed to this pattern. Anna, a younger sister with older brothers in a traditional working-class family, learned early on to accommodate. Bob, the only son in his upwardly striving family, said he was "spoiled rotten" and always got his way.
>
> I commented that their relational skew seemed to operate like "the subtle pull of gravity." Bob nodded. "Right. It's like the norm is in my head. It's real comfortable." They laughed together. Anna added, "Well, since we've been out of our families for over a decade, maybe it's time for change!"

Skewed communication processes and power dynamics often come to the fore at a major life transition, triggering a relationship crisis, as in this case (see Chapter 9). Discussing the patterns in their larger social context without blame helped the couple to work toward more balanced negotiation, with Anna asserting her needs more effectively, and Bob being more considerate and mutually accommodating. Increased reciprocity can greatly strengthen a relationship and the ability to navigate transitional challenges collaboratively.

Managing Conflicts

In crisis or with cumulative stress, decision-making processes often don't proceed smoothly and may involve intense conflict, pain, or anger. We can help families normalize tensions as common in such situations, with the likelihood that most families do rebound over time. Tolerance for conflict allows for overt disagreement and acknowledgment of differences, with resolution through agreement, compromise, or new framing of the problem. Mixed feelings and conflict are to be expected as a part of all relationships. Families handle them by expanding their perspective to consider many aspects of their situation, and acting *on balance*—for instance, to serve the greater good of the family or the long-term best interests of children.

The best predictor of relationship success is not the absence of conflict, but its management: how differences, which are bound to arise, are handled and resolved or repaired. Deferring conflict may be functional in the midst of crisis, but avoidance can become dysfunctional over time, heightening risks for relationship breakdown as unattended issues pile up and resentments brew (Driver et al., 2012; Johnson, 2002). Catastrophic fears from traumatic past experience can lead to unspoken family rules to avoid all conflict. However, this protective strategy heightens risks that tensions will build up and later explode.

In couple relationships, escalating cycles of criticism and stonewalling, generating contempt and despair, have a corrosive effect (Driver et al., 2012). Turning away from connection leads over time to withdrawal, loss of hope of repairing the relationship, and marital dissolution. Conflicts, even if upsetting at the time, can be necessary and beneficial to a relationship if they are repaired. They also need to be offset by positive emotional expression, particularly by affection, humor, positive problem solving, agreement, assent, empathy, and active nondefensive listening. Varied conflict styles can be functional, especially if partners are matched in style preferences.

Relationships are strengthened by dialogue rather than gridlock over perpetual issues or problems that can't be solved. As Gottman's research found (Driver et al., 2012), more positive affect during discussion deescalated the conflict. The ratio of positive to negative interactions was at least 5:1 in stable and happy couples. With perpetual problems, couples aimed to establish a dialogue that communicated respect and acceptance of the partner, humor, affection, even amusement, and active coping with unresolvable situations.

With both conflict-avoidant and high-conflict couples, interventions need to increase skills for handling conflict to stop the corrosive process leading to relationship disintegration. Several couple intervention approaches have been developed that help partners to fight constructively, manage negative emotions, and respond compassionately to each other (e.g., Markman et al., 2010). Such approaches provide ground rules and coaching to handle conflict and control runaway processes: partners may call "time out" when needed; escalating conflicts are slowed down; arguments are kept constructive; withdrawal is avoided; and involvement must be maintained. Couple therapy can build relational resilience by providing a safe context where partners can become more respectful of differences and more skillful in managing and resolving conflict.

Focus on Goals, Take Concrete Steps, Build on Success, and Learn from Setbacks

To gain resilience, the belief in active mastery must be put into practice. It's important to focus on a positive vision or goal and to take concrete steps toward realistic, achievable objectives. Celebrating milestones toward more distant goals boosts morale. With each small, shared success, family members' confidence and competence grow, enabling them to meet larger challenges. Setbacks and frustrations are inevitable. The acceptance of mistakes allows family members to flounder or fail without being attacked, ridiculed, or defined as inadequate. Accountable for their own part when something has gone wrong, they learn from their experience not to repeat mistakes. Indeed, failed experiences can become instructive as family members recalibrate efforts or try a new tack to solve problems. As Albert Einstein remarked, "Anyone who has not experienced failure has not known success."

From Reactive to Proactive Approach: Prevention, Planning, Preparedness

When potential problems loom on the horizon, families do best if they approach them proactively, discussing them in a clear and open way, and addressing practical, emotional, and relational aspects. Through planning and preparedness, a crisis may be averted and few problems will pile up over time or complicate efforts to deal with major issues that arise.

Because most families seek help in crisis, intervention approaches tend to be crisis reactive, helping families recover. A family resilience approach shifts the focus from reactive to proactive, strengthening family resourcefulness to meet future challenges. It's important to encourage families to look ahead, learning from their experience, to plan and prepare to prevent past problems from recurring. Looking forward, they can more readily avert hazards and surmount likely obstacles. We can suggest they might devise a "Plan B" to keep in their relationship "vault" in case their aspirations must be revised. This proactive stance increases a sense of security for family members who, while hoping for the best, are prepared to meet life's disappointments and unanticipated turns in the road. Fortunately, there are many, varied pathways in resilience.

In sum, as family process research has documented, clear communication, open emotional sharing, and collaborative problem solving are vital communication processes that facilitate family resilience. Because not all problems can be solved, resilient families find aspects of the situation where they can take action. We can foster family resilience by encouraging the communication correlates of the facilitative beliefs described in Chapter 3. As families gain a perspective on a crisis or setback as a meaningful, manageable challenge, collaborative communication processes facilitate their best efforts. Regardless of the specific problems a family may be struggling with, it is crucial to strengthen communication processes to relieve family stress and enhance resourcefulness.

PART III

PRACTICE APPLICATIONS

CHAPTER 6

Assessing Family Resilience

Useful Maps for Practice and Research

The map is not the territory.
—GREGORY BATESON (1979, p. 30)

Maps are valuable for orienting us in unfamiliar and challenging territory, noting landmarks, offering guideposts, and suggesting pathways in our journey toward our destination. In clinical and community-based practice with families facing adversity, their problem-saturated life situations skew our attention and make it difficult to identify strengths and resources to guide paths toward positive goals. This chapter offers several useful maps to orient and guide resilience-oriented family assessment and practice. First, the key processes in family resilience, presented in Chapters 3–5, are summarized and organized in a framework designed to bring coherence to intervention planning. Next, the use of a few resilience-oriented genograms, timelines, and questionnaires is discussed and illustrated. Finally, strategies and challenges in family resilience research are briefly addressed, with reflections and recommendations.

KEY PROCESSES IN FAMILY RESILIENCE:
A MAP TO GUIDE ASSESSMENT AND INTERVENTION

In all family assessment, we must be mindful that no "single thread" distinguishes well-functioning families, as several decades of family research

101

have established (Lebow & Stroud, 2012). When diagnostic formulations reduce the richness of family interaction to simplistic labels, such as "an enmeshed family," or "an alcoholic family," they stereotype and pathologize families. Instead, we need to consider the many interwoven strands in family functioning and assess strengths and vulnerabilities on multiple system dimensions in relation to the challenges each family faces, its resources and constraints, and the influence of social and temporal contexts.

The growing body of research on resilience and well-functioning families can inform intervention and prevention approaches to strengthen family processes for resilience. As practitioners and researchers, we must be aware of our own subjectivity in mapping a territory we—or others—inhabit. From my survey of the research literature and my own clinical research and practice, I identified nine key transactional processes (Walsh, 2003) and organized them in three domains (dimensions) of family functioning, as described in Chapters 3–5. This framework was constructed to serve as a flexible map to orient clinical and community-based practitioners to important elements in family functioning and bring coherence to intervention planning. Just as Sprenkle, Davis, and Lebow (2009) have identified core components of family therapy processes in effective interventions, practitioners can focus on core components in family processes that contribute to effective family functioning. By targeting key processes we can strengthen family resilience as presenting problems are addressed. Table 6.1 outlines these nine processes and their subcomponents. A brief summary is provided below.

Family Belief Systems

Family belief systems, rooted in multigenerational, sociocultural, and spiritual influences, are transmitted through family and social transactions, stories, and legacies. They powerfully influence how members view their adverse situation, their suffering, and their options. These shared constructions organize family approaches to life challenges, and they can be fundamentally altered by such experiences. Adversity generates a crisis of meaning and potential disruption of integration. Family resilience is fostered by shared beliefs that increase effective functioning, strengthen bonds, and expand options for positive adaptation and growth. Clinicians can facilitate families' efforts at making meaning of their adverse situation, gaining a hopeful, positive outlook and active agency, and drawing on transcendent or spiritual values and connections for inspiration, transformation, and positive growth.

TABLE 6.1. Key Processes in Family Resilience

Belief systems

1. Making meaning of adversity
   - Relational view of resilience—versus "rugged individual."
   - Normalize, contextualize distress: common, understandable in adverse situations.
   - Sense of coherence: view crisis as a shared challenge; meaningful, comprehensible, manageable.
   - Facilitative appraisal: explanatory attributions; future expectations.

2. Positive outlook
   - Hope, optimistic bias; confidence in overcoming challenges.
   - Encouragement; affirm strengths and build on potential.
   - Active initiative and perseverance (can-do spirit).
   - Master the possible; accept what can't be changed; tolerate uncertainty.

3. Transcendence and spirituality
   - Larger values, purpose.
   - Spirituality: faith, contemplative practices, community; connection with nature.
   - Inspiration: envisioning possibilities, aspirations; creative expression; social action.
   - Transformation: learning, change, and positive growth from adversity.

Organizational processes

4. Flexibility
   - Rebound, adaptive change to meet new challenges.
   - Reorganize, restabilize: continuity, dependability, predictability.
   - Strong authoritative leadership: nurture, guide, protect.
   - Varied family forms: cooperative parenting/caregiving teams, household.
   - Couple/coparent relationship: mutual respect; equal partners.

5. Connectedness
   - Mutual support, teamwork, and commitment.
   - Respect individual needs, differences.
   - Seek reconnection and repair grievances.

6. Mobilize social and economic resources
   - Recruit extended kin, social, and community supports; models and mentors.
   - Build financial security; navigate stressful work–family challenges.
   - Transactions with larger systems: enlist institutional, structural supports.

Communication processes

7. Clarity
   - Clear, consistent messages (words and actions).
   - Clarify ambiguous information; truth seeking.

8. Open emotional expression
   - Share painful feelings (sadness, suffering, anger, fear, disappointment, remorse).
   - Share positive feelings and interactions (love, appreciation, gratitude. humor, fun, respite).

9. Collaborative problem solving
   - Creative brainstorming; resourcefulness.
   - Share decision making; repair conflicts; negotiation, fairness, reciprocity.
   - Focus on goals; concrete steps; build on success; learn from setbacks.
   - Shift from reactive to proactive stance: prepare for future challenges.

1. Making Meaning of Adversity

A *relational view* of resilience encourages families and couples to approach adversity as a shared challenge. Their joint struggles, efforts, and pride in prevailing strengthen their bonds.

By *normalizing* and *contextualizing* distress, family members enlarge their perspective to see their difficulties as understandable in light of their adverse situation. The tendency toward blame, shame, and pathologizing is reduced when problems can be viewed as human dilemmas, with distress seen as common among those in similar predicaments—and as normal responses to abnormal or extreme conditions. Family resilience is also fostered by an evolutionary sense of time and becoming—a continual process of growth, challenge, and change over the life course and the generations. This family life cycle perspective helps members see disruptive events or transitions as milestones or turning points in their shared life passage and links them with past and future generations.

In grappling with adversity, families can be helped to gain a shared *sense of coherence* by recasting a crisis as a challenge that is meaningful to tackle and by making it comprehensible and manageable. This involves members' efforts to clarify the nature and source of problems, their options, and future expectations. Family members try to make sense of how things have happened through causal or explanatory attributions, and they look to their future with hopes and fears. Practitioners can support members' realistic appraisal of their situation and their possibilities; facilitate restoration or reconstruction of meaning following devastating events; and encourage active agency in coping and adaptive strategies.

2. Positive Outlook

Considerable research documents the strong neurophysiological effects of a positive outlook in coping with stress, recovering from crisis, and overcoming barriers to success. *Hope* is essential to the spirit: it fuels energy and efforts to rise above adversity. Hope is a faith-based, future-oriented belief: no matter how bleak the immediate prospects, a better future can be envisioned. In problem-saturated conditions, practitioners need to rekindle hope from despair. Hope for a better future for their children can keep struggling parents from being defeated by their present life circumstances.

It's essential for professionals to hold an *optimistic bias* with conviction in every family's worth and potential. Repeated experiences of futility and failure can lead people to stop trying and become passive and pessimistic, generalizing the belief that nothing they do will matter. Despair can rob them of meaning, purpose, and a sense of future possibility. A positive outlook supports their best efforts, fosters well-being, and can reduce risk and maximize chances of success.

By *affirming family strengths and potential* in the midst of difficulties, we help families to counter a sense of helplessness and failure while reinforcing their shared pride. We help them build confidence and competence through experiencing successful mastery and learning that their efforts can make a difference.

Initiative and perseverance—hallmarks of resilience—are fueled by a "can-do" spirit in family members' shared confidence and mutual encouragement through an ordeal: "We'll never give up trying." This conviction bolsters their efforts to do their best and makes them active participants in a tenacious search for solutions.

Mastering the art of the possible is vital in resilience. Practitioners can help families take stock of their situation—their challenges, constraints, and resources—and then focus their energy on making the best of their options. Efforts are supported by accepting—coming to terms with—what is beyond their control or can't be changed. When immediate problems are overwhelming, or larger social conditions are daunting, family members can be encouraged to start with aspects they can do something about, instead of feeling trapped or helpless. This does not mean accepting harsh or unjust conditions, but rather not being defeated by a sense of powerlessness and instead mobilizing efforts to take steps toward a positive aim. Although past events can't be changed, they can be recast in a new light that fosters greater comprehension, learning, and healing. It is also crucial for families to tolerate uncertainty, since many situations may remain ambiguous or outcomes unclear.

3. Transcendence and Spirituality

Transcendent values and practices provide meaning and purpose beyond a family's immediate plight. Most families seek strength, comfort, and guidance in troubled times through connections with their cultural and faith traditions. Rituals and ceremonies can facilitate passage through difficult transitions and linkage with a larger community and common heritage.

Spirituality, a dimension of human experience, comes to the fore in suffering, healing, and resilience. Religious beliefs, such as punishment for sins or loss of faith with injustice, may contribute to distress; religious doctrine may be used to justify harm to others. As a large body of research documents, spiritual resources are wellsprings for resilience, most commonly tapped through moral values, faith in a higher power, rituals and contemplative practices (e.g., prayer and meditation), and/or congregational involvement. Many find spiritual nourishment outside religious structures through deep personal faith or secular humanism, in connection with nature, in expression through the arts and music, and in social activism.

The paradox of resilience is that the worst of times can also bring out the best in the human spirit. A crisis can deepen spirituality and yield transformation and growth in unforeseen directions, as found in research on posttraumatic growth. The experience of adversity and suffering can inspire bold and creative action. It can awaken family members to the importance of loved ones or spark them to heal old wounds and reorder priorities for more meaningful relationships and life pursuits. Many emerge from shattering experiences with a heightened sense of purpose in their lives, gaining compassion for the plight of others and spurring commitment to social, political, or environmental action to alleviate suffering, injustice, or harmful conditions. Professionals can support family efforts to envision a better future through their concerted efforts and, where hopes and dreams have been dashed, to imagine new possibilities, seizing opportunities for invention, transformation, and positive growth.

Family Organizational Processes

Families with diverse structures, households, and resources must organize their living patterns and relational networks in varied ways to meet life challenges. Resilience is strengthened through transactional processes that promote flexibility, strong connectedness, and mobilization of social and economic resources.

4. Flexibility

Flexibility, a core structural process in resilience, involves adaptive change to deal with adversity. Rather than simply "bouncing back," like a spring, to a preexisting shape or norm (a mistaken view of resilience), this involves recalibrating and gaining strength to overcome the challenges. After major crises or loss, families may not be able to return to "normal" life as they knew it, but must construct a "new normal" to move ahead. Practitioners can support their efforts to navigate new terrain, realign relationships, and reorganize patterns of interaction to fit altered conditions.

At the same time, families need to buffer and counterbalance disruptive changes and *regain stability*. Children and other vulnerable family members especially need assurance of *continuity, dependability, and predictability* through turmoil and in the wake of separation or loss. Restoring daily routines and creating meaningful rituals can assist in such times.

Authoritative leadership, firm yet flexible, is generally most effective for family functioning and child rearing. In highly stressful conditions, it is most important to provide *nurturance, protection, and guidance* for children and other vulnerable family members. This may require stronger parental control and monitoring in high-risk environments. Families with complex structures and members living apart may need help to forge *cooperative coparenting and caregiving teamwork* across households and distance. Couple and coparental relationships work best with mutual respect and equal partnership in sharing joys and responsibilities.

5. Connectedness

Connectedness (cohesion) is essential for effective family functioning in adversity. A crisis or persistent multi-stress conditions can fragment family cohesion, with members disengaged and unable to rely on each other. Resilience is strengthened by *mutual support, collaboration, and commitment* to weather troubled times together. At the same time, individual needs and differences are respected. In adverse situations, members may have varied coping styles or timing needed to process events, depending on such factors as the meaning and impact for each or the age of a child.

When family members are separated, for instance with foster care, parental absence, or community disruptions, it is important to sustain vital connections through visits, photos, keepsakes, letters, and Internet contact and in links to extended kin and valued cultural and spiritual resources. These are all *relational lifelines* for resilience.

Intense pressure in times of crisis can exacerbate relational tensions and spark misunderstandings, conflict, and cutoffs. Yet a crisis, such as a life-threatening event, can become an impetus for reconciliation of wounded bonds. Therapists can facilitate *reconnection* of estranged relationships and *repair* of grievances.

6. Mobilizing Social and Economic Resources

In troubled times, it is important for families to *mobilize extended kin and other social and community resources* for practical and emotional support. The crucial influence of role models and mentors on the resilience of at-risk youth is well documented. Families that are more isolated or underserved can be helped to navigate social systems to access needed services.

It's crucial to *build financial security* in families facing sudden or persistent economic hardship. Persistent unemployment, job instability, chronic illness, loss of a breadwinner, or a major disaster can deplete a family's economic resources, with cascading effects. Serious financial strain contributes to family violence and dissolution, and heightens the risk of problems for children in single-parent households. Multi-stressed families may need help *navigating conflicting pressures of job and family responsibilities.*

Family *transactions with larger systems* are also vital lifelines for resilience. Just as individuals need supportive relationships, families need supportive institutional policies, structures, and programs in workplace, health care, and other larger systems. Community-based coordinated efforts, involving local agencies and residents, are essential to meet such challenges as neighborhood crime or a major disaster and to lower the risk of future threats. Multilevel systems approaches with at-risk youth may facilitate family transactions with school, workplace, health care, and/or justice systems, depending on their relevance in strengthening resilience.

Communication/Problem–Solving Processes

Communication processes facilitate resilience by bringing clarity to adverse situations, encouraging open emotional sharing, and fostering collaborative problem solving and proactive planning. It must be kept in mind that cultural norms vary widely in terms of informational sharing and emotional expression.

7. Clear Information

Clear and congruent messages facilitate all family functioning. In highly stressful situations, communication easily breaks down. Ambiguity and uncertainty fuel anxiety and block understanding of what is happening and what can be done. Well-intentioned family members may avoid painful or threatening information, wishing to protect each other from worry. Shared acknowledgment of the truth of a painful experience fosters recovery, whereas denial, secrecy, or cover-up can impede adaptation. Anxieties about the unspeakable can generate catastrophic fears and are often expressed in somatic and behavioral problems, especially in children.

By helping families *clarify and share crucial information* about adverse events, their current situation, and future expectations, therapists can facilitate meaning-making, emotional sharing, informed decision making, and future planning. Parents need to communicate their openness to discussing children's questions or concerns as they arise. They may need guidance on age-appropriate ways to share information and can expect that as children mature, they may seek greater comprehension or bring up emerging concerns.

8. Emotional Sharing and Positive Interactions

Open communication, supported by a climate of mutual trust, empathy, and tolerance for differences, enables family members to share a wide range of feelings that can be aroused by crisis situations and chronic stress. Members need to feel safe in *expressing painful emotions*, such as sadness, yearning, frustration, remorse, outrage, or anxiety, which may fluctuate over time and vary depending on different personalities, ages, relationships, and implications of an adverse situation. Individuals may express varied facets of complex emotions reverberating in a family system. Members may be out of sync over time; some may feel ready to move on before others. Parents or children may suppress their own painful feelings in order to keep functioning or to avoid burdening others. When emotions are intense, mutual blame or heightened reactivity to one another can fuel conflict and escalate. Masculine stereotypes of weakness may constrain men from revealing fear, vulnerability, or sadness. Practitioners need to provide a safe haven to facilitate constructive dialogue and process difficult feelings. For relational resilience, couples and families can be helped to understand and respect differences, and to comfort one another.

Positive interactions are essential for resilience when family life is saturated with problems, suffering, and struggle. *Expressions of love, pride, appreciation, and gratitude* counteract discouragement and strengthen bonds. *Finding humor* and laughter amid troubles or tragedy bolsters spirits. Making time and space to *share joy, fun, and pleasurable activities* revitalizes family life and offers essential respite. It's important to celebrate birthdays, holidays, and milestones, which may be overshadowed by problems.

9. Collaborative Problem Solving and a Proactive Approach

Creative brainstorming expands *resourcefulness,* opening new possibilities for surmounting adversity. *Shared decision making* and *conflict management* involve negotiation of differences, with fairness and reciprocity over time. It is important to set clear priorities and realistic goals. and then to take concrete steps toward them. Practitioners can facilitate efforts to build on small successes and use setbacks or failures as learning experiences.

A *proactive approach* is essential to meet future challenges. For resilience, families need to shift from a crisis-reactive mode to avert potential crises, prepare for anticipated problems, and rebound from unexpected bumps in the road. In striving toward a future vision, they need to strengthen supportive resources, anticipate obstacles and ways to overcome them, and take strides toward their aims. Encouraging members to have a

"Plan B" in mind can enable them to adapt readily if unforeseen challenges arise. If dreams have been shattered, families can be encouraged to survey the altered landscape and forge new pathways ahead.

Synergistic Influences of Transactional Processes in Resilience

The key processes in family resilience are mutually interactive and synergistic. For example, a relational view of resilience (belief system) supports—and is reinforced by—connectedness (organizational processes) and collaborative problem solving (communication processes). Shared meaning-making occurs through communication processes. A positive outlook both facilitates and is sustained by successful problem solving and proactive steps. A balance of process components is also needed, as in the fluid shifts between stability and change in the structural flexibility required for adaptation to new challenges. Social and community resources are not simply external factors; family processes include active engagement in transactions with the environment. A multilevel dynamic systems perspective recognizes the recursive nature of processes in resilience and the bidirectionality of influences within and between levels over time (see Figure 6.1).

Various family therapy models have focused on interactional processes in different domains (or dimensions) of family functioning (Sluzki, 1983). For instance, the structural model attends primarily to organizational patterns; cognitive-behavioral approaches address belief systems (schemas) and communication/problem-solving processes; and postmodern approaches focus on the social construction of meaning, expanding and reauthoring life stories, and steps toward a preferred future vision. Recent research has sought to identify common factors across models in effective practice (Sprenkle, Davis, & Lebow, 2009). Most integrative family therapists attend to transactional processes across the three domains of family functioning, in social context and over the multigenerational family life cycle (Lebow, 2013). Practitioners of all strength-based approaches can usefully apply the framework presented here to target and strengthen key processes for family resilience.

Ecological and developmental perspectives are essential to assess functioning in both social and temporal contexts (see Chapters 1 and 9). It is crucial to consider each family's strengths and vulnerabilities in relation to their cultural norms and values, socioeconomic location, and developmental priorities. Key processes may be organized and expressed in varied ways, depending on a family's aims and preferences, structural configuration, and available resources. The key processes in resilience can be applied

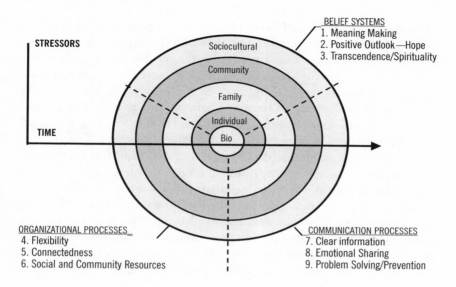

FIGURE 6.1. Multilevel recursive processes in resilience.

to diverse situations and through varied adaptational pathways as they fit family challenges, resources, and aims.

MAPPING THE FAMILY SYSTEM

A broad family resilience orientation, or meta-framework, and the key processes identified above provide a flexible map for practice and research assessment, guiding inquiry and efforts to strengthen family functioning in dealing with adversity. This approach recognizes the diversity of families, their varied situational challenges, and the viability of many pathways in resilience. It also requires attunement to the varied demands of different adverse situations over time with a major crisis event, trauma, or loss; through disruptive transitions; or with the challenges of chronic multi-stress conditions, as will be addressed in Chapters 9–14. Useful tools for family assessment are discussed here, with practice principles, guidelines, and illustrations in the following chapter.

Questionnaire Use to Assess Family Resilience

The Walsh Family Resilience Questionnaire (WFRQ; see Appendix 1) was constructed to operationalize the nine key processes and their components in the framework presented here. The self-report questionnaire items and Likert scale invite respondents to rate their perceptions of how their family deals with serious crises and/or persistent stresses. Similar to scaling questions in systemic practice, response ratings are most useful when explored more fully in interviews, both in practice and in qualitative research. For instance, a respondent (e.g., a mother) might indicate that the family draws strongly on spiritual resources in troubled times (a 4 or 5 rating). It might be important to explore in what ways religious and/or spiritual beliefs and practices are expressed in family life and how they are helpful. If a respondent rated spiritual resources as 1 or 2, it might mean that religion/spirituality is simply unimportant in their lives, not that this is a deficit. Families vary in the strengths and resources they draw on to deal with adversity. Also, since these are dynamic processes and not fixed traits, they may be increased or expanded if family members, on reflection, think they might be useful. Thus, we can think of the questionnaire as mapping a particular family profile. Yet we must be cautious not to "profile" families in a stereotypical way as resilient or not.

The scale can also be useful for rating within-family changes over time in the course of dealing with an adverse situation, such as adaptational processes after a crisis event or shifts in dealing with emerging challenges or chronic multi-stress conditions. The questionnaire can also be used in pre- and post-assessment in practice effectiveness research, offering a profile of family resilience processes at the start and end of interventions and at later follow-up. It is currently being applied in several international studies of family resilience, as discussed later in this chapter.

Resilience–Oriented Family Genograms and Diagrams

With a family resilience orientation, we search for strengths and potential alongside family problems or limitations. In assessment, it's important to gain a holistic view of the family system and its community, cultural, and spiritual connections. This includes immediate family members, extended kin, and social networks, highlighting key relationships and resources that are—or could be—important in addressing current problems and strengthening family functioning.

A *genogram* (McGoldrick, Gerson, & Petry, 2008), a systemic diagram, can be a valuable assessment tool, enabling practitioners, researchers, and family members to visualize the network of relationships and significant patterns. As a structural map of family process, it serves as a graphic representation of families and charts their interactional processes over three or more generations. Genogram construction by the practitioner or researcher, either with family members or from family data, shows the current configuration of the family system, demarcating living arrangements; noting patterns of alliance, conflict, cutoff, and loss; and identifying existing and potential resources in kin and social networks. Computerized genogram programs developed by McGoldrick and colleagues are particularly useful for depicting complex family structures and relational patterns and tracking significant past family-of-origin patterns.

A genogram can be useful for diagramming and further exploring past and ongoing issues involving the extended family that are relevant to a current problem situation. The genogram in Figure 6.2 shows the family processes relevant to presenting problems in the following case.

> Chinese parents in Hong Kong brought their 5-year-old son to a child clinic for help because he refused to attend preschool and was anxiously overattached to his mother. My genogram construction with the parents revealed that an older brother had died at the same age after contracting a virus in the preschool. When we asked how that had affected the family, we learned that the paternal grandparents had blamed the mother for the death, accusing her of insufficient care of their first-born grandson, and cut off all contact with her. The father, a loyal son, sided with his parents, withdrawing affection from his wife. Isolated in her grief, she became overprotective of the younger son. Each year on the birthday of the deceased son, she made a cake, topped with candles for the age he would have been, and shared it with the younger boy.

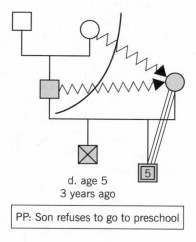

d. age 5
3 years ago

PP: Son refuses to go to preschool

FIGURE 6.2. Genogram showing extended family dynamics in presenting problems (PP) and connection to past loss.

Traditional clinical assessments and genogram construction tend to focus predominantly on problematic family members and relational patterns, which can skew intervention to overfocus on family dysfunction. A resilience-oriented approach does note problem areas and risk factors but prioritizes a search for positive influences—past, present, and potential. Who is—or could be—helpful, supportive, and caring? In what ways? Who might contribute strengths and resources in a team effort? Who would members like to be better connected with? Where resources have been lost, how might they be replenished? How might we repair conflictual or estranged relationships that could become resources? We identify potential role models and mentors in the kin network. We are especially interested in hearing about resourceful ways family members have dealt with past adversity, such as stories of grandparents' "can-do spirit" through migration or economic hardship to inspire efforts in mastering current challenges.

It is important to ask family members how they define their family. Who do they include? Who is significant? What roles do they play? How are they supportive or troublesome? Who are they cut off from? Legal and blood definitions of family or social norms may constrain clients from disclosing some relationships, as with a cohabiting or same-sex partner. The role (or potential contribution) of a nonresidential parent may be overlooked in a narrow focus on a single-parent household. A genogram can be informative in identifying potential resources for an isolated elder, such as a niece or nephew living nearby.

Because family structures and important bonds are so varied, it is important to map all significant relationships within and beyond the immediate household: nonresidential parents, partners, and extended kin (formal and informal), including grandparents, aunts and uncles, godparents, and cousins. Many people, especially single parents and individuals living independently, knit together their own nurturing bonds for resilience with intimate partners, relatives, and close friends whom they consider family, kinfolk, or kindred spirits.

The role of pets (and service animals) should be included in any assessment. A growing body of research documents the relational significance of companion animals as important bonds for resilience in families, and especially for children, adults on their own, and the elderly (Walsh, 2009a, 2009b).

One family experienced a cascade of stressors with a contentious parental divorce and the mother's remarriage. The 10-year-old daughter, Megan, was struggling to adapt as her father cut off all contact and support and she had to adjust to a new stepfamily; a move to a

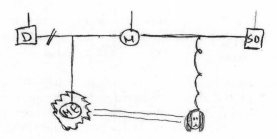

FIGURE 6.3. Genogram drawn by 10-year-old Megan showing the importance of her bond with her dog in adapting to parental divorce, her father's cutoff, and her new stepfamily.

new neighborhood, school, and peers; and the loss of her close friends. As I was gathering information and sketching a family genogram with the mother, I invited Megan to draw her own genogram, including everyone important to her. As Figure 6.3 shows, Megan ("Me") highlighted her closest bond—with her dog Sparky. Her drawing opened our conversation about all the ways this bond supported her though the hard times.

Genograms were an important tool in our family resilience training component for the Los Angeles GRYD (Gang Reduction and Youth Development) prevention program for youth at high risk of gang involvement (see Chapter 8). Our approach aimed to reduce negative influences and support positive youth development by refocusing on family strengths and potential, engaging parents and extended family members to collaborate in a supportive team effort. A resilience-based genogram was developed to guide those efforts by case managers providing counseling (see Appendix 2). Genogram construction with the youth and their families engaged their interest in learning more about their relationships and their history. The goals were:

- To increase understanding and positive connections with the family's history and network of relationships in order to strengthen positive youth identity and differentiation from negative influences.
- To identify and recruit family members who could be "relational lifelines" for positive youth development, providing active investment and problem solving to support youth efforts to decrease problem behaviors, resist gang involvement, and strive toward a positive future life vision.

Initially, we had to overcome larger systems barriers including a narrow focus on youth problem behavior, risk factors, and family deficits, as in the following case.

The counselor had been working individually with 10-year-old Rafael and was pessimistic about any positive contribution his family might make. The initial family genogram and assessment report were loaded with problems and risk factors. The negative influences stood out: The father, now out of the home, had been abusive; he and Rafa's older brother were both currently gang members. The worker reported that the mother was absent from home after school and "failed" to monitor Rafa's activities or provide structure for homework. He was falling behind in school, cutting classes, and hanging out in the streets with peers.

Searching for strengths and resources in the family, we explored the mother's hopes and dreams for Rafa and his sisters, her own life challenges, and potential resources in her extended family. She clearly loved her children and wanted to support the program efforts so Rafa could have a better future.

While the initial assessment had focused on the negative influences of Rafa's father and older brother, I noted on the genogram that the mother's older brother, Jorge, was a former gang member, had served time in prison, and was now back in the community. I was interested in learning more about him. The mother was happy to report that he was gainfully employed, with his own small mechanics' shop, and had turned his life around. We invited Jorge to join our next session, recruiting him to take on an active role in mentoring his nephew. He was enthusiastic about doing so, especially since he was Rafa's godfather and eager to help him take a better path in his life.

The structure of daily family life also needed to be strengthened. Having lost her oldest son to a gang, the mother worried constantly about Rafa, distressed that her job schedule and long commute kept her away from home when he needed supervision. We noted on the genogram that her sister, a single parent, lived nearby with her children. Although she had not wanted to burden her sister, who had her own troubles, we invited them to come together to the next session. We encouraged them to team up, finding ways to combine and trade off child care arrangements, provide mutual support, and strengthen family structure and bonds with children in both households. An after-school tutor was also involved to strengthen Rafa's proficiency and engagement in schoolwork. The mother's desire to find a less stressful job close to home was supported, encouraging her active initiative.

Challenges and resources in a family's social/economic/political ecology should be considered in all assessment and noted on any family diagram. Outside stressors impact everyday family life. In the case above, the mother, presumed to be uncaring and neglectful, was loving and deeply concerned but hampered by job and financial demands.

Collaborative Helping maps, developed by Madsen (2011) to guide thinking and action in family-centered services, was also a valuable tool in our GRYD program. The simple assessment diagram shifts attention from risk and problem reduction to positive aims and potential strengths and resources to mobilize. On a grid, workers identify: (1) a positive future vision for youth and family; (2) supports (who can help and how); (3) obstacles to overcome (reframing risks and problem behaviors); and (4) steps to take toward the preferred future vision.

Several other assessment tools can be helpful in organizing and visualizing a great deal of factual information and multiple linkages between family and broader contextual variables. The *ecomap* (Hartman, 1995), developed for use in social services, is a graphic representation of family relationships highlighting the connections between a family or household and its environment, including external systems, resources, and influences, all drawn in circles surrounding the family. It is especially useful to guide intervention with complex families in highly challenging socioeconomic contexts. A cultural genogram (Hardy & Laszloffy, 1995) and spiritual diagrams (Hodge, 2005) can be useful tools for more intensive exploration of those important influences and are especially valuable in heightening awareness and sensitivity of trainees.

In my own work on spiritual resources in families and family therapy (Walsh, 2009c, 2010, 2013b), I developed an assessment outline to explore the spiritual dimension in family life, including religious and nonreligious expression. It can be useful to guide appreciative inquiry to understand: (1) the meaning and importance of spiritual beliefs and practices in facing adversity; (2) if spiritual issues contribute to suffering or block positive growth; and (3) potential spiritual resources that might support healing and resilience, fitting each family's orientation and preferences (see Appendix 3).

Falicov (2012, 2013) has developed MECA, a valuable multidimensional framework for assessment and intervention with immigrant and transnational families. She has designed two accompanying tools, MECAmaps and MECAgenograms, to include specific influences in four domains of family life: ecological context, migration/acculturation, family life cycle, and family organization. Consistent with a strengths-based approach and similar to a culture-centered genogram, they enable visualization of family life in light of multiple complex variables. They are useful in identifying risks and strengths, locating past and present role models, and stimulating discussion of members' stories of struggle and triumph, their hopes

and despair. The process of building a MECAgenogram, as with other diagrams, actively engages adults and children in discovering aspects of their
lives not often shared, gaining greater comprehension of the many inter-
secting influences, and building connection and collaboration in surmounting their challenges.

Addressing Family Challenges over Time: Risks and Resilience

A basic premise guiding this systems-based approach is that critical events
and stressful chronic conditions impact the whole family. In turn, family processes influence the recovery and resilience of all members, their
relationships, and the family unit. Therefore, how a family confronts and
manages disruptive experiences, buffers stress, effectively reorganizes, and
reinvests in life pursuits will influence adaptation for all members. Interventions aim to build family resources to deal more effectively with stresses
and to rebound strengthened, both individually and as a relational system.
Efforts to bolster the family's ability to master immediate problems also
increase its capacity to meet future challenges.

To promote resilience in vulnerable children and families, Rutter
(1987) identified four general protective mechanisms that can be strengthened through interventions. Applying his schema to family systems, we
can specify ways in which key processes in family resilience can be mobilized:

1. Decrease risk factors.
   - Anticipate and prepare for threatening circumstances.
   - Reduce exposure or overload of stress.
   - Provide information; alter catastrophic beliefs.
2. Reduce negative chain reactions that heighten risk for sustained
   impact and further crises.
   - Buffer stress effects; cushion impact, overcome obstacles.
   - Alter maladaptive coping strategies.
   - Withstand aftershocks, prolonged strains; rebound from set-
     backs.
3. Strengthen protective family processes and reduce vulnerabilities.
   - Enhance family strengths, opportunities, and abilities for suc-
     cess.
   - Mobilize and shore up resources toward recovery and mastery.
   - Rebuild, reorganize, and reorient in aftermath.
   - Anticipate, prepare for both likely and unforeseen new challenges.

4. Bolster family and individual pride and efficacy through successful problem mastery.
    - Gain competence, confidence, and connectedness through collaborative efforts.
    - Manage challenges over time for sustained competence under duress.

Families don't simply react to stressful life events; their active approach to potential stressors can either buffer or intensify their impact (Patterson, 2002). Did they notice and prepare for potential threats? How effectively did they mobilize resources to head off a crisis or lessen its impact? Strains can be compounded by catastrophic fears and maladaptive coping processes, which can contribute to individual and relational distress. Often family members and counselors become so focused on presenting symptoms that they may not connect them to stressors in the family system and reverberations for each member, as in the following case.

> Over the past 2 months, Jimmy, age 11, had frequent school absences and failing grades. School authorities presumed that he was out in the streets and that the family, living in a low-income housing project, was dysfunctional and uncaring when no one responded to their calls and notes. When a family counselor in our program made a home visit to assess the situation, she learned that Jimmy and his two siblings lived with their grandmother, their legal guardian since their mother's death 4 years earlier. She had been hospitalized recently with a serious liver disease and kidney failure; now at home, she required dialysis several times a week. Jimmy, who had been very close to his mother, was now extremely anxious that he might also lose his grandmother. He was missing school to watch over her. Moreover, the burden of responsibility for four children heightened risk for the grandmother's fragile health. No one talked about the grandmother's condition, the threat of another loss and dislocation for the children, or what arrangements could be made for their care in the event of her further disability or death. As Jimmy said, "It was all just too scary."

Genogram construction, as shown in Figure 6.4, was especially useful in visualizing this complex family situation, gaining coherence, and identifying potential resources. In relation to Rutter's (1987) model, above, the counselor took several steps to help the family with its crisis situation. Most immediate was the need to decrease the risk factors, reduce negative chain reactions, and shore up resources for the grandmother's health and the children's care.

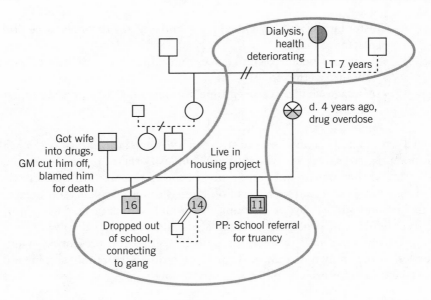

FIGURE 6.4. Genogram of the complex family situation of Jimmy, referred to counseling for truancy.

The grandmother's cohabiting partner had not been involved in the children's care, but now, worried about her health, he agreed to take a more active role to relieve her burden. A maternal aunt, contacted to be part of the team effort, arranged for Jimmy to do homework with her son after school, offering additional respite. The children's father, blamed for the mother's drug-related death and cut-off by the grandmother, was contacted to assess his current ability to assume a parenting role. His deep remorse at his wife's death had sparked him to give up drug use and get his life in order. Now stable and employed, he yearned for contact with his children. The counselor facilitated his reconciliation with the family. With steps to restore trust and monitor safety, he became actively involved with all three, each of them at risk and needing his positive investment. As the immediate stress was reduced, all members were benefiting from the strengthened family network. Counseling addressed the children's anxieties about losing their grandmother, comingled with loss issues from their mother's death. Attention turned to their future hopes and concerns, and possibilities for residence with their father.

This case illustrates how resilience-based interventions target core elements in the three domains of family functioning: meaning and mastery of the

crisis; reorganization of family structural patterns; and more effective communication and problem solving. As in this case, most serious life crises
aren't limited to a single moment in time, but involve a complex set of
changing conditions with a past history and a future course (Rutter, 1987).
Thus, efforts to strengthen resilience attend to coping and adaptation processes over time. A developmental perspective is essential (see Chapter 9).

Timeline Construction: Tracking Stressors and Distress over Time

As in the cases above, resilience-oriented assessment involves inquiry to
assess both risk and protective variables. It is important to identify highly
stressful events in family life (Lavee, McCubbin, & Olson, 1987). It is useful to construct a timeline to track distress in the family with past, recent,
ongoing, and threatened stressors (McGoldrick et al., 2008). We can then
explore their impact and family coping and adaptive strategies. A simple
vertical or horizontal line can be drawn, with significant events and changes
noted chronologically. Concurrence of distress with significant events or a
pileup of stressors can readily be seen (Walsh, 1983). A timeline is an essential tool in noting the following:

- Recent or threatened stress events, their meaning, and impact.
- Pileup of stressors and cumulative impact.
- Loading from past experiences: success or complications with simi-
  lar stressors.
- Family coping processes and potential resources.

We explore, for instance, how the timing of a family member's emotional or behavioral problems might be connected with highly stressful
events. Frequently, child behavior or school problems coincide with anxi-
ety-provoking transitions or losses, such as parental separation, incarceration, migration, or military deployment, which also involve family boundary shifts and role realignment (see Chapters 9 and 11).

A family resilience perspective attends to evolving family challenges
and responses over time. To meet the demands of different phases of adaptation, families need to draw upon varied strengths to approach an impending crisis proactively, manage disruption during the crisis period, rebound
in the immediate aftermath, and, where necessary, reorganize and rebuild
their lives over the long term. In an acute crisis families need to rally, but
once urgent needs subside they need to shift gears to resume everyday family life and attend to other priorities. Recurrent or persistent stressors pose

different psychosocial challenges over time. Some situations require a long-term adaptation to a "new normal"; others require families to repeatedly shift over a roller-coaster course, while still others require adaptation to progressive decline, as in the varied trajectories of chronic illnesses (Rolland, 2012). Challenges associated with adversity interact with other salient issues in individual and family developmental passage. They are strongly influenced by past experiences with adversity in the multigenerational family network. A holistic assessment of families aims to clarify members' challenges, resources, and constraints and to understand their past experiences, their current dilemma, and their future hopes and dreams.

Variations on a basic timeline can highlight crisis events, such as the color-coded timeline trauma genogram (Jordan, 2004). Saltzman and colleagues (Saltzman, Pynoos, Lester, Layne, & Beardsley, 2013) designed an innovative parent timeline integrating assessment and intervention in a resilience-based intervention program—FOCUS—that has been used with highly stressed military families (see Chapter 13) and with families contending with illness, death of a family member, and a range of trauma and loss experiences. In a structured narrative timeline activity, parents individually share their experiences with each other across key periods, including events before, during, and after deployments and, frequently, high-stress or formative experiences earlier in their relationship or family history. Such events may include relocations, family deaths, illnesses, injuries, or other potentially traumatic events that may present situations for misunderstanding or estrangement between the parents.

Figure 6.5 illustrates the parent timelines for one military family. Deployment and home periods are marked along the horizontal axis. Particularly stressful events are noted across time, such as a family move, a painful good-bye, death of a combat buddy, and a delayed homecoming, followed by the children having problems and parents arguing. The vertical axis shows each parent's perceived intensity (emotional temperature) of distress from these events. The mapping leads to discussion of the impact of stress events and how the family might deal with them more effectively. A children's activity, a graphic "time map" (illustrated in Figure 6.6), is done in concert, enabling the scaffolding of family-level sharing of experience. The graphs also yield quantitative data for FOCUS intervention research.

Families understand their life situations better than outside experts do, yet due to heightened distress and focus on immediate problems, they may not see connections to various stressors in their lives. Practitioners should inquire routinely about recent and anticipated change events, the family's approach and response, and the impact, noting complications that pose risks for immediate or long-term dysfunction. Intervention efforts

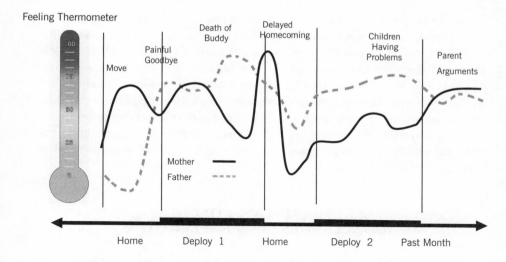

FIGURE 6.5. Parent timelines in FOCUS family resilience oriented intervention. Copyright by William R. Saltzman. Reprinted by permission.

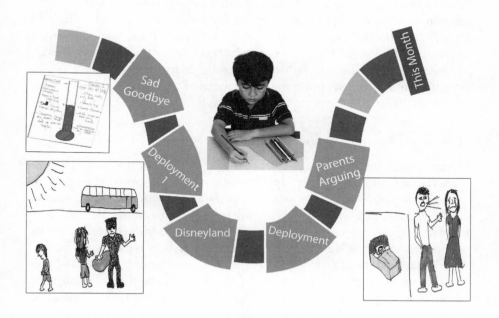

FIGURE 6.6. Child time map in FOCUS family resilience oriented intervention. Copyright by William R. Saltzman. Reprinted by permission.

should be attuned to each family's challenges and the resources that can be mobilized to meet them. We can help families assess their crisis situation and identify ways to reduce risks, thereby rendering challenges less threatening and more manageable. For instance, parents and other caregivers can be helped to provide strong leadership, guidance, nurturance, and protection in situations of disruption or loss. In anticipation of a crisis, through its midst, and in its aftermath, our aim is to strengthen transactional processes that foster coping, recovery, and resilience, enabling the family and its members to integrate their experience and move forward in life.

RESEARCH APPROACHES, CHALLENGES, AND REFLECTIONS

There has been a recent proliferation of interest worldwide in research on resilience at individual, family, and community levels. The UN Office for the Coordination of Humanitarian Affairs (OCHA) has developed a new global tool to measure the ability of a system to withstand stresses and shocks in an uncertain world. Researchers and intervention programs have drawn on early conceptual work by McCubbin, Patterson, and colleagues (e.g., Chapin, 2011) and on the family resilience framework presented here (e.g., Coulter, 2011; Coyle et al., 2009; Lietz, 2013; Saltzman, Lester, Pynoos, & Beardslee, 2012; Saltzman et al., 2013; Yang & Choi, 2002), most often as a broad conceptual map for qualitative inquiry and mixed-methods research.

Research Strategies and Challenges

Over several decades, family systems research on core processes in well-functioning families has utilized varying strategies, from self-report of individual members' perceptions of their family functioning in interviews or questionnaires (increasingly web-based) to observational studies in controlled research settings or natural home environments (see review by Lebow & Stroud, 2012). Family resilience researchers typically focus on a particular adverse situation, such as the series of studies by Greef and colleagues on the death of a parent or a child, divorce, and mental or physical disabilities (e.g., Greef & Human, 2004; Greef & Joubert, 2007; Greef & Van der Merwe, 2004; Greef & van der Walt, 2010). Studies often compare family resilience data to self-report scores on general family functioning scales, using the McMaster group's Family Assessment Device (FAD; Ryan,

Epstein, Keitner, Miller, & Bishop, 2005) and Olson's Circumplex Model and FACES inventories (Olson & Gorell, 2003; Olson, Gorell, & Tinsel, 2006).

There is widespread interest in development of simple questionnaires to assess individual and family resilience. However, efforts to date have suffered from conceptual and methodological weaknesses. Those designed to measure individual resilience have been unable to establish stable psychometric properties and have questionable item construct validity, sampling methods, and data analysis, failing to capture the complex and contextually contingent nature of resilience (Windle, Bennett, & Noyes, 2011). Similar conceptual and methodological problems have arisen in several attempts to construct family resilience questionnaires to date.

My own questionnaire (the WFRQ) is currently being applied in several research projects internationally (e.g., Taiwan, China, and Italy) studying family resilience in varied situations of adversity, such as the death of a child, chronic illness, immigration, disaster recovery, and conditions of extreme poverty. Attributes in resilience may also vary in salience in different developmental and social contexts. Thus, psychometrics related to questionnaires such as the WFRQ are inherently complex. In particular, establishing a stable factor structure may be an elusive aim, given the recursive and overlapping nature of transactional processes and the need to fit the context contingency of resilience. Questionnaire adaptation is encouraged so that particular questions can be translated and framed to fit varied cultural and socioeconomic contexts, linguistic differences, target populations, and types of adversity under study, especially whether acute crisis or chronic condition. Different patterns may emerge in dealing with different challenges. We must be mindful that any questionnaire is a map, and different mappings are to be expected to fit varied terrains.

No Single Model: Context Matters

The very flexibility of the construct of resilience complicates research efforts (Barton, 2005; Luthar, 2006). Unlike a static, singular model, typology, or set of traits, resilience involves dynamic, multilevel systemic processes over time (Masten & Monn, 2015), and are contingent on the impact and demands of specific adverse conditions and a family's composition, future aims, and available resources.

The diversity of contemporary families must be taken into account. Household living arrangements and broader relational patterns differ with varied family structures, major transitions, and developmental phases. When individual survey respondents are asked for their perspective on their family's functioning in dealing with their life challenges, who are they referring to as "family" and what is the respondent's position in the family? Study priorities, subject pool, and respondent definition of family should be clarified (e.g., current household or family network of relationships; couple relationship; coparental or single-parent family unit with children; complex family structure and households). It is crucial to know important characteristics about the family, their socioeconomic location, and the adversity faced.

Luthar (2006; Luther & Brown, 2007) has called for more concerted attention to context and different levels of inquiry in designing research. Some processes promote resilience across context, while others may be more context specific. Beyond generic influences, such as good communication, some might be highly influential in some risk settings but not in others. Some families are strong in dealing with an acute crisis but buckle under prolonged strains with chronic conditions (Rolland, 2012). More within-group studies are needed to consider these processes, disentangling their relative significance in particular contexts. Different strengths might be more or less helpful in dealing with situation-specific challenges, such as the death of a child, a parent's recurrent cancer, a natural disaster, a divorce, or the ongoing complex trauma of families in war zones or refugee camps. Financial stability supports resilience and financial insecurity is a risk factor for divorce and child maladaptation, yet many families that struggle financially are highly resilient in their functioning, drawing on relational and spiritual resources.

Cultural differences can be significant. For instance, in research on posttraumatic growth (PTG) in a U.S. sample, Tedeschi, Park, and Calhoun (1996) found five significant dimensions: greater appreciation of life and changed sense of priorities; warmer, more intimate relationships with others; a greater sense of personal strength; recognition of new possibilities or paths for one's life; and growth in spiritual (or existential) matters. Later studies identified different factor structures in diverse cultural contexts, such as for Bosnian war refugees, suggesting the universality of the phenomenon of PTG but the culture-specific nature of its dimensions. See Berger and Weiss (2008) for extension of PTG research to families.

Questionnaire rating scales may also vary. Some applications of the WFRQ (e.g., in Indonesia) used ratings of "how true/false in your family" rather than "how frequent," because local people were unaccustomed to think in terms of frequency. Other researchers (Kirmayer, Sehdev, Whitley, Dandeneau, & Isaac, 2009) have found a 4-point rating scale to be preferable to a 5-point scale in some cultural contexts, as with indigenous tribal groups in Canada, because respondents normatively select a midpoint (3) if offered that option. Given the many research complexities, I encourage ongoing consultation for researchers interested in applying my framework in studies of family resilience and strive to facilitate networking among researchers.

Caution is also advised not to construct lists of factors that tend to reify resilience as a set of additive, fixed, and deterministic traits. Because of the dynamic and variable interconnections among key processes in resilience, they can be better understood through narrative and phenomenological study approaches (Barton, 2005).

Collaborative approaches to research and practice typically employ qualitative methods through grounded inquiry in interviews and naturalistic observation, often combined with quantitative methods. The WFRQ can be useful as a guide for further elaboration and exploration of responses in in-depth interviews. The questions and their response can facilitate exploration of ways in which key processes are expressed, may be constrained, may not be relevant or useful in a particular family situation, or might suggest potential resources to develop.

Mixed methods, combining quantitative and qualitative approaches, can best advance understanding of family resilience (Black & Lobo, 2008; Card & Barnett, 2015; Lietz, 2006, 2007). Dynamic, multilevel models of longitudinal data analysis are promising quantitative approaches (Masten, 2014). A relational developmental approach rather than an individualistic or linear mode of adaptation is key to understanding resilience. Rather than seeing resilience as residing in the person or the family, a relational view sees it as a product of human transactions across multiple system levels, considering the bidirectionality of influences over time (Lerner et al., 2013; Sameroff, 2010). A dynamic process framework for systems grasps the complex nature of family life in current social contexts and does not try to resolve it using mechanistic concepts and data analysis.

Only a few studies have examined the evolving challenges and processes in family resilience over time (e.g., Conger & Conger, 2002; Saltzman et al., 2012, as described above and in Chapter 11). For instance, in a mixed-method study, Lietz and Strength (2011) used a narrative and qualitative approach to study family resilience processes in response to child separation due to maltreatment and later reunification, describing progressive stages in the child's adaptational processes over time. More multilevel longitudinal study is called for (Masten & Monn, 2015). Weine's targeted ethnographic studies of populations in war-torn regions and refugee resettlement (e.g., Weine et al., 2004) offer a superb model of multilevel systemic research yielding valuable recommendations for developing family-focused mental health preventive intervention.

Reflections on Research and Practice Paradigms

Many family systems therapists, and postmodernists in particular, have raised concerns about empirical measurement of complex family processes, preferring the richness of qualitative interviews and ethnographic studies to explore multiple, subjective perspectives and experience, particularly in meaning-making processes. The goal of qualitative research is to develop detailed, multilayered "thick descriptions" of the nature and meaning of events, situations, and experiences from the family members ("insiders") (Geertz, 1986). While qualitative methods are often criticized for the inherent biases in their socially constructed inquiry and analysis, quantitative methods' claims of objectivity are questionable. No research is free from preconceptions or blind spots, even with sophisticated computerized data analysis. All researchers need to consider their values, assumptions, preferences, and biases in the construction of instruments, framing of questions, choice of methods, and interpretation of data. We all need to be aware of our subjectivity in mapping family processes and strive to understand the fullness of the experience of adversity in family life.

As Stillman and Erbes (2012) note, many practitioners face the conundrum of being advised that they cannot practice (or be reimbursed for) an approach that is not an "empirically validated treatment." Such scientific methods are grounded in positivist assumptions and manualize a set of rules, procedures, and techniques that are generalized across populations and life situations and then applied to everyone. Postmodern approaches seek to elucidate local experiences that apply to those who construct them and live them, stressing the need to stay connected to the ideas and practice principles of these approaches and to remain flexible to multiple ways of practicing, centered on client experience. This involves taking in their feedback and adapting, to be attuned to their values and situations, and to ways that were helpful and that fit for them.

In sum, as in the resilience-based approach presented here, this requires an assessment process that is principle-based, person- and family-centered, flexible, and open to the organic nature of practice. In the pilot study of Stillman and Erbes (2012) they preferred the terms *observation scale* and *observer* in place of *rating scale* and *rater*, to better follow witnessing principles in the interviews and not the measurement of performance. Important principles include seeing the position of the interviewer (researcher) as influential yet decentered; externalizing the problem as separate from the person as well as supporting a person's ability to act on his or her own behalf (personal agency); questioning the effects of culture and society; and eliciting and identifying preferred stories that have been subordinate to problematic stories in the person's life (White & Epston, 1990). These principles allow for rich alternative story development and the opportunity to share these developments in important relationships. The family resilience framework presented here aims to be consistent with these principles.

Practicing Resilience in Family Resilience Research: Mastering the Art of the Possible

Just as resilient families "struggle well" to overcome multi-stress challenges in complex situations, researchers need to practice resilience in overcoming the many conceptual and methodological challenges to advancing our knowledge and practice. Table 6.2 summarizes important principles and variables to keep in mind in any assessment.

Although it may not be feasible to directly assess or control all variables, it is advisable to focus on those most relevant to the population, type of adversity, and study aims. A systemic lens helps to keep researchers mindful of the broad and interdependent family, social, and developmental contexts. Like families, research efforts are more likely to succeed with a team approach, integrating multiple perspectives and striving to gain a sense of coherence. This involves "mastering the art of the possible": focusing on what can be learned, accepting what is beyond control or comprehension,

---

TABLE 6.2. Family Resilience Assessment: Important Variables

- Resilience as a flexible construct:
  - Dynamic multilevel systemic processes over time

- Many varied pathways in resilience:
  - No single model; not a set of traits

- Context contingent: useful strengths and resources may vary, depending on:
  - Challenges of varied adverse situations
    - Crisis event, short-term impact versus long-term effects
    - Multi-stress situations—concurrent stressors; pileup; cascade effects
    - Disruptive transitions
    - Chronic conditions—persistent/recurrent/emerging challenges
  - Family structure (two-parent, single-parent, stepfamily, couple without children)
  - Household(s)—living arrangements
  - Extended family, social, and community support
  - Ecological context—social/economic resources, barriers, disparities
  - Cultural values and norms; language and meaning systems
  - Family values, aims, and preferences
  - Life cycle timing and ramifications

---

and tolerating considerable uncertainty. Doing research, indeed, is akin to living our complicated lives.

Advances in research on human resilience—in individuals, families, and communities—have transformative potential for social policy, intervention, and prevention programs with vulnerable and at-risk populations. This valuable research can inform and redirect funding and service priorities from how families fail to how families, when challenged, can succeed. To move beyond the rhetoric of promoting strong families we need to better understand and support key processes in intervention and prevention efforts. Continuing and future work can clarify the most useful components of family functioning in varying adverse conditions and with different populations.

Caution is advised that assessment of family resilience not be misapplied to judge families as "not resilient" if they are unable to rise above extreme trauma or harsh conditions. Key transactional processes can strengthen a family's resilience but may not be sufficient to overcome powerful biological or environmental influences. As we will see in the following chapters on practice and program applications, a multilevel systemic assessment is important in clinical and community-based work in a variety of formats (individual, couple, family, and multifamily group modalities) and in mobilizing vital community resources and larger systems supports.

CHAPTER 7

Practice Principles and Guidelines to Strengthen Family Resilience

> The horizon leans forward offering you space to place
> new steps of change.
> —MAYA ANGELOU, "On the Pulse of Morning" (1993)

A family resilience framework draws on strength-based systemic approaches to increase family capacities to overcome adversity. This chapter presents core practice principles and guidelines, and suggests useful strategies and techniques, with case illustrations. Chapter 8, which follows, describes a range of clinical and community-based practice and programmatic applications, with recommendations for more responsive family-centered service delivery and for prevention efforts to increase resilience in couples and families. We also consider there the resilience needed by helping professionals in our challenging work and practice environment and the unexpected benefits of vicarious resilience.

CORE PRINCIPLES AND GUIDELINES FOR STRENGTHENING FAMILY RESILIENCE

A family resilience approach to practice has much in common with current family systems models: emphasizing a collaborative process and seeking to identify and build on strengths and resources (Walsh, 2014b). It is distinct in focus on the impact of traumatic events, disruptive transitions, and highly stressful conditions on family functioning and the distress of

131

members. This approach is also broadly inclusive of sociocultural, developmental, and multigenerational influences in vulnerability, risk, and resilience. Intervention efforts aim to enhance family coping, mastery, and growth in dealing with life challenges. Core principles in this family resilience approach are summarized in Table 7.1.

Here, below, useful inquiry, strategies, and techniques are suggested for practitioners to facilitate the key processes in family resilience, as described in Chapters 3 to 5 and summarized in Chapter 6.

Making Meaning of Adverse Experiences

It is crucial to explore the meanings that adverse situations hold for each family, and to be mindful not to make assumptions based on our own experience or concerns. We might ask: "What stood out for you as most challenging in your experience? Most upsetting? Most remarkable or reassuring?" "What was the impact for the family? For various members?" "How have you tried to deal with the challenges?" Such inquiry acknowledges the unique experience of each family and the subjective views of members on what is most meaningful, troubling, or remarkable.

It's especially important to assist families in helping children and vulnerable members make sense of a crisis or threat and to provide reassurance that they will be well cared for. Family members do best when they understand more fully what's happening, how it came about, the future implications, and what steps they can take to cope and adapt. Resilience is fostered as we help them gain a shared sense of coherence, rendering their crisis experience more comprehensible, manageable, and meaningful.

Compassionate Witnessing: Stories of Suffering and Struggle

As family members grapple to make meaning of their adverse situation and come to terms with their challenges, practitioners need to be fully present, showing genuine interest and concern about their experience. Often, people in their lives turn away, uncomfortable or uncertain how to respond. We need to listen openheartedly to very painful accounts of what has happened and to their ongoing struggles. It important to convey our assurance that we can bear to hear about their suffering and that we will provide a safe haven to contain and process intense feelings. At the same time, we need to notice, ask about, and highlight sparks of loving care and resilience.

> One couple came for counseling after the tragic death of their baby, Sophie, just 10 months old. In contrast to common gender-based differences in couples dealing with tragedy, Ivan, a Croatian immigrant, was emotionally distraught and requesting help for himself; Nora, his

TABLE 7.1. Family Resilience Framework: Principles for Practice

- Relational view of human resilience
  - Family and social bonds; community, cultural and spiritual resources
- Shift perspective from family deficits to strengths, resources
  - Challenged by adversity; potential for repair and positive growth
- Grounded in developmental systemic theory
  - Biopsychosocial–spiritual influences (bidirectional, ecological view)
  - Multilevel dynamic processes over time
- Crisis events, major stressors impact family system
- Family processes in approach/response influence adaptation of all members, relationships, and family unit
- Contextual view of crisis, distress, and adaptation
  - Family, larger systems/institutional supports; sociocultural influences
  - Temporal influences
    - Timing of symptoms vis-à-vis crisis events
    - Pileup of stressors, disruptive transitions, persistent adversity
    - Varying adaptational challenges over time: immediate to long-term
    - Individual and family developmental priorities, multigenerational patterns
- Varied pathways in resilience—no single model fits all families and situations
- Interventions have prevention value: in strengthening resilience, families become more resourceful, proactive in meeting future challenges

American wife, said she was coping well and didn't need therapy. But she agreed to come for couple sessions to support Ivan.

Ivan began by explaining that he came for therapy because he had suffered terribly in the past, through the brutal war and atrocities in Croatia, and had fallen into a dark hole in the aftermath. He said that losing his child was even more devastating and he wanted to get help so he wouldn't fall into an even deeper pit. We spent the next few sessions going over the events of the past year and all their loving efforts, which he related through tears. After a normal birth, doctors discovered a rapidly growing brain tumor at a 6-month checkup. They underwent grueling ordeals of surgery, radiation, and chemotherapy, but were unable to save Sophie's life. He didn't regret all the treatments; he was glad they had done their best. But the loss of her precious little life, after all that, was more than he could bear.

The following week the couple went to visit close relatives and friends in another city. In our next session, Ivan was distraught: he was furious at them. After dinner, sitting around over coffee, one person finally mentioned their loss. Ivan asked if he would like to see a photo of Sophie and handed it to him. His friend was so uncomfortable he only mumbled, "Oh, how sad." He quickly passed the photo to the person next to him, who glanced at it and passed it on. And so it went around the room, in awkward silence until someone changed the subject. The couple left early, feeling totally isolated in their grief.

I said I would very much like to see photos of Sophie, if they would bring them to the next session. Ivan replied, "I have them right here on my iPhone!" and eagerly pulled it out. He had photos from her birth—and a photo taken every single day in her struggle to live. I moved my chair up close to the couple.

I told them I was interested in starting with her birth and early months and hearing about their joyful times. They shared moments of their delight in Sophie and how beautiful she was, how full of life. I held the iPhone with Ivan as we then scanned through the many photos from the diagnosis through the treatments, tracing their journey. I asked him to pause at photos that stood out and were most meaningful for them and to tell me about those times. I listened intently and shared my observations. In one photo, Sophie lay in a hospital bed, hooked up to tubes and monitors; in another her head was bandaged after surgery. I acknowledged how hard that must have had been, pausing as they recalled that experience. I then also noticed how beautiful her eyes were as she gazed directly into the camera. Ivan remarked, yes, he thought she was trying to reassure them, not to be so worried, that she was pulling through. In one photo, she had lost her hair; I asked if they had saved any of her beautiful curls, and Nora smiled and nodded. In the last photo, Ivan was lying in bed, holding tiny Sophie on his chest, his arms encircling her. I commented on his loving embrace and the peaceful smile on her face. I was quiet as Ivan and Angela sobbed and held each other for quite some time. As we ended the session, I commented on Sophie's remarkable strength in enduring all her painful treatments, and I told them how much I admired their loving care of Sophie and their continuing support of each other their through their darkest times.

That session marked a turning point in the couple's journey in recovery. In the following weeks, Nora started a scrapbook, including Sophie's hair and some of their favorite pictures. Ivan became more animated and resumed his old activities, returning to his neighborhood soccer games, where teammates welcomed him back.

Clarifying Ambiguity

Often, many aspects of an adverse situation are unclear; information may be insufficient, inconsistent, or difficult to comprehend. In a crisis, things may be in flux. It is important to ask about family members' understanding of their situation: what they, themselves, experienced, what they have been told by experts or others, and what they each believe to be the case. Often family members hold quite different perceptions and assumptions as a challenging situation becomes increasingly stressful and tensions heat up. In one family, conflict erupted over concern about the mother's medical condition. She had recently been diagnosed with lupus, and her doctors had given little information to her or the family about her prognosis, how the disease might progress, or what might be done to best manage her chronic illness. Some family members worried that she was working too hard and that it would kill her; others thought she was doing too little and playing on everyone's sympathies. Amid all the bickering, she finally took to her bed—fearful and unsure about what to do, and feeling unsupported by her family.

Helping family members to gain and share crucial information eases anxieties and supports active coping. We can encourage and assist them in locating reliable sources, such as health care or public authorities, and reputable Internet sites. We can coach members in navigating larger systems (Unger, 2010), such as pressing medical or legal professionals to help them sort out complicated or conflicting information about their case. A family consultation can be useful to share information gathered and plan next steps.

We can also coach clients on seeking out information about past traumatic experiences, bringing greater clarity and peace of mind, as in the following case:

> Dennis was having recurrent nightmares about the death of his brother Al ten years earlier in a car crash. He now worried constantly about the safety of his own son—named Alan after his brother—and imagined every sort of traffic accident. The circumstances of Al's death were ambiguous; his parents had arranged a closed-casket funeral, and no one in his family had wanted to talk about it. In our work together, I encouraged Dennis to locate his brother's friend who had been in the car and had survived the accident. At first he was pessimistic about finding him, saying it was "like a needle in a haystack." Urged to ask others and search online, he reached the friend within a few weeks. The friend was open and informative: Their buddy driving the car had been drinking and swerved out of control, crashing into a tree. Al had died instantly of a skull fracture. The friend, only slightly injured, had stayed with him. It brought Dennis considerable solace to learn more about the accident and the care shown to his brother. It also reduced his global anxiety that "anything could happen at any time" to his son. Drawing lessons from the incident, he drove more cautiously himself, and he taught his son never to drink and drive.

Normalizing, Depathologizing, and Contextualizing Distress

A normalizing orientation heightens our appreciation of each family's unique set of experiences and beliefs, as well as commonalities with other families in similar life circumstances. We can offer new perspectives to help family members see individual symptoms, strained relationships, or breakdown in family processes as understandable and common under the stressful circumstances the family is facing.

In a culture that readily finds fault with families and touts the virtues of self-reliance, parents commonly feel deficient when they have a problem they are unable to solve. Often they are referred for family therapy because they are told (or it is implied) that the family is the *real* problem. Their worries about blame, shame, and failure—often not understood by professionals and labelled "resistance"—contribute to reluctance to seek therapy and to early dropout. It is crucial to explore any blaming and stigmatizing experiences families may have had in contacts with other mental health professionals, schools, or courts. Families then expect professionals to judge them negatively and may mistake a silent or neutral stance for confirmation of that view.

A therapist's engagement with a child or adolescent with problems must be coupled with respectful connection with parents or caregivers and appreciation of their experience and best efforts. A fundamental tenet of strength-based approaches to family therapy is that most families do not seek suffering or intend harm to their members. Most parents want desperately to do the best for their children, yet they may need help finding viable solutions to their distress. We need to disengage assumptions of pathology from the rationale for involvement in therapy and make it clear that we regard family members as valued partners and essential resources in addressing their problems.

The aim of normalizing is to depathologize and contextualize family distress. It is not intended to reduce all problems and families to a common denominator, and it should never trivialize a family's unique experience or suffering. We must be careful neither to oversimplify the complexity of family life nor to normalize truly destructive family patterns. Violence and sexual abuse should never be normalized as acceptable, even though they are all too common. Likewise, respect for diversity is not the same as "anything goes" when family processes harm any member. Family therapists have moved beyond the myth of therapeutic neutrality to address serious ethical concerns and therapeutic responsibility.

Reframing and Relabeling

Through such techniques as reframing and relabeling, a problem situation can be redefined in order to cast it in a new light more amenable to positive change. In the early days of family therapy, strategic therapists used techniques such as paradoxical intention as clever tactics to outwit families (Goldenberg & Goldenberg, 2013). When used genuinely and respectfully, reframing techniques, such as positive connotation, can offer a useful new perspective, generate hope, help to alter a destructive or blaming process, and overcome impasses to change. Problems can be depathologized when viewed as common reactions under highly stressful conditions. Symptoms of acute traumatic stress are normal responses to abnormal, traumatic events (see Chapter 11). Problem behavior can also be seen as a survival strategy—an attempt to live with an unbearable situation or to prevent a feared outcome. We note the helpful intentions, albeit misguided ways, of caring members trying to help one another.

A problem presented as "inside" an individual, such as a personality trait, can be redefined behaviorally in context. For example, a label of "bothersome nag" may be recast in terms of a mother's tenacity in her struggle to get an unresponsive school system to provide needed services for her struggling child. In a vicious cycle, the more she complains, the less responsive the school becomes, viewing her as the problem. By recasting the set (Watzlawick, Beavin, & Jackson, 1967), the mother's efforts are validated and more effective dialogues can be facilitated.

Narrative reauthoring serves as a means to expand and reframe problem situations through language and perspective—to view them in more empowering terms that facilitate problem resolution (Freedman & Combs, 1996). In Michael White's technique of externalization (White & Epston, 1990), the therapist recasts a problem (often a child's behavior problem) as an external force that is wreaking havoc in family members' lives. The therapist aligns with the child and family as partners who together will defeat this negative force, leaving the child and family feeling victorious.

Clinicians must be mindful that a new perspective may not be sufficient to surmount overwhelming obstacles. Knowledge, skills, and opportunities to succeed are also required to respond to powerful external forces, such as a changing job market. When conditions are beyond control and can't be changed, such as an incurable illness, our efforts involve "mastering the possible": making the best of the situation.

Using Respectful Language and Constructs

For effective intervention, we need to learn the language and perspective of family members in order to appreciate their experience. We need to understand the values and expectations that influence their approach to handling their problems and their difficulties in making needed changes. Narrative therapists have heightened our awareness of the power of words: they may reflect pessimism and foster blame, shame, guilt, and failure; or they can express hope, pride, and confidence about ability and potential.

The health care system in the United States is so oriented around individual pathology and disease that in most cases, for even partial coverage of payment for couple or family therapy, one member must be labeled with a psychiatric diagnosis—and more serious pathology documented for more than a few sessions (American Psychiatric Association, 2014; Frances, 2013). While family resilience-oriented practice is grounded in a biopsychosocial orientation, we broaden our understanding of problem situations in relation to transactional processes, stressful events, and contextual influences. Systemic descriptions focused toward solutions and positive aims open up more possibilities for change. We eschew demeaning labels for persons (e.g., "she's a borderline") and pejorative assumptions about "dysfunctional families." Because the very language of therapy can pathologize a family, we take great care in framing problems, questions, and responses in a way that is respectful of distressed individuals, their families, and their situations.

Encouraging a Positive Outlook: Rekindling Hope

While being empathic with the struggles of our clients when they are despairing, it is important to rekindle their hope, because hope fuels efforts to succeed. For example, I may say, "I understand that you're experiencing a lot of pain and conflict right now. I'm also convinced that you have many strengths as a family. I believe that beneath the turmoil and upset, you care deeply about each other. One sign of that caring is that you made an effort to come in and meet to solve your problems. I'm quite hopeful that if you will work together as a team on these issues, you can make things better. I'll be glad to work with you, to support your best efforts."

When clients have lost hope, we might ask, "Can you recall a time when you felt more hopeful about your situation? What was helpful? Who supported that hope? How?" "How might you harness that positive energy now?" Conversations can explore what might be learned and applied to the present dilemma, as well as what could help the family regain hope. What might a partner, parents, or others say or do that might reinvigorate them? Often one spouse will turn to the other and say, "I just need you to hold me and tell me you love me. That will keep me going through this crisis." A parent may need to be told she or he is appreciated. A family bear hug at the end of a session can bolster everyone's spirits.

Kaethe Weingarten (2004, 2010) has written about "doing hope," in many ways, big and small. She views hope not only as an emotion, but also as a practice, noting that feeling follows action. The practice of hope provides a profound spiritual satisfaction, almost contentment. It connects one to the webs of meaning and relationship that make life purposeful and meaningful. But what we do depends on our position in relation to hope. Those who are hopeless and those who witness their despair have different tasks. If hopeless, we must resist isolation. If witness to despair, we must refuse indifference. Neither is easy.

Weingarten encourages us to practice realistic hope; it is not the same as blind optimism. Doing hope requires that we recognize the complexities and contradictions of lives and acknowledge doubt and despair. The challenge, she asserts, is to look at the messiness of a situation without losing hope. When clients spiral downward, losing all hope, it is crucial that therapists not spiral down with them. One worker told a beleaguered family that he understood how it was hard for members to feel hopeful at that moment. He acknowledged their daunting challenges and setbacks, and then reminded them of the efforts and gains they had made, sharing his confidence that they could weather the current crisis. He told them, "I realize that you have lost hope right now—so let me lend you some of mine until you regain yours."

Refocusing from Complaints to Aims

Distressed couples and families can become caught up in a vicious cycle of negativity, focused on each other's deficiencies and constantly finding fault. Despite our inclinations to support a child and to interrupt scapegoating, therapists must be cautious not to adopt a critical stance toward a critical parent or spouse; this only adds to cycles of blame. Asking a parent, "Why are you so hard on your child?" or commenting to a wife, "It seems like you can't see anything good in your husband" criticizes them for being critical. Instead, it's important to understand the stress, pain, and frustrations underlying such criticisms, and to help family members refocus from complaints (what's wrong) to positive aims (what would be better) and how they might achieve them. What would improve an unbearable situation? How would a couple's relationship need to change for the better for a spouse on the edge of divorce to reinvest? What would a more satisfying family life look like? What changes would they need to make to achieve it? What commonalities can help them to bridge their differences?

After hearing family members' complaints in an assessment interview, it's important to acknowledge parents' frustration and to ask what they hope to *gain* through counseling. We shouldn't assume that the desired change is simply to resolve the presenting problem. I'm frequently surprised, as I was in this case:

> In a family evaluation, the parents, Manny and Sylvia, presented a tirade of complaints about their son's bad behavior, including failing grades and stealing money from his mother's savings, stashed under the parents' mattress. I asked about their attempts to deal with the situation, and the father's furious response. I acknowledged the frustration and worry they must feel. When I asked what they most hoped

to gain in our work together, I expected to hear that their son should shape up. Instead, I was surprised when Manny replied, his voice choked up, "I'd like to learn how to show love to my kids." Moved by his response, I asked to hear more about that. Manny responded, "My dad had a temper—he only knew how to yell." I asked what that had been like for him as a kid and noticed how attentive the children were, realizing that he had felt as bad with his father as they did with him now. I asked what that experience had taught him. He replied, "I don't know any other way, but I'd like to do better by my kids."

Here again, in linking past experience with present distress, a future vision can become a positive force to break destructive patterns and achieve healthier relationships. It was also crucial to explore the contextual stresses in the recent problems. Manny, a mechanic, had recently lost his job; they were late on paying the rent and other bills. For Sylvia, this precarious financial situation tapped into catastrophic fears from her childhood experience, when her unemployed father had abandoned the family, and her mother had to go on public aid. She became tearful in recalling how tough those years had been. Manny softened and took her hand, saying, "That's why she took it so hard when her small savings were missing—she lost her security." They hugged, as we expanded our frame to refocus in the next session on their goals: ways to regain their security and share more love in the family.

Bringing Out the Best: Identifying, Affirming, and Building Strengths

All competence-based approaches, at their core, aim to bring out the best in people (Waters & Lawrence, 1993). When we can see and appreciate their best, it can help them to do their best. We can affirm strengths by finding something worthy to commend about each family member. Although no family is strong in every area, all families possess strengths and resources. Amid very real limitations, we can foster resilience by noticing members' assets and potentials, and by finding ways to nurture and praise their positive intentions, efforts, and achievements. They may believe that they are drowning in an ocean of inadequacy, but everyone has "islands of competence" that are, or could be, sources of pride and accomplishment.

A cartoon I love depicts a dog gazing fondly at his owner, with the caption "I think you're wonderful!" We cherish that unconditional positive regard in our bonds with pets (Walsh, 2009b). As therapists, we do need to express our positive regard for all family members, but simply telling them we think they are terrific will ring hollow. It's important to link our praise to their qualities and behaviors that we genuinely admire, from their accounts and our own observations.

Overcoming Culture-Based Gender Barriers

When problems arise in a family, women are more likely to seek professional help, to acknowledge distress, and to feel at fault. Professionals often need to work harder to engage men in therapy, because stereotyped images of masculinity cast vulnerability and the need for help as signs of male weakness and inadequacy. We can encourage men's involvement by tapping into their deep desire to be responsible and loving spouses and parents and strong role models for their children. We can help couples and single parents to transcend traditional gendered role constraints to develop more functional patterns that fit their situations, needs, and preferences.

Therapists need to be sensitive to ethnic or religious values that uphold the role of fathers as head of the family while not sanctioning the denigration of women or girls in the family. Men in traditional cultures are often more reluctant to come for therapy if they anticipate shaming experiences, especially in front of other family members. Resilience-oriented practice, because it is so respectful of all clients, is more likely to successfully engage men. When we focus on their strengths and potential, in my experience, they are also more likely to acknowledge any faults, fears, and vulnerabilities and be open to positive change efforts. We can then reframe their openness as a sign of their strength.

Crediting Positive Intentions

Resilience-based practice approaches help family members to develop in ways that bring forth their deepest desires for mastery and belonging. I prefer to err on the side of assuming that members' intentions are positive, or at least benign, even when their actions may be ineffective or hurtful. For example, we can affirm a father's desire to be a better parent, aligning with his healthier aspirations to help him gain control over his explosive temper. The assumption of a positive intent behind or alongside problematic behavior helps family members to become less defensive and more open, and to strive for their best.

Praising Efforts and Achievements

It's important to notice and appreciate the efforts family members are making in very difficult situations, even when they are not successful. It is more effective to ground praise in small, concrete examples of caring efforts and actions they have demonstrated, such as making it to a parent–teacher meeting despite bad weather. In every session, alongside problem solving, we must make sure to ask how new endeavors are going (e.g., a parent's job training program) and to applaud progress. Every family member has some talent or special interest to express. It is so important to let them know we care about their lives and pursuits beyond their problems. Again, the praise offered must be genuine and connected to their words and deeds.

Wherever possible, we can try to shift a vicious cycle to a virtuous cycle. For example, even though an overstressed mother at times loses control or lashes out at a child, I may share my observation of other signs that she loves the child and has the capacity to be nurturing. I may praise the parenting skills and bonds I observe in a session, such as tenderness in cradling her infant, and point out how responsive the baby is to her loving care. She may initially respond with disbelief ("I am? She is? Really?") and then caress the child, who then breaks into a smile. So often family members comment that coming to sessions has helped them realize they're really not as bad off as they thought.

We can honor the relational base of resilience as we celebrate individual success. I once gave a long-stemmed rose to a hardworking single mother on the occasion of her daughter's graduation from college, to honor her important contribution to her child's success. Another time, I took a photo of beaming immigrant parents and their son, holding up his GED certificate. At the end of therapy, I gave them each a framed copy of the photo, so that they could always keep in mind—in good and bad times—the son's hard-won achievement and the parents' pride and love.

Drawing Out Hidden Resources and Lost Competence

When families are in distress, their view becomes problem-saturated. They most often seek help when they have reached an impasse, coping and problem-solving efforts are exhausted, and they feel overwhelmed and inadequate. Their abilities to solve their problems may be hidden, inaccessible, or forgotten. Family members benefit from therapeutic conversations that bring into awareness untapped resources or unnoticed strengths. We can help them to regain lost competence and to recognize loving concern that may be overshadowed by their current distress. Solution-focused and narrative therapists search for *exceptions* to a problem situation—positive interactions or abilities shown at other times or in other parts of their lives that can be drawn upon now (Freedman & Combs, 1996). For instance, asking spouses about their ways of finding pleasure together before troubles arose can help to rekindle lost intimacy or bring to the foreground positive aspects of their lives that may have been trampled on by persistent adversity.

Highlighting Strengths in the Midst of Adversity

As in solution-focused therapies, it is useful to ask about positive exceptions *apart from* presenting problems, or happier times before troubles arose. Because a resilience-oriented approach focuses on the experience of adversity, it is even more important to search for strengths *in the midst of* challenging situations. For example, we might commend family members' perseverance in their struggle to overcome a financial setback and discuss how they manage to keep up their efforts and spirit.

Adversity can bring out the best in family members. Yet, in distress, they may not see or access these strengths. By highlighting them, we help families to recognize their own resources and potential. In doing so, we increase their confidence that they can draw on these strengths when future need arises. As we support their efforts to manage a crisis well, family members often discover resources they never knew they had and build new competencies. A husband may develop new tenderness in caring for his wife, now disabled after a serious accident. A father who may have been uninvolved with his children can learn new parenting skills and achieve closer bonds when forced to manage on his own as a single parent. We search for strengths in the hard times, striving for meaning making and mastery.

> Ray and Barbara sought help for intense conflict in the seventh month of her second pregnancy. The therapist's attempts to refocus on happier times, and future visions for the new baby, fell flat. As a consultant, I explored the meaning of this pregnancy. I learned that Ray and Barbara had lost their first baby and now were fearful that the worst would happen again. They tried to push that experience out of their minds and avoided talking about it. Yet they were quite anxious and found themselves arguing over plans for the baby's room, and Ray kept putting off assembling the crib. I asked them to share their memories of the first pregnancy—from their initial hopes and dreams, their preparations, and the anticipatory joy of family and friends through to the unexpected, shattering loss on what should have been their happiest day. The tears came anew as they recounted the details of the birth, the hushed voices of the medical staff in the delivery room, and their utter devastation in learning that the baby would not survive. In the wake of that loss, each partner had tried to process the events and the grief separately, but they had never shared their pain. Now their unspoken fears blocked them from investing in plans for the child soon to arrive.
>
> Acknowledging their sorrow, I shared my admiration for their love and their courage in trying anew for a much-desired child. I

encouraged their mutual support in the weeks leading up to the birth. We also discussed how they might communicate their wishes and needs to friends and family members, who, in their anxiety, either distanced or hovered nervously around them.

We also explored their contacts with health care professionals. Much anxiety came from ambiguous generalities from a doctor who told them only that there was nothing to worry about this time. They were encouraged to meet together with a genetic counselor to gain a fuller comprehension of their situation. She clarified that the new baby's fetal development was normal. In more fully sharing and integrating their past crisis with their current concerns, Ray and Barbara approached the impending birth joyfully.

Helping Families Live with Uncertainty

Many families need help in tolerating protracted uncertainty. When past events or future expectations remain murky, we can help family members to clarify as much as possible about the situation and find a way to live with persisting ambiguity. In many cases, we need to help a family cope with uncertainty about the future course and outcome of a precarious situation, such as the threatened loss of their home due to job and financial insecurity. After a major disaster, it may be many months or much longer before families know if they can move back and whether their homes and communities can be rebuilt.

Seizing Opportunities

As therapists and families work to solve presenting problems, we can seize opportunities for personal and relational growth out of the crisis that brings them for help. We can help clients cast their problem situation in a new light that opens possibilities. When facing a crisis, it's helpful to look back to past family experiences with adversity for lessons that can be drawn about both helpful and unhelpful responses. In the aftermath of a crisis, family members can explore what can be learned from their situation. There may be important lessons about risk and vulnerability, or about the need to anticipate pitfalls and take more precautions in the future. In building resilience, we help families strive to integrate the fullness of their crisis and recovery experience.

Often something valuable is gained from a crisis that might not have been learned or achieved otherwise. Adversity may bring a startling recognition of the importance of relationships that had been taken for granted or written off. A disruptive family relocation can also be a milestone for taking time out to reassess life and relationship priorities, or to affirm and strengthen commitments. A crisis can lead family members to question, review, and redirect their lives. A woman who had oriented her life around her husband was devastated when he left her. Therapy facilitated her life transformation from an initial sense of emptiness to the development of new talents and confidence in her own identity and ability to lead a fulfilling life on her own. We can open these pathways to growth out of shattering loss.

Exploring the Spiritual Dimension in Suffering, Healing, and Resilience

Exploring faith beliefs and practices should become part of all efforts to help families dealing with adversity (Walsh, 2009d). We shouldn't presume that spiritual matters are unimportant if not voiced or if clients are not religious. Just as we would inquire respectfully about cultural beliefs and practices, we need to show comfort and interest in exploring the spiritual aspect of painful experiences. As we expand our vision of psychotherapy as both a science and a healing art, our change efforts must take the human spirit into account, conceptualizing adverse experience holistically, including biopsychosocial–spiritual dimensions. We need to explore how spiritual concerns may contribute to suffering, and how spiritual connections, fitting our clients' value systems, can be powerful resources in recovery, healing, and resilience. (See "Exploring the Spiritual Dimension in Family Life," Appendix 3.)

One mother's self-destructive drinking was fueled by the belief, rooted in her childhood Christian upbringing, that the death of her newborn daughter was God's punishment for not having baptized her son. Although she had not practiced her religion in years, this conviction seized her mind in her tragic loss. She had not shared her belief and guilt with her husband, who was raised Jewish and was very close to his family. When they married, they had both thought religion was unimportant in their lives. It was crucial to open discussion with the couple, facilitating their reconsideration of religion for themselves and for their children's upbringing.

Building Empathic Connections and Appreciation

We work with families most effectively when we build empathic connections with and between members. Often therapists find it hard to be empathic with a parent who at first strikes us as harsh and abrasive. Yet a mother's hard edge, for instance, might be seen in terms of the feistiness she developed in order to keep her family afloat through tough times and her ex-partner's bouts of drinking. We can identify with her struggle as a single parent and appreciate her toughness, given her many challenges.

Epston (2012) offers the idea of *mother appreciation parties* in families where a parent has been undervalued, misunderstood, or maltreated. He describes a case where a son screams at his mother and berates her as stupid, just as his father had done before the mother left him. As the therapist invites the son to listen to his mother's account of their family life, he comes to realize that she took verbal and physical violent abuse his father intended for him, out of her loving desire to protect her son. In the son's next session, he said he wanted to show his mother how much he appreciated all she had done but didn't know how. He enthusiastically took up the idea of a secret mother appreciation party and planned it with the involvement of an aunt and other relatives. Epston, supporting his efforts, suggested that he might give a speech of appreciation at the party and helped him to craft what he wanted to say. At a follow-up session with the mother and son, she expressed her appreciation for his recent efforts to be helpful and respectful and said that the surprise party, with her son's moving speech, was the best day of her life.

Family members gain greater compassion for one another when they are asked to share their life stories, the painful experiences they have suffered, and the sparks of resilience they have shown in weathering those ordeals. A mother who is resented for overprotecting her daughter can be seen in a new light—as trying to spare her the harm that she had endured in childhood sexual abuse. The confusion of a father who is at a loss in dealing with a teenager is clarified when he describes how his own father wasn't there for him; we can be empathic with the challenge of becoming a good father without having had a positive role model. We might also ask who else in his family network had been a good father or surrogate, such as an uncle or grandfather, and explore their qualities that he might aspire toward. Viewing current dilemmas in the light of life experience can make them more understandable, and flawed individuals, such as his father, can be seen with compassion, as struggling as best they could.

The following case presented intergenerational tensions common in immigrant families (Falicov, 2013):

> Stavros brought his 17-year-old only son, Stavros Jr., for therapy to "straighten him out." An immigrant, Stavros was furious that his son had left their church, was hanging around with "no-good" friends, and was on the verge of school dropout. Steve (as the son preferred to be called) sat respectfully quiet in the session, yet defended his friends and was obstinate that he didn't care about school or religion. Steve felt constantly pressured by his father to succeed academically and go

to college to get a good job. He looked down on his father's work history of low pay and long hours, and felt badgered to make up for the father's "failure" in life.

I asked Stavros whether he had ever shared his full life story and the difficulties of immigration. In a hushed voice, he revealed that he felt ashamed of his humble beginnings in the United States and his poor English. Encouraged to tell his story, he described the brutal military regime that he had fled; he was forced to leave school at 17 with his brother to escape being drafted. Although he had excelled in school, when he arrived in this country he took the only work he could find, as a janitor, and added odd jobs in order to send money back to his aging parents. Like many immigrants, he realized that he would have to start from scratch and struggle for a living, but his determination was kept strong by his hope that his efforts would enable his children to have a better life. Things became even harder when Steve's mother died after a long illness when the boy was 12. Spending nothing on himself, Stavros secretly put away a few dollars whenever he could for his son's college education. He was so proud to have such a smart son. How could Steve not care about his future?

Steve, although initially claiming a lack of interest in his father's story, listened intently. His voice broke as he said he hadn't realized what his father had been up against, how much courage it had taken to do all he did, and how he had struggled for the sake of his parents and his son. Steve began to see his father not as a failure, but a hero. Moreover, he hadn't been aware of his father's pride in him; he had only felt his disapproval and disappointment. For his part, Steve needed his father to be more tolerant of his friends, activities, and beliefs, so different from the father's experiences and world view in the old country. Through their conversations over several sessions, and the therapist's reframing, Stavros was able to hear how Steve's differences were less a rejection of his father and more about seeking to find himself in another culture. Stavros reflected, sadly, that in demanding that Steve do everything *his* way, he had become no different from the military dictator he had fled. Father and son were helped to find a better balance. While coming of age, Steve still needed his father's encouragement and support in making his own choices for a good life. Cast in a new light, the very possibility of choice meant that Stavros had truly succeeded in his dream of a better life for his son. He had given him the gift of freedom.

In addressing Stavros's harsh and overbearing treatment of his son, it was crucial to learn (and to help his son appreciate) how he came to that position, and to understand its protective function. I admired his concern for his son's future so that Steve would have a better opportunity for success in life. Reaching greater mutual understanding with his son enabled him to be less controlling and more accepting of Steve's autonomous strivings. In turn, Steve became less likely to make bad choices for himself out of angry defiance. To foster family resilience in cases such as this one, it's essential to help members reach a new understanding and esteem for one another.

Encouraging a Positive, Future-Oriented Vision

People coming for help are often stuck in a vision of their lives that is narrow and joyless, filled with adversity, suffering, and fear. Approaching clients about their hopes and dreams encourages them to imagine a more satisfying future and seek to achieve it (Madsen, 2009).

For instance, families approaching later life can be encouraged to consider and prepare together for such challenges as retirement, transitional living arrangements, and end-of-life decisions—discussions that are commonly avoided. Future-oriented questions can also open up new possibilities for later-life fulfillment. One son was concerned about how each of his parents would manage alone on the family farm if widowed, but he dreaded talking with them about their death. Finally, on a visit home, he got up his courage. First he asked his mother, tentatively, whether she had ever thought about what she might do if Dad were the first to go. She replied, "Sure—we've never talked about it, but I've thought about it for years. I'd sell the farm and move to Texas to be near our grandkids." Her husband scratched his head and replied, "Well, if that ain't the darnedest thing! I've thought a lot about it too, and if your mother wasn't here, *I'd* sell the farm and move to Texas!" This conversation led the couple to make plans to sell the farm, which had become increasingly burdensome, and move to Texas, where they enjoyed many happy years.

In work with distressed couples and families, a positive, future-oriented focus shifts the emphasis of therapy from problems to possibilities, from "What went wrong?" to "What can be done for enhanced functioning and well-being?" Together, we and our clients can then envision possible options that fit their situation, and reachable aims through shared, constructive efforts. This involves imagination, a hopeful outlook, and initiative in taking actions toward desired goals.

When the Past Intrudes on the Present and Future

A future-oriented focus is valuable even when a current crisis reactivates past traumatic experiences, as in the following case:

Joanne and Ralph were seen in family consultation after their 22-year-old son, Joey, had a serious drug overdose on the eve of his wedding.

In exploring their feelings about their son's leaving home and getting married, Joanne said it harder for her than it had been with their other children, but she didn't know why. I noted that Joey had been named after her, and asked about her own experience of leaving home and getting married. Joanne told of running off to marry her husband against her father's strong objections. She had been furious at his opposition, and he, in turn, had refused to speak with her again. He died 6 months later of a heart attack without reconciliation. At this point in her story, Joanne became tearful and said, "Somehow it feels the same now."

It was crucial to inquire beyond the obvious dyadic relationship between Joanne and her father to explore other system patterns that might also be fueling current difficulties. Joanne had been very close to her mother, who, once widowed, spent the rest of her life depressed and lonely. Asked if she ever worried that history might repeat itself, Joanne began to cry, saying that she worried constantly about her husband's health and his overweight condition. In recent months he had complained of chest pains but had refused to see a doctor. Joey's leaving aroused her fear that something terrible would happen to Ralph and she would end up like her mother.

With Joanne's catastrophic expectations and her lack of a model for later-life marriage (Ralph's mother had also been widowed), she and Ralph had never discussed any dreams or plans for their future together after launching their children. Brief couple therapy focused on envisioning their future possibilities. Ralph had a medical workup and started to take better care of himself. They celebrated their son's wedding and then spontaneously took a "refresher honeymoon" on their own.

In helping a family to move forward, it's important to make overt the covert connections between the past, present, and future so that family members can more fully understand current distress and integrate their experiences. They can't change the past, but we can help them learn from it to chart a better future course.

Accepting Human Limitations with Compassion

The Navaho say that the way to tell a rug has been made by human hands is by its flaws. As helping professionals, we can cultivate acceptance of imperfections within families—as well as our own limitations—by viewing flaws not as defects, but instead as part of being human. If a family member has been wounded by life struggles, we need to diminish blame and shame and, instead, foster compassion.

Our therapeutic approach is grounded in the recognition that mistakes and failures are inevitable in life and can be expected in challenging endeavors, especially under stressful conditions. We can help family members to own errors and to view them as valuable learning experiences, rather than as demoralizing defeats. It's also important, to the extent possible, to attribute mistakes to factors that members can change, such as making greater effort or setting more realistic goals, rather than to their own innate deficits, such as telling a child she is just not smart enough. This is most challenging, yet essential, when youth and families have experienced many difficulties and have come to feel beaten down by repeated setbacks. We can also broaden their perspective to help them recognize the structural barriers in their environment that constrain them.

Involving Families in Healing from Individual Trauma

Even when a crisis strikes an individual and family members are not directly touched by the event, a systemic approach considers how all are affected by it and how the family response influences recovery. Other members may not currently be showing distress but may hold hidden concerns and be at heightened risk for later problems. A family resilience approach draws members together for mutual support and healing. All can benefit from family interventions and become better resources for one another.

> Heather, a high school freshman, had been sexually assaulted by a 17-year-old football player at an unsupervised party. Her family, wanting to help her recover, arranged for her to have individual therapy. At home, they said nothing about the incident so as to not upset her, even though it preoccupied their thoughts. They tried to lift her spirits by being cheerful and acting "normal," as if nothing bad had happened. Her therapist was very caring, yet after 2 months she remained withdrawn from family and friends and took a handful of pills in a suicide attempt. Heather had misinterpreted her family's silence and "phony" cheer as covering over condemnation of her for the incident.
>
> A family session was held, where Heather's parents revealed deep concern for her well-being and regret that they hadn't known how to show their support. None of her family members blamed her for the assault; instead, they blamed themselves and each other. Her parents fought over the decision to let her go to the party. Her older brother, Brian, felt especially guilty because he knew the boy's bad reputation and felt he should have protected his sister. Other concerns surfaced as well: Heather's 11-year-old sister silently worried that it could happen to her; could boys and friends be trusted?
>
> A relational resilience approach brought a cascade of positive benefits. Heather's healing was facilitated by open, honest communication

with her family. Also, the guilt, regret, and concerns of other family members could be addressed. Family members became better able to show their support; they mobilized to take action with Heather in filing sexual assault charges. Brian and Heather together organized a crisis hotline that any students feeling at risk in a social situation could use to call for a ride home. The parents organized a parents' association meeting at the school, where the family therapist and the school counselor were invited to discuss information about rape and the important roles family members can play in recovery and prevention. Families were encouraged to network better to ensure safety at social events. The initiatives generated by this crisis fostered a sense of empowerment and healing for Heather and her family, strengthening their bonds and sense of community. Although Heather had been reluctant for schoolmates to learn of the assault, her friends rallied to support her and praised her courage in coming forward on a concern shared by many girls.

Even when an individual suffers a traumatic experience, the impact of the crisis reverberates through the network of relationships. Family sessions can be essential for both individual and collective healing. This case also illustrates two common findings in the resilience research. One key to resilience involves mastering the art of the possible: acknowledging what can't be changed (the assault that occurred) and putting efforts and actions into possible options (mobilizing to bring the assailant to justice and prevent future harm). A related key to resilience involves transcendence from personal tragedy and suffering to efforts to prevent harm for others. The inspiration to organize a hotline is empowering as it benefits other teens in high-risk situations.

Encouraging a Team Approach for Competence, Confidence, and Success

Just as negative interactions can have a destructive cascading effect, small successes have a positive ripple effect, increasing family members' confidence and ability to master more difficult challenges. To foster family resilience, we need to create a therapeutic climate that maximizes the possibilities for members to collaborate successfully and to experience achievements as largely due to their shared efforts and abilities. Small successes can be sources of pride and accomplishment to build on. These affirming beliefs and experiences generate realistic hope and optimism that they will be able to master their challenges through a team approach.

Several guidelines are useful to strengthen family teamwork for competence, confidence, and success. First, we can encourage all members' sense of responsibility and pride in their contribution to the process. We can recognize their efforts and offer to facilitate more effective joint strategies for coping and problem solving. Second, it's important to help families initiate and follow through on concrete, achievable steps toward objectives, and to persevere when challenges loom as overwhelming and goals seem remote. As my colleague Carol Anderson told families in her psychoeducational model with persistent mental illness, "Yard by yard, it's just too hard; inch by inch, it's a cinch."

Second, it's crucial to attribute successes to family members—not the therapist's expertise—so they come to believe that their collaborative efforts can make a difference. As good coaches affirm after a winning game, the victory goes to the team. As they become successful more often, they will come to believe that these shared efforts can make a difference. Experiences of success in one arena of life can generalize to enhanced coping with other life challenges (Rutter, 1985).

MANY PATHWAYS IN RESILIENCE

Families most often come for help in crisis. When they are overwhelmed and their presenting problems skew therapeutic attention toward deficits, a resilience-based framework offers a positive and pragmatic focus for intervention. This approach normalizes distress as understandable in the context of a family's life challenges. It generates hope in the future while grounding changes in specific actions toward reachable aims. Table 7.2 summarizes major practice guidelines to strengthen family resilience.

In our work with struggling families, we must be mindful that in most adverse situations, resilience does not mean bouncing right back or always maintaining competence, cheerful optimism, and steady progress. Dealing with adversity may be a matter of taking three steps forward, two steps back—and then taking a breath and attempting to move forward again. Family members are bound to have times when they falter or need respite, when they take a wrong turn, or when they sink into despair. When they experience setbacks, we may need to first help them catch their breath, and then encourage them to rebound, persist in their efforts, or seek a new pathway. We cannot solve their problems, but we can accompany them on a stretch of their journey.

My colleague Carlos Sluzki once offered the apt metaphor of climbing a mountain to describe the process of therapy. He noted that you don't go straight up to the top, but you make a plan that fits the contours of the mountain, the rigors of the climb, and your own skills. As on a mountain

TABLE 7.2. Practice Guidelines to Strengthen Family Resilience

- Honor the dignity and worth of all family members.
- Convey conviction in their potential to overcome adversity through shared efforts.
- Use respectful language, framing to humanize and contextualize distress:
  - View as understandable, common in adverse situation (e.g., normal reactions to abnormal or extreme event or conditions).
  - Decrease shame, blame, stigma, pathology focus.
- Provide safe haven for sharing pain, concerns, challenges.
  - Show compassion for losses, hardships, suffering, and struggle.
  - Build communication, empathy, mutual support among members.
- Identify and affirm strengths, resources alongside vulnerabilities, limitations.
- Draw out, increase potential for coping, mastery, healing, and growth.
- Mobilize extended kin, social, community, cultural, and spiritual resources—build "relational lifelines," support networks, teamwork; recruit models, mentors.
- View crisis and challenges as opportunity for learning, change, and positive growth.
- Shift focus from problems to possibilities.
  - Reorient life priorities, deepen bonds, engage in meaningful pursuits.
  - Future vision; hopes and dreams.
- Integrate adverse experience—including resilience—into individual and relational identity and life passage.

road with hairpin turns, you choose a challenging yet doable climb, first to one side and then back across a little higher, forging a zigzag path ever closer to the summit. At each plateau, you can pause and gaze out over the horizon to appreciate the distance you've come. At some points, you need to double back or find new ways to go around huge obstacles. You make a base camp for rest and refueling en route, find shelter from a storm, and gather strength for the next phase of the journey. Should the next stretch prove too arduous, you can return to the base camp to refuel and regroup, then try again on the same path or forge a new one. This image resonates with my experience of the therapeutic journey—and the journey we take in life. We may not reach the goal we first set out toward, and we may travel in unforeseen directions, forging new and varied pathways. Along the way, we can find meaning and joy in the journey and gain new perspectives at each plateau we reach.

CHAPTER 8

Applying a Family
Resilience Framework
in Community–Based Services

The road to success is always under construction.
—ANONYMOUS

A family resilience framework is especially valuable in community-based intervention and prevention services. This chapter describes several training and programmatic applications developed through the Chicago Center for Family Health (CCFH) to address a wide range of adverse situations. Attention is also given to strengthening the resilience of helping professionals to prevent burnout and compassion fatigue in highly stressful work, and the vicarious resilience professionals experience in drawing out our clients' resilience.

BROAD APPLICATIONS
OF A FAMILY RESILIENCE FRAMEWORK

A family resilience orientation can serve as a broad meta-framework for the training and practice of mental health, health care, social service, and pastoral care providers, and for the design and delivery of community-based programs. It can be applied usefully with a wide range of crisis situations, disruptive transitions, and prolonged life challenges. Interventions utilize principles and techniques common among many strength-based family systems practice approaches but attend more centrally to the impact of significant stressors and aim to strengthen the family resources and potential for positive adaptation. This approach also affirms that families may forge varied pathways for resilience over time, fitting their adverse situation and their values, resources, and challenges. Using varied formats, including brief consultation, family counseling/therapy, and multifamily groups, this collaborative resilience-oriented approach strengthens family functioning, relational bonds, vital community connections, and resources to meet future life challenges.

Family resilience-oriented practitioners serve as compassionate witnesses and facilitators, helping family members share with each other their experience of adversity, overcome silence, secrecy, shame, or blame, and build mutual support and teamwork in their efforts. Appreciative inquiry that attends to family strengths in the midst of suffering readily engages families, who are often reluctant to seek mental health services out of concern that they will be judged as disturbed or deficient. Instead, family members are respectfully regarded as essential members of the healing team for recovery and resilience. Where they have faltered, they are viewed as struggling with an overwhelming set of challenges, and their best intentions are affirmed. Intervention efforts are directed at mastering those challenges through their shared efforts.

In community-based services, a resilience-oriented systemic assessment may lead to individual, couple, family, and multifamily group modalities, as well as larger workshop formats and community forums. Putting an ecological view into practice, family-centered collaborative efforts may combine multilevel approaches and involve peer groups, the workplace, schools, faith congregations, and community agencies, as well as health care, justice, and other larger systems. Effective programs need to be flexible and creative in their approaches to involve families. While these programs must be structurally sound to be effective, it is their process, the ability to engage and encourage families, that is most important.

Resilience-based family interventions can be adapted to varied formats, from family consultations or conferences to brief counseling or more intensive family therapy. Psychoeducational multifamily and couple groups emphasize the importance of social support and practical information, offering concrete guidelines for crisis management, problem solving, and stress reduction as families navigate through stressful periods and face future challenges. Therapists, coaches, or group leaders facilitate discussion, help families to clarify specific stresses they are dealing with, and support their efforts to develop effective coping strategies, measuring success in small increments and maintaining family morale. Brief follow-ups and cost-effective workshops or forums can support families at various steps or transitions along their journey, helping them to integrate what has happened and meet anticipated challenges ahead.

A family resilience framework has broad utility for practice application with families facing a wide range of adverse situations:

- Recover from crisis, trauma, and loss events (bereavement, war-related trauma, major disaster).
- Navigate disruptive transitions (e.g., job loss, migration, separation, divorce, stepfamily integration).
- Overcome challenges of chronic multi-stress conditions (e.g., serious illness, disability; conditions of poverty).
- Overcome barriers to success (e.g., at-risk youth, school dropout).

FAMILY RESILIENCE-ORIENTED PROGRAMS AT THE CHICAGO CENTER FOR FAMILY HEALTH

Over the past 25 years, the family resilience framework described in this book has guided the development of professional training, consultation, and services at the Chicago Center for Family Health (*www.ccfhchicago. org*), a nonprofit advanced training institute affiliated with the University of Chicago. Cofounders and codirectors, John Rolland, MD, and I formed a network of talented clinical faculty members interested in advancing family systems training and practice. Our faculty, bringing together varied couple and family therapy models and areas of expertise, all share a strength-based, collaborative approach, responsive to family diversity and committed to serve disadvantaged and marginalized populations and social justice concerns.

Building partnerships with community-based organizations has been at the heart of our mission to train and support health care, mental health, and human service professionals, particularly those who work with low-income and minority families, LGBT (gay, lesbian, bisexual, and transgender) clients, persons with disabilities, and other vulnerable groups. Toward this end, we have offered workshops and intensive certificate programs and partnered with local health care centers, schools, and human service agencies to provide specialized staff training, organizational consultation, and program development. Our systems approach has also been usefully applied in the fields of pastoral counseling, family law, and family business.

Our overarching mission is to advance family-focused, resilience-oriented policies, services, and practices to strengthen resilience in youth, couples, and families facing serious life challenges. Programs have been designed and implemented to address a wide range of adverse situations, as summarized in Table 8.1, with program coordinators noted.[1]

Several of these applications are discussed in the following chapters, which address family life cycle challenges such as divorce, complicated family bereavement, major trauma and disasters, chronic illness, multi-stressed families, and reconnection and reconciliation. In the 1990s, a resilience-oriented training and counseling program addressing the challenges of LGBT clients was developed in partnership with Howard Brown Hospital and Horizons Community Services (Bruce Koff, Coordinator). Multilevel approaches, such as the successful Family–Schools Partnership Program (Kelly, Bluestone-Miller, Mervis, & Fuerst, 2012) work with larger systems with at-risk youth and families. Four programmatic descriptions are offered here to illustrate the potential utility of this approach in community-based services to families facing varied situations of adversity.

The Families, Illness and Collaborative Healthcare Program

CCFH's Families, Illness and Collaborative Healthcare Program (FICH), grounded in a resilience-based, developmental systems orientation, centers on Rolland's integrative family systems illness model for collaborative health care (Rolland, 1994, in press; Rolland & Walsh, 2005, 2006). This approach helps families and couples challenged by major health conditions to live and love well in the face of physical limitations and loss. It normalizes painful and disruptive illness-related experiences and builds on family strengths and resources to optimize healthy functioning and the well-being of all members. The approach includes as equal partners the biomedical and psychosocial service providers, patients, their families, and other caregivers. Caring for families in a way that focuses on prevention and maximizes their own resources has been shown to be more successful and cost-effective (Campbell, 2003; see Chapter 12).

---

[1] CCFH faculty members who have been instrumental over the years in program development, training, and consultation services include Bessie Sultan Akuamoah, LCSW; Michele Baldwin, PhD, LCSW; Mary Jo Barrett, MSW; Cheryl Berg, LCSW; Robin Bluestone-Miller; Pamela Brand, PsyD, LMFT; Gene Combs, MD; Mona Fishbane, PhD; Jill Freedman, LCSW; Ruth Fuerst, LCSW; Katherine Neill Goldberg, MA; Deane Graham, LMFT, LCPC; Miriam Gutmann, MD; Lynn Carp Jacob, LCSW; Michael Kelly, PhD; Bruce Koff, LCSW; Jay Lebow, PhD, LMFT; Ronna Lerner, LCSW; William Martin, LCSW; Bonnie Mervis, LCSW; Michelle Adler Morrison, LCSW; David Schwartz, PhD; John Schwartzman, PhD; Nancy Segall, MA, LCSW; Len Sharber, MDiv, LCSW; Kate Sori, PhD, LMFT; Michele Scheinkman, LCSW; Robert Sholtes, MD; Susan Sholtes, LCSW; Virginia Simons, LCSW; Sant Singh, MAS, MA, FIC, LCSW; Karen Skerrett, PhD, RN; Thomas Todd, PhD; Lorena Valles, LCSW; Stevan Weine, MD; and Steven Zuckerman, PhD, LMFT.

TABLE 8.1. CCFH Resilience–Oriented, Community–Based Program Applications

Recover from crisis, trauma, and loss

- Family adaptation to complicated, traumatic loss (Walsh)
- Mass trauma events; major disasters (Walsh)
- Relational trauma (Barrett, Center for Contextual Change)
- Refugee families (Rolland, Walsh, Weine)
- War- and conflict-related recovery (Rolland, Weine, Walsh)

Navigate disruptive family transitions

- Divorce, single-parent, stepfamily adaptation (Jacob, Lebow, Graham, Simons)
- Foster care (Engstrom)
- Job loss, transition, and reemployment strains (Walsh, Brand)

Overcome challenges of chronic multi-stress conditions

- Serious illness, disabilities, end-of-life challenges (Rolland, Walsh, R. Sholtes, Zuckerman)
- Poverty; ongoing complex trauma (faculty)
- LGBT issues, stigma (Koff)

Overcome obstacles to success: at-risk youth

- Child and adolescent developmental challenges (Lerner, Schwartz, Gutmann, Martin)
- Family–school partnership program (Furst and team)
- Gang reduction/youth development (GRYD) (Rolland, Walsh, and team)

Training offerings, including workshops, brief intensives, and an advanced certificate program, were designed to address the challenges of work with chronic and life-threatening illness, disability, and loss for health and mental health care professionals in a range of practice settings. The program features a nationally highly regarded 1-year FICH Doctoral Fellowship, in partnership with Advocate Illinois Masonic Medical Center, Department of Family Practice.

The FICH Program has partnered with community-based health, mental health and social service organizations in numerous training and consultation projects and in promoting systemic change by incorporating resilience- and family-oriented practices in leadership development and program planning and implementation.[2] In one illustrative project, Dr.

---

[2]Numerous consultation and training services over the years have included partnerships with the Kovler Diabetes Center at the Pritzker Medical Center of the University of Chicago; Children's Memorial Hospital/Lurie Children's Hospital at Northwestern Feinberg School of Medicine; the End-of-Life Coalition and regional hospice programs; the Why Me? and Gilda's Club cancer support programs; and the NorthShore University HealthSystem Integrative Medicine Program and Center for Compassion in Medical Care.

Rolland developed the Resilient Partners Program for couples facing the challenges of multiple sclerosis (MS), in collaboration with the National Multiple Sclerosis Society, Illinois chapter (Rolland, McPheters, & Carbonell, 2008). The program offered two formats: four weekly multicouple group meetings and a 1-day workshop. The majority of couples had been living with MS for at least 5 years. Many attendees had participated in support groups for either patients or spouses, yet strikingly, this was the first time they had the opportunity to meet as a couple with other couples living with MS. They all remarked on how valuable it was to focus specifically on the challenges for their relationship over time. Because of the large number of MS-affected families in the Chicago region, we were able to offer illness phase-specific groups and groups tailored to specific life phase challenges for younger couples, many involved in child rearing, and for mid- and later-life couples often coping with greater levels of disability and caregiving demands.

Stresses of Job Loss, Transition, and Prolonged Unemployment

Job and income loss, as well as anxiety and uncertainty about prolonged unemployment, can be highly stressful for the entire family and heighten risks for a cascade of other losses and homelessness. The severe strains often fuel depression, substance abuse, intense marital conflict, relational abuse, and family breakup. Spousal and parental roles are disrupted. Single-parent families may lose their only income source. Cumulative stresses over many months or longer, in turn, reduce the ability of spouses and family members to support worker efforts, through retraining and job search, for successful reemployment.

One multiyear CCFH family resilience-based program was directed toward the adaptation of displaced workers and their families when jobs were lost due to factory closings or company downsizing. Operation Able, a community-based agency in Chicago specializing in job retraining and placement services, contacted us to develop family resilience-based services in partnership with them. In one case, over 1,800 workers lost their jobs abruptly with the closing and relocation of a large clothing manufacturing plant. Most were ethnic/racial minority individuals and/or immigrants with limited English and lacked education and skills for employment in the changing job market. All were essential breadwinners for their families; many were single parents. Agency staff sought our approach because their individually focused services were not addressing the family strains generated by the job loss, which, in turn, hampered vital family support needed by the displaced worker.

Family resilience-oriented workshops were designed to address the personal and familial impact of losses and transitional stresses, attending to family strains, reorganizing role functions, and rallying family members to support the best efforts of the displaced worker. Workshop participants and leaders together identified discussion themes relevant to their challenges and focused on keys to resilience. For instance, they discussed constraining beliefs (e.g., "No one will hire me"; "I feel worthless to my family without a job and paycheck"). Facilitators shifted focus from perceived deficits to identify skills and strengths, such as pride in doing a job well, and dependability and loyalty in work and family life.

Parental roles needed to be realigned. For men whose sense of worth was diminished with the loss of the traditional male "breadwinner" role it was crucial to broaden their perceived and actual contributions to their families. It was important for them to hear from family members the ways they were valued. The job transition also presented the opportunity, with greater availability, to spend more time with their spouse and children and expand helpful contributions in family life. Fathers experienced new competencies and benefits through greater sharing of household and child-rearing responsibilities. Single parents, depressed and depleted, were encouraged to reach out to "lifelines" in their kin network. For instance, they might involve their children's aunts, uncles, and godparents by offering mutual support, such as exchanging child care time for respite from burdens.

A "can-do" spirit was contagious in the group process, turning a vicious cycle of discouragement and despair to a virtuous cycle of hope and determination to succeed. The genuine interest and respect families showed each other, all experiencing tough times, decreased the stigma and shame many felt in their situation. The biweekly family workshops offered the displaced worker encouragement to take initiative and persevere in job search efforts. They celebrated small successes and commiserated around disappointments, strengthening bonds ands mutual support. The ability to find humor and laugh together in the midst of their challenges was uplifting: One mother, anxious before a job interview, reached up to fix her hair and felt an earring missing—she then realized she had hooked both earrings on the same ear. Family members brainstormed simple ways to build in "family fun time" and agreed to show daily appreciation of each other despite stresses. Families needing more intensive help were offered family counseling.

Based on the success of that project, a similar resilience-based mothers' group was developed for young single mothers seeking employment for the first time. Most had to overcome vulnerabilities and multiple barriers to sustained employment, many involving their families and household (see Chapter 13, on multi-stressed families). These mothers are too often seen through a deficit lens as unmotivated and underfunctioning. In contrast, our resilience approach viewed these mothers as underresourced and overwhelmed by persistent stressors in all aspects of their lives. We addressed challenges in finding and managing child care arrangements around new employment demands. We also worked with larger systems to change workplace policies and practices that derailed child care plans and family life, such as part-time, irregular, and uncertain shift schedules. Counseling assisted parents in mastering particular challenges associated with raising a special needs child, caring for disabled elders, stabilizing a chaotic household, or ending a troubled relationship with a boyfriend who heightened risks of substance abuse or violence. Potential kin and social supports, including religious/spiritual resources, were identified and tapped. The resilience-based orientation shifted the mothers' outlook from hopeless despair to affirm their strengths and potential. It encouraged their active initiative, perseverance, and mastery of the possible in their efforts to make a better life for themselves and their children.

Community-Based, Resilience-Oriented Multifamily Groups with Bosnian and Kosovar Refugees

A project developed by the CCFH in collaboration with the Center on Genocide, Psychiatry, and Witnessing at the University of Illinois demonstrated the value of a community-based family resilience approach. In 1998–1999, we designed and implemented resilience-based multifamily groups for Bosnian refugees, and the following year for Kosovars. Both groups had suffered multiple trauma and losses of loved ones, homes, and communities in Serbian ethnic cleansing campaigns. Our family resilience approach was sought out because many of the refugees were suffering deep emotional wounds but were not utilizing mental health services, which were viewed in the refugee community as pathologizing, particularly with psychiatric labeling of posttraumatic stress disorder (PTSD), diagnosis as a mental disorder, and narrow treatment focus on individual symptoms. Our resilience approach countered stigma and shame as it mobilized families to foster healing and adaptation.

The program, utilizing a 9-week multifamily group format, did not use the language of psychotherapy. Rather, the group for Bosnian families, serving cookies and a huge pot of coffee, was called CAFES Coffee And Family Education and Support). For the Kosovars, it was called TAFES— because they loved their tea. Families readily participated because it tapped into their strong family-centered cultural values and was located in a neighborhood storefront where residents felt comfortable. The group offered a compassionate setting for families to share stories of suffering and struggle through multiple transitions, traumas, and difficulties in adjustment. It also drew out and affirmed family strengths and resources, such as their courage, endurance, and faith; strong kinship networks; deep concern for loved ones; and determination to rise above their tragedies to forge a new life. The focus of family sessions wove between sharing past experiences and grief and tackling practical demands and challenges in their new environment. To foster a spirit of collaboration and to develop local resources, facilitators from their communities were invited to co-lead groups and remain available if urgent needs arose. This approach was experienced as respectful, healing, and empowering (Weine et al., 2005).

Resilience-Oriented Family and Community Services in War-Torn Regions

The success of the resilience-based multifamily groups for Bosnian and Kosovar refugees led to a multiyear project to develop community-based, resilience-oriented, family-centered training and services in Kosovo. The aim of this project was to enhance the capacities of Kosovar mental health professionals and paraprofessionals to address the overwhelming service needs in their war-torn region by strengthening family capacities for coping and recovery. The Kosovar Family Professional Educational Collaborative (KFPEC) was a partnership between mental health professionals in Kosovo, headed by Dr. Farid Agami, through the University of Pristina, a team of family therapists,[3] through the auspices of the American Family Therapy Academy, the CCFH, and the University of Illinois. In describing the value of this approach, the team coleaders, Rolland and Weine (2000), noted:

> The family, with its strengths, is central to Kosovar life, but health and mental health services are generally not oriented to families. Although "family" is a professed part of the value system of international organizations, most programs do not define, conceptualize, or operationalize a family approach to mental health services in any substantial or meaningful ways. Recognizing that the psychosocial needs of refugees, other trauma survivors, and vulnerable persons in societies in transition far exceed the individual and psychopathological focus that conventional trauma mental health approaches provide, this project aims to begin a collaborative program of family focused education and training that is resilience-based and emphasizes family strengths. (p. 35)

---

[3] The KFPEC's American family therapy team included Stevan Weine, MD and John Rolland MD (Coordinators); Carol Becker, PhD; Ellen Pulleyblank Coffey, PhD; Melissa Elliott, RN; James Griffith, MD; Judith Landau, MD; John Sargent, MD; Carlos Sluzki, MD; Jack Saul, PhD; Kaethe Weingarten, PhD. The Kosovar professional team was led by Ferid Agani, MD.

In many international assistance programs, experts arrive with enthusiasm but leave without sufficient ongoing efforts or collaboration to build local capacities to address long-term challenges. In contrast, this project was carefully planned and implemented collaboratively with Kosovar professionals, with sustained contact and periodic return training sessions over the next several years, each geared to emerging local needs and priorities. Over an initial 12-month period, the American family therapy team conducted weeklong training sessions in Pristina, with visits to affected rural areas. The consultants, sharing a strengths-based, collaborative, family resilience-oriented meta-perspective, encouraged Kosovar professionals to adapt this framework and develop their own practice applications to best fit local culture and service priorities. Readings found to be valuable (including chapters from the first edition of this book) were translated into Albanian. Between visits, contact was sustained through the Internet and collaborative writing projects.

The approach emphasized the importance of meeting with families to hear their stories, bearing witness to atrocities suffered, and eliciting the strengths and resources that helped them to cope and move forward. In one family, the mother had listened to gunshots as her husband, two sons, and two grandsons were murdered in the yard of their farmhouse. Team members talked with her and her surviving family members in their home about those events and asked about what has kept them strong:

> The surviving son replied: "We are all believers. One of the strengths in our family is from God. . . . Having something to believe has helped very much."
>
> Interviewer: "What do you do to keep faith strong?"
>
> Son: "I see my mother as the 'spring of strength' . . . to see someone who has lost five family members—it gives us strength just to see her. We must think about the future and what we can accomplish. This is what keeps us strong. What will happen to him [pointing to his five-year-old nephew] if I am not here? If he sees me strong, he will be strong. If I am weak, he will become weaker than me."
>
> Interviewer: "What do you hope your nephew will learn about the family as he grows up?"
>
> Son: "The moment when he will be independent and helping others and the family—for him, it will be like seeing his father and grandfather and uncles alive again." (Becker, Sargent, & Rolland, 2000, p. 29)

In this family, the positive influence of belief systems and communication was striking, in particular, drawing strength from their Islamic faith and the inspiration of strong models and mentors, and stories conveyed to the next generation.

Many families forged resilience through their connectedness, collaboration, and adaptive role flexibility: "Everyone belongs to the family and to our homeland, alive or dead, here or abroad. Everyone matters and everyone is counted and counted upon." The consultants observed that when cooking or planting everyone moved together fluidly, in a complementary pattern, each person picking up where the previous person left off. They noted that although their grief was immeasurable, "A hidden treasure in the family is their adaptability to fill in each of the absented roles" (Becker et al., 2000, p. 29).

Growing out of that program, other collaborative projects were developed and continue, with an emphasis on the treatment and prevention of substance abuse and AIDS and on adolescent developmental challenges, in the broader context of high unemployment and human rights violations, which increase with the chaos and breakdown of social systems and economies in postconflict regions. And yet, the spirit of resilience persists in creative efforts to build a new community-based family-focused mental health care system for Kosovo (Pulleyblank-Coffey, Griffith, & Ulaj, 2006).

Promoting Positive Development of Youth at High Risk of Gang Involvement: Family–Centered Training Component (GRYD Prevention Program)

Gang prevention programs in the United States rarely involve families, deterred by prevalent assumptions in the juvenile justice field that families of high-risk youth are too dysfunctional, unmotivated for change, and not worth the investment. Yet studies have found that families matter: parental warmth, higher levels of supervision, and monitoring practices are related to lower youth conduct problems and gang involvement (e.g., Gorman-Smith, Henry, & Tolan, 2004). Families are our primary bonds, meeting needs to belong and feel nurtured, protected, valued, and supported in our best efforts. Efforts to strengthen those bonds in more vulnerable families and communities can offset the pull of gang involvement.

We were fortunate to work for 2 years with a unique program developed by the Los Angeles Deputy Mayor's Office for Gang Reduction and Youth Development (GRYD), in a city plagued by gang-related drugs and violence. The deputy mayor, Guillermo Cespedes, designed a multilevel systemic model for intervention and prevention. The prevention program involved 150 case managers assigned to 1,000 youth ages 10–14 who had been identified at high risk for gang involvement. (For research evaluation, a comparison group of 500 high-risk youth received only standard community-based agency services.) Interventions included individual and group counseling, activities, and family sessions. Cespedes, who had been trained in family therapy and community work early in his career, recognized the vital importance of a family component to counter the pull of gangs for struggling youth in hazardous neighborhoods. And it made no sense *not* to involve families, since the program youth were living at home.

Researchers with the program initially recommended the use of an evidence-based family intervention model. However, Cespedes was dismayed by their top-down, problem-focused approach, dispensing cookie-cutter methods to trainees to fit the intervention protocol. He most objected to the proposed consultant's requirement to bring in his own staff to run the program to assure fidelity in adherence to the model, replacing the GRYD program staff—all very competent, ethnic and racial minority, master's-level professionals who understood the local inner-city residents and their challenges. There was also a disparaging view of the case managers, most with limited formal professional education, failing to appreciate their work and life experience in the neighborhoods they served and their strong dedication to helping youth rise above the hazards.

In contrast, Cespedes believed that it was essential to have a strengths-oriented approach, flexible and responsive to workers' and clients' needs and challenges. He contacted CCFH Codirectors John Rolland and me to develop and coordinate a family resilience-oriented training program, appreciating our flexible, principle-based framework grounded in the conviction that highly vulnerable youth and their families have the potential to improve their lives if we identify and build on their strengths.

Our collaborative team approach was designed to respect and draw on the local knowledge and both the practice and life experience of the GRYD training staff, agency directors, and case managers. We engaged families as experts on the nature of their challenges and in support of their best hopes for their children (Fraenkel, 2006). Our approach aimed to shift attention from the prevailing focus on problems and deficits to view youth and their families as "at promise" instead of "at risk," with the potential for achieving positive growth and successful lives by strengthening supportive relational bonds. Youths' behavior and future aspirations were addressed in the context of their living situation, including consideration of family, peer, community, and larger socioeconomic influences and cultural and spiritual resources.

In order to be adaptive to local needs and concerns, we were asked to design and schedule training sessions addressing focal priorities, and yet flexibly alter them in response to feedback, making modifications as we went along. As Cespedes put it, "We need to build the plane as we are flying it"—and that was what we did.

To provide this training, we assembled a team of highly seasoned family therapy trainers who had extensive experience working with low-income and ethnic minority communities and doing collaborative work with agency case managers and staff. Dubbed by the GRYD staff as the "Dream Team," our training team members included Harry Aponte, William Madsen, Jorge Colapinto, Andrae Brown, Nancy Boyd-Franklin, Celia Falicov, Tom Todd, John Rolland, and myself. Each of us brought particular areas of focus and expertise, including our family resilience framework; genogram application and extended family resources; Madsen's (2011) Collaborative Helping maps; family structural skill building; workers' use of self; immigrant family challenges; drawing on cultural resources; and supervision training.

The training program focused on two strategy components that had been defined by the GRYD staff to meet their broader program aims.

Vertical Strategy Component

Based on a multigenerational life cycle model, resilience-oriented genograms were developed by the GRYD staff with our input (see Chapter 6 and Appendix 2). All workers and their supervisors first completed their own family genograms to learn and appreciate their utility. Coaching techniques were used to connect youth and their parents/caregivers to relational resources, or "lifelines" for resilience. The vertical strategy explored multigenerational family history to (1) draw out stories of resilience in dealing with past adversity, and (2) identify positive models and mentors in the current extended family system to support long-term family resilience and engagement with at-risk youth for their successful development. We identified and involved family members who are—or could become—invested in the youth to support their best efforts, believe in their potential, and encourage them to make the most of their lives. Resilience-oriented genograms and Madsen's Collaborative Helping maps also provided tools that youth and families could use to develop a stronger sense of identity, connectedness, and competence, increasing their ability to overcome the challenges and barriers confronting them.

Horizontal Training Component

This component focused on the household unit to strengthen the parental/caregiver functioning and to increase youth and family problem-solving abilities. Specifically, training provided the staff with skills to (1) identify problem behaviors and transactional patterns associated with risk factors; (2) gather information about problem definition and already-attempted solutions; and (3) develop with each youth and family both a future vision and strategies to engage in and follow through with. We shared the conviction that fostering positive beliefs and behaviors, strengthening family structural functioning, and building relational support toward desired aims would be more effective for positive youth development than focusing narrowly on reducing the youth's problematic and self-defeating behaviors. Instead, those behaviors and risk factors were tackled as obstacles to overcome on pathways toward preferred life dreams (Madsen, 2009, 2011; see Chapter 6 for the use of resilience-oriented genograms).

Family structural processes were also addressed. This training component aimed to increase both parental/caregiver nurturing and authority, particularly in monitoring and supervising the youth's daily activities, while decreasing parental use of harsh and coercive control. Active family support of school success was also essential.

The training program centered on a 9-month series of 2- to 3-day workshops for all participants (150 case managers, neighborhood agency directors, and GRYD staff). Workshops included:

- Presentations of practice-relevant knowledge and skills, with handouts and supplemental readings in PDF format.
- Case-based family-centered consultation for presentations by agency staff (strategy teams) to consolidate training component skills.
- Small-group and whole-group discussions of applications and challenges.

To reinforce learning and application, periodic web-based small-group case consultation sessions were held at agencies with distance training consultants through Skype. These sessions also strengthened collaborative teamwork by staff at local agencies. Regular contact among training team members and with the GRYD staff facilitated ongoing feedback and tweaking of the training sessions to adapt the program elements and schedule to fit emerging challenges and best meet objectives. This flexibility, at times challenging, proved to be a strength of the program and contributed to the satisfaction of staff and trainees and their growing competence and confidence in their work with youth and their families.

Throughout GRYD's intervention and prevention programs, attention was given to broader community, cultural, and spiritual resources for resilience. Their highly successful "Summer Night Lights" initiative transformed neighborhood parks from dark and foreboding havens for gang activity and drug sales into brightly lit gathering places for youths, families, and their communities to come on summer evenings, much like a town plaza. There they could enjoy ethnic foods from local vendors and take part in games, sports, and other activities. In coordination, the police department staffed officers to assure safety and interact with residents, building mutual trust. This initiative has significantly reduced gang-related crime and violence as it provided summer jobs for youth, and strengthened community connectedness (*www.grydfoundation.org/summer-night-lights*).

RE-VISIONING COMMUNITY SERVICES TO STRENGTHEN FAMILY RESILIENCE

A family resilience practice approach is both pragmatic and growth oriented: it targets key family processes to strengthen family functioning and resourcefulness as presenting problems are addressed. Core principles include collaboration and teamwork; multilevel systemic, community-based interventions; flexible service delivery; and prevention/early intervention. Just as there are many varied pathways in resilience, a family resilience meta-framework can be applied with a variety of systems-oriented practice models and modalities.

Collaboration and Teamwork

A family resilience approach strives to build teamwork among family members in surmounting their life challenges. In crisis, mutual support is most likely to break down as members hunker down in isolated, self-reliant modes of coping. When we encourage mutual support, empathic communication, and shared problem solving among family and community members, bonds are strengthened as problems are tackled together. Couple and family meetings, as well as community forums, set a collaborative context. More explicitly, we invite members to think of themselves as partners or teammates, who become more resourceful through shared efforts.

In service delivery, collaborative team approaches across disciplines, both within and across systems, respect the role and expertise of each team member. This facilitates integrated client- and family-centered care and overcomes fragmented and unresponsive services, especially in complex systems. Health and human services have tended to be problem centered, narrowly focused on a symptomatic individual, perhaps involving a partner, parent, or caregiver, while the family network—including other strains and potential resources—remains a dim backdrop. When services are family centered, efforts can be better coordinated and proactive in helping all family members through concerted efforts.

Multisystemic, Community-Based Interventions

For families in extreme circumstances to sustain themselves and overcome their challenges, environmental support can be vital. Therapists are urged to expand their focus beyond the interior of the family to build linkages between individuals, families, their social networks, and larger systems. For instance, CCFH faculty, led by Ruth Furst, developed the Family–Schools Partnership Program in several Chicago public schools, aiming to reduce the high rates of school failure and dropout of at-risk youth and to promote their resilience and success. Such partnerships, encouraging positive, proactive involvement of families with school professionals, can make all the difference. A community-based family resource perspective is vital in work with multi-stressed, vulnerable families (see Chapter 13). Interventions aimed at enhancing positive interactions, supporting coping efforts, and building extrafamilial resources work in concert to reduce stress, enhance pride and competence, and promote more effective functioning.

Flexible Service Delivery

Our health care and social service delivery systems must be more flexibly organized to be responsive and proactive to family challenges over time. Recovery from crisis or loss and adaptation to multiple challenges can't happen all at once in four to six sessions. This does not mean vague, open-ended contracts with unlimited therapeutic horizons. One colleague worried that attending to adaptations over time would mean that once a family is seen for help, they remain in treatment for life. Part of the problem lies in the traditional view of psychotherapy. A resilience-based approach more closely fits the model of preventive family medicine, the ongoing role of a family doctor, and the concept of healing. When we think of our physical health, we don't think of ourselves as patients in perpetual medical treatment. We see our physicians both in crisis and for periodic checkups, and, optimally, we develop a health- and prevention-oriented relationship with them (or their clinical setting) over time.

A resilience-oriented approach broadens the conception of family therapy to include counseling, brief consultations, and psychoeducational groups. A systemic framework guides intervention priorities: Meetings might be held at different points with a family unit, subgroups, couples, or individual members, and therapy might even include meetings with informal kin or friends when these help to build support networks. Their community linkages are actively encouraged, such as with a family's faith congregation. We need to re-vision the traditional therapeutic contract and the rigid schedule of weekly sessions until termination so that interventions can fit varied challenges and adaptive processes over time.

A Psychosocial Road Map to Guide Practice

The family systems–illness model developed by Rolland (1994, 2012; see Chapter 12) has potential value in a range of adverse situations as a useful psychosocial road map to guide intervention and foster family coping and resilience. Family challenges and intervention priorities may vary in relation to the crisis patterning in terms of onset (acute vs. gradual), course (brief, recurrent, constant, progressively worsening), outcome, degree of functional impairment, and uncertainty about the future trajectory. Stressors can be approached as ongoing processes with landmarks, transitions, and changing demands. Different phases in events unfolding over time pose challenges that may require different family strengths. A brief crisis requires immediate mobilization of resources; then, after the initial period of disequilibrium, a family may be able to reorganize and resume accustomed patterns of living. With long-term or permanent change or with persistent adversity, a family may need to grieve the loss of its precrisis identity and alter familiar patterns, as well as hopes and dreams, to accommodate a new set of circumstances. This psychosocial road map can guide consultations and periodic family "psychosocial checkups" to strengthen the family's capacity to manage stress-related crises or sustained efforts over the long haul.

Practice efforts can focus on building strengths to meet the immediate psychosocial demands of a disruptive transition, such as divorce, and can prepare for the anticipated course ahead. CCFH divorce mediation and postdivorce training and services drew on findings of longitudinal research that tracks families from predivorce strains through several years postdivorce (Hetherington & Kelly, 2002), identifying processes that promote resilience (see Chapter 9). Such research informs efforts to help parents approach separation decisions and custody, residential, and visitation options planfully to reduce risk and facilitate children's positive adaptation. After a divorce, we can be proactive in helping parents to anticipate and manage transitional distress and complications that commonly occur over time (e.g., decisions about a child's education or religious training, changes in residence, or remarriage and stepfamily formation). We link families with collaborative divorce specialists, postdecree mediation, or other appropriate services to address challenges that arise.

Just as families need to pool resources in times of crisis, more intensive professional help is needed at such times. Likewise, just as families can shift balance to more separateness in stable periods, more intermittent therapeutic contact can sustain family functioning during plateaus of adaptation. In an initial crisis phase (which may last from a few weeks to several months), sessions can be held weekly, or more frequently if the situation is urgent. Family members can be seen separately and in different combinations—for instance, a depressed adolescent can be seen both privately and with the family. Over time, progress can be sustained by meeting at less frequent intervals (e.g., biweekly or monthly). Sessions can be scheduled for predictable stress points, such as stepfamily formation. Help can also be available as needed when unexpected problems or new disruptions occur.

Systems-Oriented Approaches: Many Pathways in Fostering Resilience

Just as there are many pathways in healthy family functioning, our view of family therapy must be expanded to a variety of systems-based approaches and modalities to strengthen and support families. When combining individual and conjoint sessions, careful planning, timing, and focus are important, with attention to issues of confidentiality and triangulation. In varied formats, valuable information, coping skills, and support can bolster families in crisis or coping with persistent stresses and challenges. Multifamily groups offering psychoeducation and a support network are particularly helpful for families facing a wide range of adverse situations. Research on successful family coping relevant to their situation can inform interventions and can be shared among families, Many are eager for information and guidelines to clarify ambiguities and manage stresses. New resources are gained and distress normalized through shared experiences with other families dealing with similar challenges. Families respond positively to the energizing group aim of strengthening resilience.

Prevention: From Crisis Reactive to Proactive Services

In accord with emerging priorities for mental health and health care, resources must be directed to cost-effective prevention services. Most programs for children and families in distress are reactive, focused on salvaging victims from the wreckage. It makes more sense to offer proactive, wellness-based services—to bolster those at risk or in acute distress *before* problems become entrenched and multiply. Programs providing

information, resources, and opportunities for skill and knowledge development, in an ongoing rather than a crisis-triggered manner, are both effective and cost-effective (Dolan, 2008).

Resilience-building family intervention can serve as a psychosocial
inoculation to boost immunity or hardiness in facing adversity. By strengthening resilience in families before crises erupt, we can decrease their vulnerability, fortify their capacity to cope with stress, and increase their
resources to meet new challenges. We can develop crisis prevention skills
by strengthening family functioning and mobilizing supportive resources in
kin and community networks.

Preventive interventions may be offered before, when, or after a problem develops. Primary prevention and family life education are strategies
for creating support and empowerment for individuals and families at risk
(Harris, 1996). For instance, the Chicago-based programs Family Focus
and Ounce of Prevention work with new teen parents to support healthy
parent–child relationships, early child development, and parents' own educational, job, and social functioning. There is need for a wide range of
family-focused prevention and early intervention services in natural community settings such as schools and neighborhood centers. Family therapists and other professionals can offer information and family coping
strategies through community consultations, forums, and public speaking
events. Preventive actions at larger system levels can lower vulnerability
and risk by modifying hazardous environmental conditions.

Secondary prevention involves early intervention in an early phase
of crisis or initial adjustment to a stressful transition. Tertiary prevention
involves actions taken later in the course of persistent problems to prevent
further recurrence or exacerbation. From a resilience standpoint, *all* therapeutic efforts can also be preventive if we help distressed families develop
strengths to avert future crises and support well-being and positive growth.
The treatment and healing of a knee injury offers a useful analogy. Physical therapy not only aids in recovery but also strengthens the resilience of
muscles in the vulnerable area so that future injury can be prevented and
healthy functioning sustained. Many brief crisis intervention approaches
are helpful for short-term recovery, but unless family resilience is strengthened, future crises are likely to overwhelm a vulnerable family, requiring
further rounds of crisis intervention in revolving-door emergency treatment. If we organized family-centered mental health services for psychosocial care like the preventive models of family medicine or dentistry, a great
deal of suffering could be avoided.

In sum, resilience-based services foster family empowerment as they
bring forth shared hope, develop new and renewed areas of competence,

and build mutual support. We enable families not only to resolve presenting problems but also to become more proactive to meet future challenges more effectively. Every intervention is thus also a preventive measure.

STRENGTHENING THE RESILIENCE OF HELPING PROFESSIONALS

As helping professionals, we all need resilience to meet the demands of our challenging work in our practice environment. Burnout is common in chronically stressful jobs and underresourced agencies, schools, medical settings, and other larger systems. Constant demands and an overload of cases and recordkeeping sap energies. Compassion fatigue is experienced in working with many clients in crisis, those experiencing ongoing trauma, and those overwhelmed by multi-stress conditions.

The Human Connection

The focus of much professional training and research emphasizes strategies and tactics for change. Yet the therapeutic relationship has stood out as a common factor in research on the effectiveness of various approaches to psychotherapy over the years (Lebow, 2012; Sprenkle et al., 2009). This relationship is founded on open communication and a trusting climate that fosters clients' ability to reflect on and express a wide range of ideas, feelings, and opinions. Recent narrative approaches emphasize the healing power in therapeutic conversations. Our empathic listening, genuine interest, and respectful curiosity encourage family members to tell their stories and consider new perspectives on their troubling situations.

Our human connection with families is vital in a resilience-oriented practice approach. For clients to be open and receptive to change, helping professionals must be genuinely interested in their life stories and concerned about their well-being. We must be understanding of their predicament, empathize with their pain, and encourage their best strivings. We need to be comfortable in being fully engaged, modeling by example in our transactions and sharing (as appropriate) what we've learned from our own experiences with adversity.

The "courageous engagement" of therapist and clients—a wonderfully apt phrase offered by Waters and Lawrence (1993)—is at the heart of competence-based work and collaborative efforts to build resilience. We, as therapists, as well as our clients, need courage to question and challenge constraining beliefs; to support attempts to move from a helpless, victimized position; and to encourage our clients to bring out their best through the worst of times. It requires courage to expect more from them to take risks for better relationships and life goals. When we work from this perspective, our clients are better able to take steps toward positive change and to live with greater ease in situations that are unchangeable or uncertain.

Relational Lifelines for Resilience

Our own resilience as helping professionals is relationally based, nurtured and sustained through collaboration with colleagues, supportive work systems, and satisfying personal relationships. As caseloads increase in numbers and complexity while staff resources are cut back, the risk of professional burnout is heightened. I encourage students and therapists to create supportive professional networks and to seek out learning and enrichment experiences at each phase in their careers. Postgraduate family therapy training centers can offer a revitalizing professional home, nurturing contact, and growth through participation in workshops, courses, and case consultation groups. Collaborative consultation teams or partners are ideal for building camaraderie, competence, and confidence. Ongoing group experiences offer mentoring relationships, collegial support, and skill enhancement. A monthly peer consultation group can sustain professional growth and connectedness.

In practice settings where teams are not feasible, a "buddy system" can readily be formed. Trusted colleagues can serve as professional lifelines: mutual resources and consultants when clients are in crisis or a professional is undersupported and discouraged. My close colleagues and I continue to turn to one another, and we always find our spirits renewed and our creative energy rekindled as a result.

A colleague once asked me to observe a session with a client after he had nearly fallen asleep in the last session. He was upset that he was becoming bored and irritated with Gloria, a middle-aged mother who was trapped in despair since her husband had left her 2 years earlier. Intending to show empathy for her plight, my colleague sat quietly nodding, trance-like, as she went on and on about her troubles, recounting everything bad that always happened to her in life. As his thoughts drifted and he looked away, Gloria increased the intensity of her drama to reengage him, which only irritated him more. This relational impasse repeated itself week after week.

As my colleague and I reflected together on the situation, it became apparent that by concentrating so intently on Gloria's sad story, he was unwittingly reinforcing her passive, victimized position, her global pessimism, and her belief that others could only care about her if she evoked their sympathy. For change to occur, he needed to show genuine interest in Gloria as a lovable person who deserved a better life for herself and her children and could achieve it. As the focus of the therapeutic conversation shifted to noticing and affirming her strengths, she came alive, and he had no difficulty sustaining his investment in helping her rebuild her life after the devastation of the divorce. A resilience-promoting therapeutic relationship seeks to repair the damage from traumatic experience, to expand the client's vision of what is possible, and to support actions and relational resources in pursuit of those dreams.

Waters and Lawrence (1993) encourage therapists to see our clients' struggles and confrontations as the mythic "hero's journey"—a view consonant with the resilience approach. They note Joseph Campbell's observation that the heroes of myths are all on a quest against the odds to slay a dragon or other foe, as in the biblical story of David versus Goliath. The hero comes to participate in life courageously and decently, in the way of nature—not in the way of personal rancor, disappointment, or revenge. When we take such a view of our clients, we can more easily appreciate the positive, competent aspects of their life journeys and our own efforts. Waters and Lawrence state:

> In our work, this goal of a courageous engagement with life guides us more than a desire to avoid the "negative" aspects of symptoms. In therapy, our clients are the heroes attempting to "slay their dragons," but if we lose sight of that and become preoccupied with their dysfunction, victimization, or handicap, we are less helpful to them. We must see that at their core is their desire for mastery and belonging. They become heroes when they—and we—have the courage to struggle against those obstacles and transform the possibilities of life. (1993, p. 58)

Compassion Fatigue and Vicarious Resilience

Among the most highly stressful work situations are those helping individuals, families, and communities who have experienced trauma, torture, and other atrocities (see Chapter 11). The cumulative emotional strains from bearing witness to extreme suffering, powerlessness, and disruption often place helping professionals—including medical personnel, therapists, counselors, humanitarian workers, human rights activists, first responders, and even journalists—at risk for vicarious trauma and, over time, symptoms of burnout or compassion fatigue. Compassion fatigue, a concept developed by Figley (2002), involves the convergence of traumatic stress, secondary traumatic stress, and cumulative stress/burnout in the lives of helping professionals and other care providers. Listening and responding empathically to intensely traumatic accounts and ongoing posttraumatic struggles can affect helpers in negative ways.

Vicarious resilience involves the positive benefits commonly experienced by professionals, as well, when they expand their focus to explore their clients' resilience in coping and overcoming adversity. This concept, developed by Hernandez and colleagues (Hernandez, Engstrom, & Gangsei, 2010; Hernandez, Gangsei, & Engstrom, 2007), was based on their interview studies with mental health professionals working with survivors of torture, political violence, and kidnapping. Workers reported that when they drew out people's stories of their resourcefulness, such as remarkable courage, endurance, heroism, and generosity, alongside accounts of their suffering and struggles, they were deeply inspired in their own work and personal lives.

The data revealed a complex array of elements contributing to therapists' professional and personal empowerment through interaction with clients' stories of resilience. The most common benefit cited was witnessing and reflecting on human beings' immense capacity to heal. They also reported learning from their clients the power of hope and commitment and the value of spiritual resources, a dimension they had not appreciated from their mental health training but now included in their practice. In their work, they gained efficacy in the use of self and in developing time, setting, and intervention boundaries that fit helpful interventions in context. They also learned the value in using community interventions. Supporting Weingarten's (2004) work on witnessing violence, the therapists reflected that, at their best, they were able to perform their work from a position of compassion, awareness, knowledge, and effective action.

These effects of vicarious resilience generalized beyond their work situation to significantly shape their perceptions of themselves, their relationships, and their environment. The experience led them to reassess the significance of problems in their own lives. They gained tolerance for frustrations and increased their ability to reframe and cope with negative events. Therapists also experienced clarification and strengthening of their own values and perspectives regarding violence and the importance of social and legal validation and reparation as key processes in recovery and resilience. Working with multiple systems and witnessing transformations in clients' lives inspired some professionals to expand their trauma work into teaching, writing, research, and activism.

MENDING THE SOCIAL FABRIC:
TRANSFORMING BROKEN SERVICE SYSTEMS

Systems-oriented professionals, I firmly believe, have an ethical responsibility to direct our energies beyond our office walls toward repair of the social fragmentation that heightens risks for individual and family breakdown. As we help families withstand the onslaught of social and economic pressures in their lives, we must also work to eradicate destructive social forces that heighten risks and undermine resilience. This involves active investment in larger system change and in social movements—lending our expertise to help mend the frayed social fabric. Collaborative professional and family consumer advocacy can strengthen efforts to overcome barriers and promote family-centered policies that enable families to thrive.

The resilience of helping professionals is essential to overcome the barriers of the for-profit health care system in the United States, which limits access and availability of psychosocial care to at-risk and distressed families in all segments of human services. Despite these daunting challenges, systems-based, family-centered services will continue to be in demand, because of their useful application to a broad range of problems and the cost-effectiveness of interventions that strengthen the family as a functional unit. We need to articulate the importance of family systems-based services and marshal research evidence in support of its effectiveness. Helping professionals across disciplines must put aside turf rivalries and band together in collaborative efforts to transform larger systems that threaten our common mission to foster the well-being of families. The keys to resilience for our clients are also keys to our professional resilience.

Balancing Our Professional and Personal Lives

We are also challenged to achieve a healthy balance in our professional and personal lives. The risk of compassion fatigue and the potential for spillover of painful and threatening issues come with the territory of our chosen work. The professional and the personal each hold meanings for the success of the other if we apply them wisely and stay aware of our clients' and our own life situations, our commonalities and differences. The safe boundaries and hierarchies of more traditional psychotherapy can become blurred in more collaborative therapeutic relationships. But the gains can be worth the challenge if we recognize our own limits and take care of ourselves (Barrett & Stone Fish, 2014).

In our personal lives, we all need lifelines for resilience. It is essential to reach out to others and deepen our intimate bonds; enjoy extended family and social connections; and tap cultural and spiritual resources for nourishment—including nature, the arts, and music—so that we find respite, joy, laughter, and meaning in various aspects of our lives. One oncology professional, when overcome with sadness, visits the maternity unit to see the newborns; another therapist enjoys the immediate pleasures in tending a garden; another plays soccer on weekends. I find peaceful contemplation in daily walks with my dog—and love best our walks along the beach in summer, sharing her sheer joy as she dashes in and out of the water chasing the shorebirds that always fly away. We each nourish our resilience as we become more fully engaged, compassionate, and grateful in our helping relationships and also with our families, friends, and our wider circle of connection.

PART IV

FACILITATING FAMILY RESILIENCE THROUGH CRISIS, TRANSITION, AND PERSISTENT CHALLENGES

CHAPTER 9

Challenges and Resilience over the Family Life Cycle

A Developmental Systems Perspective

The present is the ever-moving shadow that divides
yesterday from tomorrow. In that lies hope.
—FRANK LLOYD WRIGHT

Our efforts to understand and strengthen family resilience require attention to the temporal context of major stressors in relation to individual and family life cycle passage. A family developmental perspective, based in a multilevel systems orientation, is needed to address highly stressful family challenges and pathways in resilience over time. A relational perspective assumes the centrality of relationships in human development. Accordingly, a relational approach to resilience facilitates the study of processes and outcomes associated with mutual adaptive functioning and development. Research on risk and resilience can inform efforts to strengthen family processes in navigating disruptive family transitions and mastering developmental phase-related challenges.

The family life cycle is becoming ever more lengthened, varied, and fluid, as described in Chapter 2. Abundant research reveals that children and families can thrive in a variety of stable family structures. Yet over time, adults and their children are increasingly likely to transition in and out of varied households and kinship arrangements, adding complexity to all relationships. Multi-stress environmental conditions further strain and destabilize low-income and minority families and those on the margins of society. Because chronic and recurrent stresses heighten risks for maladaptation and child problems, families need to buffer disruptive transitions, construct new workable strategies, and weave together supportive kin networks for resilience in their life passage.

A DEVELOPMENTAL SYSTEMS PERSPECTIVE

The Family as a System Moving through Time

The family is a transactional system evolving over the life course and across the generations. Families construct and reweave a complex web of kinship ties within and across households, linking past, present, and future as they move forward in their life passages. Individual and family development co-evolve over time. Relationships with parents, siblings, spouses, children, and other family members grow and change, boundaries shift, roles are redefined, and new members and losses require adaptation (Hetherington, 2003).

A developmental systems perspective considers family functioning in terms of basic transactional processes in and between human systems and their social ecology, dependent on the mutual interaction of biopsychosocial variables over time. As recent epigenetic and socioneurobiology studies confirm (Cozolino, 2014; D'Onofrio & Lahey, 2010; Feder et al., 2009; Spotts, 2012), individual predispositions may be enhanced or countered by interpersonal and sociocultural influences throughout life. Key relationships and experiences, in turn, can affect future generations through epigenetic processes.

Thus, a developmental systems approach views family functioning in relation to the evolving needs and priorities of members and in sociocultural and temporal contexts. Through multilevel dynamic processes over time, families forge varied coping styles and adaptational pathways that fit individual and family values, priorities, challenges, and resources.

Chronological Time, Social Time, and Historical Time

Our expectations for normal development and family life—both typical and optimal—are largely socially constructed, influenced by subjective world views and by the larger culture and our historical time (Walsh, 2016a). Family and social time clocks are influential in setting expectations and goals in life and contribute to feeling successful and in sync with one's age peers (Neugarten, 1976).

Chronological ages tend to be associated with normative milestones, such as reaching maturity, marrying, having children, and retirement.

Transitions to the next decade in life—turning 30, 40, or 60—can hold heavy meaning. Yet with medical advances and biological and social changes, traditional mileposts have been shifting and age-appropriate norms blurring. A variety of reproductive strategies now assist older adults in having children. Most adults ages 65–75 are healthy and productive, do not consider themselves "elderly," and are expanding later-life possibilities (Walsh, 2012b).

Varying ethnic and societal norms influence family life cycle expectations, intertwined with socioeconomic factors that impact career and marital options, family stability, and life expectancy. Gender, class, ethnicity, race, and religion structure our developing relationships and our role expectations for marriage and family life. Multigenerational legacies also influence family world views, including members' expectations about life passage and their hopes and dreams.

Normative (typical, expectable) passage over the life course is also profoundly influenced by the historical era in which individuals grow up, come of age, and grow old. Each generational cohort is distinct as it evolves through time, influenced by the social, economic, and political tides of its era (Elder & Shanahan, 2006). Major societal and global events such as war or famine impact various age cohorts differently, shaping their identity and life aspirations. The recent economic downturn and job market transformations have severely impacted the career establishment, marriage prospects, and child-rearing plans of today's emerging adults. They also threaten the job and financial security of older adults in their later years.

BEYOND NORMATIVE MODELS
OF HUMAN DEVELOPMENT:
A SOCIAL CONSTRUCTIONIST LENS

In the mid-20th century, influential models of human development and the family life cycle were developed from an Anglo-American perspective, reflecting cultural ideals and typical patterns in that era (Walsh, 2012c). Normative studies were standardized on white, middle-class, intact families headed by a heterosexual married couple with traditional gendered breadwinner/homemaker roles. That model of family life became reified as a universal standard, essential for healthy family and child development.

Likewise, those formulations sanctioned and privileged a standard sequential progression of stages in individual, marital, and family development over the life course. Those who followed other pathways tended to be stigmatized and pathologized, with their lives regarded as deviant, deficient, incomplete, harmful, or even sinful. Single women and those without children have been viewed as having incomplete lives; "childless" couples considered selfish; stepparents regarded as not "real" or "natural" parents; and gay parenting assumed to harm children.

Individual models of healthy life span development were largely based on male standards and generalized from small studies of more affluent, educated men. Separation, autonomy, and career success—values associated with masculinity—were primary markers of positive development and adult maturity. The prioritizing of relationships and the care and nurturing of others were viewed as the primary attributes in female development. Yet Vaillant's (2002) longitudinal studies of male Harvard graduates throughout adulthood concluded that strong relationships were the overriding key to men's positive development and life satisfaction. Feminist scholarship has heightened recognition of the value of relational connectedness and interdependency in human development, eschewing the stereotyping of attributes as feminine or masculine to expand the full potential for men and women, for husbands and wives, and for sons and daughters (McGoldrick et al., 1989).

A social constructionist lens is imperative to appreciate the multiplicity of contemporary family forms and the intersection of cultural influences, life options, and timing of nodal events that make each individual and family developmental pathway unique. Above all, as abundant research confirms, no single model or life trajectory is essential for positive development.

FAMILY CHALLENGES AND RESILIENCE

The Temporal Context of Family Resilience

Current developmental approaches to individual resilience attend broadly to dynamic, multilevel, and process-oriented variables over time, reflecting a theoretical shift toward a *relational developmental systems* framework in life course human developmental science (Masten, 2014). Advanced computer programs for data analysis address these complex mutual interactions along developmental pathways. This systems orientation encourages integration of individual and family-level approaches (Masten & Monn, 2015).

The impact of adverse situations and adaptational strategies varies over time and in relation to both individual and family life cycle passage.

1. Families navigate varied pathways to meet emerging challenges over time.
2. A cumulative pileup of multiple stressors can overwhelm family resources.

3. The impact of a crisis may vary depending on its timing in the multigenerational family life cycle.

4. A family's past experiences of adversity and response can generate catastrophic expectations or can serve as models of resilience.

Emerging Challenges and Varied Adaptational Pathways over Time

Most major stressors are not simply a short-term single event, but involve a complex set of changing conditions with a past history and a future course (Rutter, 1987; see Chapter 6). Given this complexity, no single coping response is invariably most successful; varied strategies may prove useful in meeting emerging challenges. In assessing the impact of stress events, it is important to explore how family members approached their situation, from their proactive steps to immediate response and long-term strategies. Some approaches may be functional in the short term but may rigidify and become dysfunctional over time or as conditions change. For instance, with a father's stroke, families must mobilize resources and pull together to meet the crisis, but later they need to shift gears to adapt to chronic disability and attend to other members' needs (Rolland, 2012). Family resilience thus involves varied adaptational pathways extending over time, from a threatening event on the horizon, through disruptive transitions and multiple shock waves in the immediate aftermath and beyond.

Cumulative Stresses

Some families do well with a short-term crisis but buckle under the cumulative strains of multiple, persistent challenges, as with chronic illness, unrelenting conditions of poverty, or complex, ongoing trauma in war-torn regions (see Chapters 11 and 12). Multi-stressed families, often in low-income, underresourced, single-parent households, are especially vulnerable (see Chapter 13). A pileup of internal and external stressors can overwhelm most families, heightening their risk for subsequent problems with cascading effects (Patterson, 2002).

> Brian and Jasmine, parents of three small children, were on the verge of divorce, with escalating conflict and Brian's heavy drinking. Brian was in AA and an anger management group. Brief couple counseling focused on reducing emotional reactivity in their interactions, but no family history or contextual influences had been explored.
>
> Invited in as a consultant, I asked about their family life and any recent stresses, tracking events over time. Brian choked up, relating the sudden death of his brother 2 years earlier. Brian had then struggled unsuccessfully to save their small family business. Since its failure in

the past year with their town's economic decline, he had found only part-time work and the family lost essential income and health benefits. Then, the maternal grandmother suffered a debilitating stroke; she had been their mainstay in raising their three small children, and Jasmine now needed to attend to her needs as well. The couple was reeling from crisis to crisis, with mounting pressures. They said they were just trying to keep their heads above water and had not realized or discussed the cumulative impact of it all.

It was essential to situate their current crisis in the context of the family's barrage of stressful events over the past 2 years. Resilience-oriented couple counseling helped them to contextualize their distress in light of the cumulative strains and losses and facilitated their mutual support, role reorganization, and team efforts. Extended family and community resources were mobilized to master ongoing challenges.

Multigenerational Family Life Cycle Passage

A family developmental assessment of functioning and distress attends to the multigenerational family system as it moves forward over time (McGoldrick et al., 2016). Relationships with parents, siblings, spouses, children, and extended family members evolve and change over the life course. The meaning and implications of an adverse situation should be considered for all members and their relationships. For instance, when one couple suffered a stillbirth, the impact was devastating throughout the kinship network: all had eagerly awaited this birth of the firstborn son to the first son in a large Greek extended family.

Life's many crises and transitions generate emotional disequilibrium and often require structural reorganization and relational realignments, particularly with the addition or loss of family members, and as subsystems are redefined and updated. Successful family functioning over the life course depends on strong relational connections and flexibility in structure, roles, and responses to new developmental priorities and challenges (Walsh, 2015c). As patterns that were functional in earlier life phases no longer fit, new options can be explored. With the loss of functioning or the death of significant family members, others are called upon to assume new roles and responsibilities. In doing so, they can develop new competencies and an enhanced sense of worth.

Mild to moderate disruption is commonly experienced with *normative family developmental transitions*, such as the birth of the first child (Cowan & Cowan, 2012). *Nonnormative stressors*, which are uncommon, unexpected, or untimely in chronological or social expectations, tend to be much more disruptive, especially the death of a child, the premature loss of a parent, or early spousal loss (Walsh & McGoldrick, 2013).

Stress is intensified in transition periods from one developmental phase to another as families and their members redefine and realign their relationships. Although all normative change is to some degree stressful, with highly disruptive events or multi-stress conditions even well-functioning families can falter. Transitional crises and immediate distress are common, yet they do not produce long-term dysfunction for the majority of children and their families. How a family prepares for anticipated challenges, manages disruption, effectively reorganizes, and reinvests in life pursuits will influence the immediate and long-term adaptation for all members and their relationships (Walsh, 2011).

The counterbalance of continuity and change over time is extremely important (Falicov, 1988). Shared rituals are valuable in linking past, present, and future, and in facilitating disruptive transitions, such as stepfamily formation (Imber-Black, 2012). Funeral rites and memorial events serve many important functions: they mark the death of a loved one, honor the life, sustain memories, and offer community support for the bereaved to move forward.

Well-functioning families tend to have an evolutionary sense of time and a continual process of growth, change, and losses across the life course and over the generations (Beavers & Hampson, 2003). Members experience strong intergenerational connections, with internal images updated and modified as a guiding narrative over time. This perspective helps members to see disruptive events and transitions also as milestones on their shared life passage. It helps them to accept the rhythms and flow of family life as children grow up and parents grow old, new members are born, and loved ones die.

In contrast, risk of dysfunction is heightened when members can't accept the passage of time and the continuities—or discontinuities—between past, present, and future (McGoldrick et al., 2016). Symptoms commonly occur at times of disruptive transition. Family members may lose time perspective under stress, becoming frozen in time, preoccupied with the past, or terrified to move forward into the unknown. Some live only in the present moment, without a sense of past connection or future direction; or they may attempt to escape a traumatic past through detachment from painful relationships and aspects of their history.

Legacies from the Past

Traumatic past experiences become encoded into family scripts that are often out of awareness, providing a blueprint for meaning and behavior when a family is facing a dilemma or crisis (Byng-Hall, 1995). Unresolved conflicts, secrets, and losses can reverberate underground, erupting in painful symptoms or destructive behavior, or enacted in family dramas at the next generation, as we saw in Martin's family in Chapter 1. Clinicians who are trained to search for negative family-of-origin influences need to seek out positive multigenerational stories, heroes, and legacies that can inspire hope and courageous action with current challenges.

For some, positive family ties may be overshadowed by past disappointment, conflict, or loss. Yet resilience and growth involve family members' coming to terms with their past and integrating that meaningful understanding into their current lives and their future hopes and dreams. As Bateson (1989) observed, "Composing a life involves a continual reimagining of the future and reinterpretation of the past to give meaning to the present" (pp. 29–30).

Distress is heightened when current stressors reactivate painful memories and emotions from past experiences. Family members may lose perspective, conflating immediate situations with past events, and become overwhelmed or cut off from painful feelings and connections. Past adversity, such as relational abuse or war-related and refugee trauma, influence future expectations; catastrophic fears heighten the risk of complications whereas stories of resilience can inspire positive adaptation. Reaching the age when a parent died can be fraught with anxiety, leading some to expect the worst while others start new health regimens, thereby gaining resilience (Walsh & McGoldrick, 2004, 2013). The convergence of developmental and transgenerational events should be explored (McGoldrick et al., 2016).

> One couple sought therapy because of intense fighting over the husband's vehement opposition to the wife's wishes for a second child. Genogram construction revealed that the husband's mother had died in childbirth with his younger sibling, a devastating loss he had suppressed and shared with no one. In exploring that experience, with his wife's empathic understanding, he realized his catastrophic fear of losing *her*, and their bond deepened as they charted their future course.

Assessing Family Functioning in Temporal Context

When assessing family functioning in the context of the multigenerational system over time, a timeline is useful to note the sequence of critical events or pileup of stressors and presenting problems (see Chapter 6). For instance, a son's drop in school grades may be precipitated by family tensions around his father's recent job loss. Because family members may not mention, or even notice, such connections, the genogram and timeline can guide inquiry and reveal patterns to explore. We inquire about family organizational shifts and coping strategies in response to anticipated, recent, and past stressors, particularly disruptive transitions. We explore any connection of heightened anxiety in a current crisis; such as a threatened separation, with a reactivation of past trauma or loss. It is important to identify processes that promote resilience, such as active coping and perseverance, and to draw out stories of positive adaptation in facing other life challenges.

FAMILY LIFE CYCLE PHASES AND TRANSITIONS: DEVELOPMENTAL CHALLENGES AND RESILIENCE

Individual and family development are intertwined, with each life phase posing new challenges and opportunities. The impact of adversity will likely vary for individuals, couples, and families depending on their concurrent life phase-related priorities and concerns. Shifts in family organization, roles, and boundaries are required with relationship changes and with the addition and loss of members. Individual symptoms and relational distress often coincide with major family transitions, including both predictable, normative stresses and unexpected disruptions (Hadley, Jacob, Milliones, Caplan, & Spitz, 1974). For instance, the death of a grandparent near the birth of a child poses incompatible demands for bereaved parents to attend both to grieving and to forming attachments with their newborn (Walsh & McGoldrick, 2004).

In every family, major stressors and parental life challenges intersect with needs and concerns related to children's developmental stages. A parent's serious illness, disability, and caregiving needs could derail educational or career plans for a young adult child (Rolland, 2012). For siblings at different developmental phases at the time of a family crisis, salient concerns and coping strategies will differ. Over time, as each child matures, new concerns may come to the fore. In one family, a mother's diagnosis of breast cancer aroused intense loss issues for her 8-year-old daughter; as she later approached puberty, anxiety surfaced over her own future risk of breast cancer. Families need to be sensitive to such developmental issues and the need for open, ongoing, age-appropriate communication over time.

Without prescribing a normative model of sequential life cycle stages, it is nonetheless helpful to understand salient challenges that commonly emerge for couples and families that are navigating through various life phases and transitions. Situations are more complex, with overlapping challenges, for those raising children who are at different developmental stages, such as parents of teenagers starting a second family with remarriage.

Couples over the Life Course

The transition to marriage or commitment to a life partner is more varied today, with cohabitation increasingly common before or in lieu of marriage. For many couples, marriage follows childbearing. More couples are opting not to raise children, defining their relationship as family. Many adopt a pet instead of, or in preparation for, childrearing (Walsh, 2009b).

Couples today, less bound by family traditions, are freer to develop a wide variety of intimate relationships and gender arrangements (Sassler, 2010). They increasingly marry across race, cultural background, and faith orientation. Yet negotiating family-of-origin relationships can be painfully challenging when parents disapprove of a bond.

Traditional marriage vows "till death do us part" are harder to keep over a lengthening life course (Walsh, 2012c). While divorce rates are high, it is perhaps remarkable that well over half of first marriages do last a lifetime. Couples increasingly celebrate 60 and even 70 years together. Relational resilience is required to weather the storms of life and to meet changing priorities (Fishbane, 2013; Jordan, 1992). In youth, romance and passion tend to stand out in choosing a partner. For those raising children, relationship satisfaction is linked more to sharing family joys and responsibilities. In later life, needs for companionship and caregiving come to the fore.

For couples, launching children into young adulthood involves a reappraisal and restructuring of their relationship and household as they take stock and look ahead—with good health they can anticipate another 20–40 years together. Some who have stayed in unhappy marriages while raising children decide to leave. Women now initiate most divorces in midlife, with more financial independence than in past eras. Yet numerous studies have found that marital satisfaction—which tends to be lowest for those with children in adolescence—rebounds to high levels for most after the children are launched. Adjustments with retirement require reorientation of life priorities and renegotiation of spousal household responsibilities. Most find greater relationship satisfaction in their later years, with more time for individual and shared leisure and pursuits, a sense of shared history, and bonds with grandchildren. Aging gay and lesbian persons meet needs for intimacy in varied ways, influenced by their past experiences (in eras of strong stigma and the HIV/AIDS epidemic) and their present life circumstances and social environment (Cohler & Galatzer-Levy, 2000). With growing societal acceptance, many long-term same-sex relationships are now openly celebrated in their later years.

In light of these developments over time, resilient couples approach marriage less as an institution and more as a dynamic partnership over the life course. Successful relationships require periodic renegotiation of roles, mutual expectations, and priorities as partners actively shape and reshape their bonds to fit changing needs and preferences.

Child–Rearing Phases and Developmental Transitions

Anticipated family developmental transitions are more manageable than unexpected changes, yet they are stressful because family structures must adapt to meet emerging needs and priorities. Families need to counterbalance continuity and change to provide stability through disruption and to maintain ongoing connections.

Transition to Parenthood and Early Child Rearing

For new parents, the transition to parenthood involves a structural transformation, with a shift in identity and focus as they assume new roles in child rearing. With the birth or adoption of a child, parents must reorganize their lives. For the development of secure attachments, they need to be emotionally engaged and consistently attentive to innumerable demands. Raising two or more children requires even more juggling of time and resources. All life patterns are altered for new parents: time and space, money, work schedules, and leisure.

For couples, transformations take place in their relationship as they expand their bond from dyad to triad and two-generational household and form a shared parental coalition. They need to negotiate workplace–family strains and relational imbalances as well as child-rearing values and practices, such as discipline. This transition to parenthood is often accompanied by declining marital satisfaction and a reversion to more traditional gender roles by dual-career couples (Cowan & Cowan, 2012). New attachment and attention to the newborn take priority, reducing time and energy for personal needs or couple intimacy. Common strains involve conflict over different parenting styles and role expectations, which are often influenced by family of origin, cultural, or social class norms.

For dual-earner couples, family resilience requires considerable flexibility, collaboration, and good communication in navigating the ongoing demands and unexpected challenges in child care, household management, and jobs (see Chapter 2).

In single-parent families, most children fare well when households are stable and financially secure and there is strong parental functioning. Single parents do best when they can draw on practical, emotional, and financial resources in their extended family and social networks, especially in stressful times. Grandparents often play a significant role in rearing children through stressful times and in assuming guardianship in kinship care (Hayslip & Kaminski, 2005; see also Chapter 13). The flexible involvement of formal and informal kin can provide multiple attachments and a web of support for resilience in times of crisis. With the vast majority of mothers in the workforce, the ready availability of affordable, quality child care is essential.

Sibling bonds can be an important resource for resilience (Kramer, 2010). It is important for parents to nurture positive relationships between siblings from early childhood, as longitudinal studies find them related to a host of better outcomes for teenagers and adults. Variables such as gender and age difference matter less than encouraging older siblings to model and mentor positive social behavior and to develop relationships with mutual respect, cooperation, and the ability to manage problems.

> Small children commonly use magical thinking and invent imaginary friends or siblings to help them cope with traumatic experiences. One father related the experience of his three-year-old daughter, Ella, when her baby sister went through months of treatment for a brain tumor and then died. Ella seemed to be handling it well, supported by her parents, relatives and friends, and visited her sister in the hospital, pleased to make her smile. One day, early in the ordeal, she began talking about an imaginary brother, named Mingus. She would tell her parents stories about how he had a tumor, and how she would give him shots and treatments to get better. After her baby sister died, she informed her parents that Mingus had moved out—but he was living around the corner. Occasionally she would report conversations with Mingus, and how she was glad he wasn't in pain anymore.
>
> Her father, a writer from Bosnia, had written stories about the ethnic cleansing atrocities experienced by his community. He appreciated her ability to construct imaginary narratives as a way to process mentally and emotionally all that was happening that was beyond her comprehension and control. As he dealt with his own grief over the following months, he decided to write of the experience they had all come through, saying he was doing this not for his own healing—but to bear witness to their experience and honor the baby's short life (Hemon, 2013).

Transitions with Adolescence

Family transitions with adolescence can be disruptive, requiring flexible shifts in roles, rules, and relationships to fit teenagers' changing cognitive, emotional, physical and social needs. As youth seek more autonomy, separate space, independent activities, and peer involvement, parents need to establish qualitatively different rules and boundaries than with younger children. Setting strong yet flexible rules and limits can be challenging, especially around issues of authority, privacy, and the use of cell phones and the Internet. Management of a youth's serious medical condition, such as diabetes, can be fraught with conflict over control and treatment adherence (Rolland, in press).

Yet close adolescent–parent relationships, guidance, and monitoring remain crucial to positive development, especially for those in high-risk communities (Gorman-Smith et al., 2004; Liddle, 2013; Steinberg et al., 2006; also see Chapters 8 and 13). Those who lack supportive family bonds are at greater risk for developing problems of substance abuse, pregnancy, school dropout, and gang involvement. Pernicious peer bullying or risk of sexual assault may require parental intervention. The high risk of suicide by gender-questioning or nonconforming teens is significantly lower for those with family acceptance (LaSala, 2010). Trusting bonds, reliable structure, and open communication enable adolescents to share their interests and concerns and to depend on support and a sense of security. Teenagers need the input of parents and other adult family members to learn about life, to discuss their own emerging identity issues and social concerns, and to help them make informed choices about their education and peer relations.

Parents often confront stresses on both generational sides, with financial, practical, and emotional support of their adolescents and their own aging parents. In other cases, past family-of-origin issues can be reactivated. One close father–son relationship became stormy as the launching transition approached, replicating the father's unresolved conflict with his own father around leaving home.

Launching Young Adults and Parents at Midlife

With the launching of young adults and the structural contraction of the family unit from a two-generational household, most parents adjust well to this "empty nest" transition, welcoming increased freedom from child-rearing responsibilities and reorienting attention to their own needs and priorities.

In American society, the primary developmental tasks in emerging adulthood involve establishing autonomy and forging personal life goals through education and/or initial commitments in work life and intimate bonds. Those who have had highly conflictual or abusing families may cut off contact or flee reactively into other relationships. Yet most young adults are able to separate and individuate while renegotiating and realigning their relationships for close connection and interdependence as autonomous adults. However, the harsh economic climate and financial debts incurred in advanced education have brought many young persons back home as they figure out career options. For families that have lovingly raised children with serious developmental disabilities or mental illneess, young adulthood poses daunting challenges in providing essential support while encouraging their offspring to make the most of their lives.

Families and Later Life Challenges

Despite society's ageist stereotypes, focused on deterioration and decay, most older adults remain healthy well into their 70s, experience relatively high levels of life satisfaction and emotional well-being, enjoy greater leisure, and find meaning and satisfaction in new pursuits and active involvement with friends and family (Walsh, 2012b). Neuroscience findings of neuroplasticity support the many possibilities for functioning and positive growth into later years (Cozolino, 2014). The subjective sense of future time shifts, with priorities reoriented in consideration of time left in life. For resilience in later life it is important to engage in lifelong learning, keep active, strengthen kinship bonds, rekindle old friendships, and make new ones (Walsh, 2016b).

Family bonds and intergenerational relations tend to be mutually beneficial, dynamic, and co-evolving throughout adult life (Bengston, 2001; Walsh, 2015a). Most older adults maintain close connection with their family members. Grandparenthood or other generative involvements offer a new lease on life (Mueller & Elder, 2003). Both young and old reap benefits as older persons become energized, productive, and valued for their wisdom, knowledge, and care.

Significant bonds with siblings, cousins, nephews and nieces, godchildren, close friends, companion animals, and social networks are vital for resilience, especially for those living alone or without children. In our mobile world, important relationships are often carried on at a distance and sustained through frequent cell phone and Internet contact.

In middle and later life, the family as a system, along with its elder members, confronts major adaptational challenges. Each family's approach evolves from its earlier patterns and cultural world view. Systemic processes over the years influence the ability to adapt to losses and flexibly meet new demands. Once functional patterns may no longer fit changing priorities and constraints. Changes with retirement, illness, death, and widowhood alter complex relationship patterns, often requiring family support, adjustment to loss, reorientation, and reorganization. Such challenges also present opportunities for relational transformation and growth. For instance, elders commonly become more open to expressing their love and appreciation, pride in children, and remorse for past wrongs.

Many older adults continue working past retirement age for financial security and yet often face job discrimination. Loss of needed income and benefits threatens self-sufficiency and later-life plans. With the ethos of self-reliance and stigma of dependency in our dominant culture, most older adults are reluctant to ask for or accept financial assistance from their adult children or burden them with their needs. Issues of pride and shame keep many from even acknowledging that they are financially strapped or can no longer live independently.

With advanced age, chronic illness and disability pose significant family challenges (see Chapter 12). Alzheimer's disease and other dementias, with a cascade of ambiguous losses over time, are especially anguishing for loved ones (Boss, 1999). Prolonged caregiving takes a heavy toll on the designated primary caregiver. Most are women at midlife, juggling responsibilities for elder care, jobs, and teenage or young adult children (Brody, 2004). Increasingly, caregivers for very aged elders are themselves past retirement, with limited resources.

A collaborative *caregiving team* approach facilitates resilience and avoids the disproportionate burden in our society's individual caregiver model. A family network consultation can encourage all caring members to pitch in, each contributing according to ability, proximity, and resources (Walsh, 2012b, 2016b). The sharing of responsibilities and challenges can become an opportunity to strengthen bonds and heal old rivalries (see Chapter 12).

Intergenerational relations are often strained when elders have issues around declining abilities or dependency needs (e.g., refusing to give up driving when it becomes unsafe). Even when older parents are quite frail, losing mental or physical capacities, this should not be seen as an intergenerational role reversal, nor should parents be labeled as "childlike." Just as parents care for children in earlier life phases, adult children assume filial responsibilities for their aging parents (Walsh, 2016b). Parents remain parents to their children in the generational hierarchy. The importance of dignity, respect, and meaningful involvement for elders is paramount.

A priority for the resilience of elders and their families is to draw out sources of meaning and satisfaction and to integrate the varied experiences of a lifetime into a coherent sense of self, relational integrity, and life's worth. King and Wynne (2004) introduced the concept of *family integrity*, referring to older adults' developmental striving toward meaning, connection, and continuity within their multigenerational family system. It involves gaining three competencies: (1) dynamic transformation of relationships over time, responsive to members' changing life cycle needs; (2) resolution or acceptance of past conflicts and losses; and (3) shared creation of meaning by passing on positive legacies across generations.

FAMILY PROCESSES IN DIVORCE AND STEPFAMILY TRANSITIONS

Family transitions that are unanticipated and untimely are especially disruptive in family life and heighten members' risk of emotional and behavioral problems. Here we will address the family developmental challenges, risks, and resilience with divorce processes and stepfamily integration. Later chapters in this volume will consider the death of a loved one, illness and disability, war and major disasters, migration, multi-stress conditions, and foster care, all of which require attention to loss and renewal for positive adaptation.

Divorce and Post-Divorce Processes: Risk and Resilience

Divorce, while thought of as a discrete event, entails a complex set of changing conditions over time, posing a series of challenges. Longitudinal studies have tracked family processes associated with risk and resilience from an escalation of tensions in the predivorce climate through separation, legal divorce processes, and subsequent reorganization of households, roles, and relationships (Hetherington & Kelly, 2002). While the experience can be especially painful and disruptive through the first year, claims that divorce inevitably damages children, based on small clinical samples, have been refuted in large-scale, carefully controlled research (Greene et al., 2012). Although some studies find a higher risk of problems for children of divorced parents than those in intact families, fewer than one in four children from divorced families shows serious or lasting difficulties. In high-conflict and abusive families, children whose parents divorce tend to fare better than those whose families remain intact. Moreover, financial strains and unreliable contact and support by the nonresidential parent heighten risks for postdivorce maladjustment. Although grown children may have painful memories of the divorce, most have no greater difficulty developing committed intimate relationships than those whose parents stayed unhappily married. Above all, children's healthy adaptation depends on the strong functioning of their residential parent, financial security, household stability, and the quality of relationships with and between parents before and after divorce (Ahrons, 2004).

Joint custody works well when parents can cooperate in decision making, child contact, financial support, and shared responsibilities. With serious conflict, sole custody and a primary residence are advised, with clear guidelines for support and visitation by the nonresidential parent (Kelley, 2007). An arrangement of "parallel parenting" is often most realistic. Parents each assume authority and responsibility for their own parenting, with an agreement not to interfere with the other's parental rights or to involve children in coalitions against the other. Yet strong differences in household rules and expectations can burden children shuttling between two residences. Clinicians can help parents minimize hostilities, increase mutual respect, and agree on common guidelines

Continuing bonds with important extended family members sustain a larger network of connection and support for parents and children. This is especially vital for children in cases of parental absence or restricted contact, as with migration, incarceration, or mental health, substance abuse, or safety concerns. Clinicians should evaluate the current status and potential involvement of parents who were unreliable, absent, or harmful in the past. If barriers to contact can be surmounted and a child's security is protected, many can become more supportive of their child's positive development.

Family processes over time are a roller-coaster course, with peaks of emotional tension at transition points. Parents can facilitate children's adaptation in the way they manage and communicate the decision to divorce and in their custody, financial, and visitation arrangements. Particularly important is reliable follow-through, especially in child contact and financial support commitments by the nonresidential parent. Despite marital grievances, it is crucial for parents not to triangulate children as go-betweens, in loyalty conflicts, or by demonizing the other parent. They do best when parents cooperate across households over time as each child celebrates milestones, such as birthdays and graduation, or has special needs.

Facilitating Postdivorce Healing and Reconciliation

When a marriage ends, how families handle adaptational processes over time can make all the difference for the healing and resilience of all members and their relationships. Divorce involves a complicated web of feelings and transactional processes from the first consideration of separation through failed attempts to reconcile, tangled legal proceedings, painful losses and transitional upheavals, reorganization and relocation of households, revision of life plans, and further alterations with remarriage.

Children's functioning and relationships with divorced parents often improve when no longer embedded in ongoing marital strife. In nearly half of postdivorce families, parents are able to work out amicable coparenting relationships, and many former spouses are able to sustain an informal kinship connection (Ahrons, 2004). This involves reconfiguration of family structural patterns and renegotiation of relationships. However, in a common attempt to "just put troubles behind and move on" (a mistaken view of resilience), some cut off and plunge into new relationships without tending to emotional wounds, as in the following case.

> Gary, age 45, requested help "to get my wife—I mean my life—in order." He explained that his prior individual therapy had helped him realize that his 18-year marriage was hopelessly dysfunctional (even though the therapist had never met his wife or suggested couple therapy). That had freed him to leave his marriage for a new, energizing affair. He remarried immediately on the heels of a bitter divorce; the new couple had a baby within the year. His teenage kids refused to see him and sent back his birthday presents unopened. Gary blamed his "ex" for turning them against him. Their continuing stormy relationships, with constant sniping and disputes over visitation and support, were now seriously straining his current marriage. Why, he wondered, couldn't they just get on with their lives and accept the new realities?
>
> A session with Gary's older children and their mother, Cindy, revealed their rage that he could just cast them off and instantly create a new family to replace them. The oldest daughter was particularly upset that Gary was so doting on his new son—much more involved than he had ever been with her. Cindy was furious for having sidelined her own needs over the years while Gary was building his career. With his abrupt departure, the whole family seemed suddenly ripped apart. Gary's refusal to talk about the past left the reasons for the breakup unclear. Cindy tried in vain to make sense of it all—first blaming the other woman and then blaming herself. If he could be so loving with a new wife and child, maybe it was all her fault. The daughters doubted their own lovability and their ability to trust men.
>
> It was crucial to heal the wounds of the breakup and to strive to repair grievances and cut-off relationships. In a session with Gary, he now struggled with guilt about the affair and the way he had cast them off. He was encouraged to write letters of sincere apology to Cindy and the girls, with remorse for the pain he had caused them, the way he had handled the divorce, and his hope to mend relationships. He asked Cindy if she would agree to come to a session with him and his counselor. Together, they began a painful but healing path forward and over time he regained a strong bond with his daughters.

Postdivorce reconciliation is distinct from reunion. It involves coming to terms with difficult and painful aspects of a relationship in order to integrate the experience and move ahead in life (see Chapter 14). Intense, mixed emotions are common in relationship endings. In-depth studies have found that many former partners are able to put old grievances in perspective and reconcile hurts and hostilities to the extent that they can collaborate in raising their children and can maintain cordial, respectful relations. It's also crucial for parents to clarify ambiguities that may fuel children's reunion fantasies: they will not be getting back together as a couple or a family unit, but they will always do their best to be there for the children.

With divorce, a devaluation of the relationship and the other person commonly occurs; this loosens attachments, eases the pain of loss, and diminishes the sense of shame and guilt. The adversarial legal system intensifies conflict and polarization. Divorce holds stigmatizing implications of failure and inadequacy. As each partner grapples to make meaning of the painful loss, "divorce stories" take shape. Each partner's narrative construction of the marriage and its breakdown can influence relationships for years to come. Hetherington and colleagues (Hetherington & Kelly, 2002) found that postdivorce accounts given by ex-spouses were so different that "blind" raters could not match partners in the same marriage. Stories that demonize the ex-spouse can keep individuals trapped in a helpless, victimized position or an angry, accusatory stance. Those who feel depressed, enraged, or powerless over an undesired breakup or unforgivable actions by a former partner often try to punish the other. After fighting over possessions, men commonly withhold child support payments as women withhold visitation in a vicious cycle of reactivity and mutual retaliation. Therapists and mediators can lay important groundwork at the time of divorce to prevent such avoidable fallout. Long-term follow-up studies show that most children's successful postdivorce adaptation is enhanced when both parents can remain involved with their children and cooperate as much as possible in child rearing and financial support to assure children of reliable, nonconflictual relationships with both of them.

There are many losses with divorce. Even if the partner or relationship was deeply disappointing or hurtful, divorce also involves the loss of the intact family unit and the hopes and dreams for the future of the relationships. A painful emotional divorce may delay or lag behind the legal divorce, complicating ongoing involvement with children and arousing old attachments and conflicts. One divorced man found it so upsetting to have to ring the doorbell of his former home to take his children out that he moved away and stopped seeing them. Arranging pickups and drop-offs at school or other neutral places can ease such tensions.

Ambiguous loss complicates divorce processes (Boss, 1999). In contrast to the idealization and sorrow common in widowhood, divorce tends to highlight hurts and injustices, with anger and resentment often stoked by lengthy litigation and custody battles. Unlike widowhood, in divorce the marriage and intact family unit are dissolved, yet the former partner and each parent live on, moving into separate lives and new relationships. The ex-partners are no longer a couple, and yet they remain parents to their children for the rest of their lives. As parents move on in separate lives and households, forming new attachments and families, their continuing contact around child-related issues and events can arouse painful feelings and reactivate old conflicts. Positive adaptation is facilitated by grieving what is lost (including past hopes and dreams) and dealing with hurt, anger, blame, and guilt.

The tendency to vilify an ex-spouse is as strong as the tendency to overromanticize a new partner. The blame, shame, and guilt surrounding divorce, further inflamed by an adversarial legal system, often fuel brutal character assassinations that rationalize the divorce or a desired settlement. Many individuals are so hurt or bitter in the aftermath of divorce that they lose sight of the positive aspects of their former partners and their relationships, which brought them together and may have yielded many good years. It takes maturity and generosity to resist joining in blaming indictments by well-intentioned family or friends. For postdivorce resilience, it is vital to understand the hopes and dreams, the energies and efforts that were invested in couple and family relationships alongside disappointments, hurts, and losses.

A client who is stuck in destructive, stereotypical victim–villain scenarios can be helped to revise and expand such stories to include the many dimensions of the former partner and relationship, or shared pride in their children. A therapist can encourage review of the history of the relationship, from courtship through the high and low points, noting the stressors that contributed to tensions. It's also useful for clients to gain clarifying information and perspectives from the ex-spouse, other important family members, and close friends, to comprehend more fully how the marriage ended. Shandra, feeling inadequate for not having met her ex-husband's sexual needs, was encouraged, a year postdivorce, to invite him to a joint therapy session to better understand his decision to leave. He revealed that he had come to acknowledge that he was gay and could no longer live a lie. Yet because of their families' conservative religious convictions, he had not been able to reveal it openly at the time.

Adaptation is facilitated when both ex-partners can own their parts in the breakdown of a relationship over time. A therapist can pose questions that encourage a rebalancing of negative views to include positive aspects of each other and the relationship. Helping ex-partners to make meaning of their relationship and acknowledge their role in its ending can greatly facilitate the emotional resolution of the divorce so they can move on with life without rancor or bitterness.

A sense of dislocation, loss of security, and uncertainty about the future can fuel anxiety. With a breakup, core beliefs and assumptions about oneself and the relationship are reexamined (e.g., "Who am I if not your spouse?"). A therapist's questions can also encourage future-oriented possibilities: "What strengths do you see each of you having that could help to reduce resentments and conflict?" "How might you set aside marital differences in order to coparent, for the sake of your children?" It's important to help the ex-partners accept what can't be changed and consider how they can do their best for their children's future.

With time and effort, many former spouses rise above past grievances to transform a broken marriage into caring kinship. One man, visiting his seriously ill ex-wife in the hospital, was unsure how to introduce himself to other visitors. His former wife said simply, "This is Sam; he's my children's father. We were together for many years, and now he's my good friend for life."

Reweaving Extended Family Ties after Divorce

Relational dynamics in families of origin sometimes contribute to divorce. I asked Joel, recently divorced, when his marital troubles had begun. He replied, "Even before the honeymoon!" At the wedding, his father had congratulated him on finding a woman just like his mother—whom the father had constantly berated throughout their marriage. Joel noted, "That was the kiss of death for my marriage." In conflictual divorces, the families of origin may be drawn in to support one side against the other or may be pushed to the margins. They often risk losing precious contact with grandchildren. Active efforts can be made to avoid triangulations and to sustain important extended family ties. We can encourage clients to facilitate strong connections for their children and to consider the kinds of relationships they themselves would like to maintain with former in-laws and extended family members.

One source of discomfort concerns the language and categories we use to define these relations. Some jokingly refer to former in-laws as "outlaws." "Step-uncle" seems as absurd as "ex-aunt." Many cultures don't have our problems with language and formality in regard to family reconfigurations; they value a wide variety of kinship bonds, which nourish children's lives and can be lifelines for resilience.

Stepfamily Adaptation

Over two-thirds of divorced adults go on to remarry; most others repartner. Where children are involved, this transition requires negotiation of step-relationships and realignments with the other biological parent. Adding complexity, often there are ex-spouses and children of both partners from former unions spanning several households and extended family networks.

Challenges in stepfamily formation contribute to a higher divorce rate in remarriage (Coleman, Ganong, & Russell, 2015; Pasley & Garneau, 2012). Solidifying the new couple relationship is a priority, without vilifying the ex-spouse. Children caught in a loyalty conflict commonly express their bind by resisting or turning against the stepparent. Adaptation is facilitated when the biological parent assumes the primary parenting role and the new partner take a supportive role, gradually building a trusting, caring relationship with children. Stepfamily integration typically takes several years.

With repartnering, many bring unresolved issues into the new relationships that contribute to the higher risk of divorce in remarriage. A common mistake in remarriage is the misguided attempt to cut ties to the past and seal a border around the new family unit to emulate an intact nuclear family model. Children are at higher risk of dysfunction when they are drawn into loyalty conflicts, cut off from caring biological parents, or expected to form an instant replacement bond with a stepparent. Fathers who are estranged from their children in previous unions sometimes become blocked from developing relationships with stepchildren. Working through feelings of loss and guilt and fears of attachment can facilitate both reconnection and new bonds. We can also help new partners understand children's yearning to maintain ties with both biological parents in most cases. If jealous of or threatened by a good relationship between the ex-partners, it's helpful to frame relationships as a collaborative parenting team across households. Children will more readily form positive step-relationships when they are not forced to take sides.

Because separation, divorce, and stepfamily formation are evolving processes over time, therapists need to inquire about previous family units, the timing and nature of transitions, and future anticipated changes. In particular, recent or impending changes in membership or household composition may precipitate a crisis related to presenting problems. Focusing only on the current household can result in tunnel vision, as in the following case.

A divorced father with custody of his two children, Matt, age 14, and Maggie, age 12, sought help for Maggie's stormy oppositional

behavior. In presenting the case for consultation, the therapist dia-
grammed the family structure as follows:

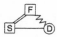

The therapist had limited the family focus to the current household
and assessed the problem as a triangle in which the father's strong
bond with Matt excluded Maggie, who then sought attention through
misbehavior. Interventions had focused unsuccessfully on increasing
the father's attachment and parenting skills with Maggie.

Unseen beyond the borders of the household and the present time
frame of intervention were critical relational complications fueling the
crisis. To facilitate developmental systems exploration, we constructed
a family genogram and timeline with the father in the next session, as
illustrated in this diagram:

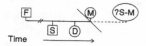

The father had divorced the mother 3 years earlier after learning she
had carried on an affair with his best friend. Furious, he fought and
won a bitter custody battle, severely restricted the children's contact
with their mother, and continued to demonize her to them. In the
midst of the divorce, he plunged into a new intimate relationship with
a woman who was now pressuring him to get married. Maggie repeatedly rebuffed her efforts to win over her affections.

In a session with the father and children, Maggie expressed strong
anger at having been turned against her mother, upset by her loss of
contact, and resentment of the "replacement" mom in the wings. The
father then admitted his own hesitation about remarriage, rooted in
his shattered trust and sense of betrayal. These relational knots needed
to be untangled and dealt with for the family to move forward from
the past. It was crucial for the father to facilitate positive connections
between the children and their mother and to deal with his own emotional divorce before moving on to a possible remarriage and the complications of new stepfamily relationships.

EXPANDING OUR DEVELOPMENTAL LENS

With the growing diversity of relationships and households in society, our
view of "family" must be expanded to fit the lengthened and varied life

course, attuning therapeutic approaches to the challenges and preferences that make each individual, couple, and family unique. We can help family members learn to live successfully in complex and changing relationship systems, buffer disruptive transitions, and make the best of stressful times.

Families most often come for help in crisis, but they may not connect presenting problems and distress with relevant stressors. A genogram and timeline help to visualize complex family systems and to track significant events and changes over time in order to understand and address problems in family developmental context (McGoldrick et al., 2008). Reactivation of past painful experiences at significant nodal points can be addressed. Recent or threatened crisis events, a pileup of stressors, and changes in family or household composition should be explored to understand their implications.

With a family developmental perspective, clinicians show interest in each family's life journey, listening to stories of crisis or hardship with compassion for the family's struggles, suffering, and losses, and with affirmation of their courage, caring, and best efforts. With a resilience orientation, it is important to rebalance a problem focus to identify and enhance strengths and resources that can facilitate positive adaptation. It is crucial to identify and draw on extended kin, social, and community networks and cultural and spiritual resources. Through interventions targeted to strengthen key transactional processes for resilience, families can become more resourceful in dealing with crises, navigating transitions, weathering persistent stresses, and meeting future challenges. We can help families find coherence in the midst of complexity and restore continuities in the aftermath of upheaval. We can encourage their efforts toward meaning, purpose, joy, and connections, with conviction in their potential to forge personal and relational growth from their life challenges.

The importance of family ties throughout adulthood has been neglected in research, clinical training, and practice, which emphasize early developmental phases: young couples and families raising children. As young adults leave home, attention follows them into their own life course and family formation, relegating the parent generation to the margins as extended kin, or into the background story of past family of origin influences. Intergenerational bonds continue to be significant and parents never cease to be parents, with their own needs and with lifelong concern for the well-being of their children and any grandchildren.

It is also crucial not to define a child or family identity by one milestone in their life passage. Pejorative labels such as "child of divorce" or "broken family" can trap those who want to move on with their lives, and they can overshadow previous or future years of satisfying relational life.

Our developmental lens needs to be expanded to the full life course and the interdependence of multigenerational connections that extend from the past into the future. The shared construction of identity and meaning is a lifelong process as individuals and their families organize, interpret, and connect experiences over time.

A facilitated *family life review* (Walsh, 2012b, 2016b) can assist families in the integration of family life phases and transitions, updating relationships and gaining appreciation of loved ones. Sharing reminiscences can be a valuable experience, incorporating multiple perspectives and members' subjective experiences of their lives over time. Recalling hopes and dreams, important milestones, and their satisfactions, pride, and regrets enlarges the family story and fosters empathic understanding. Earlier conflicts or hurts that led to cutoffs or frozen images and expectations can be reconsidered from new vantage points; misunderstandings and faulty assumptions can be clarified. As they mature, family members are often more open and honest about earlier transgressions or secrets and more readily acknowledge and regret past mistakes and hurts, opening possibilities to heal old wounds. Family photos, scrapbooks, genealogies, reunions, and pilgrimages can assist this work. Stories of family history and precious conversations can be videotaped, preserved, and transmitted to younger generations. Wisdom can be drawn from past hardships, and stories of resilience can inspire the journey ahead.

We are relational beings; most lives are enriched by a variety of intimate relationships and significant kin and social bonds within and beyond households. A family developmental framework views each family's functioning in relation to its broader sociocultural context and evolution over the multigenerational life cycle. We must be sensitive to the culture and time in which families and their members live, their history, and the contribution of critical events and structural sources of meaning.

Crisis and challenge are inherent in the human condition. Families need to counterbalance continuity and change to provide stability through disruption and to maintain ongoing connections. How the family deals with its challenges as a functional unit is critical for all members' positive development and for the future of the family. Many adaptational pathways are possible, with more resilient families using a flexible variety of strategies. Resilience involves struggling well, effectively working through and learning from adversity, and integrating the experience into life's journey.

CHAPTER 10

Loss, Recovery, and Resilience

> In coming to accept death, we can more fully
> embrace life.
> —VIKTOR FRANKL, *Man's Search for Meaning*

I recall my delight, as a child, watching our neighbors' celebration when their only daughter got married. Like other families, they planned for the perfect wedding, the bride and groom looked radiant, and everyone cheered as they drove off on their honeymoon. En route to their romantic destination, their car skidded off the icy, winding country road, ending their lives. Tragedy struck at the happiest moment for all, shattering their hopes and dreams.

Coming to terms with death and loss is the most difficult challenge families face. From a systems orientation, loss is seen as a transactional process involving those who die with their survivors in a shared life cycle, recognizing both the finality of death and the continuity of life (Walsh & McGoldrick, 2004, 2013). A significant death affects all family members, their relationships, and the family as a functional unit. A family resilience approach fosters the ability to face death and dying and for survivors to live and love fully beyond loss.

This chapter presents a framework for resilience-based systemic assessment and intervention with bereavement challenges. With a developmental perspective, loss and recovery processes are considered over time and across the family life cycle. Major family adaptational tasks are described, identifying variables that heighten risk for dysfunction and key processes that facilitate healing and resilience. Guidelines are offered for dealing effectively with complicated situations.

DEATH AND LOSS IN SOCIOHISTORICAL CONTEXT

Families over the ages have had to cope with the precariousness of life and the disruptions wrought by death. Across cultures, mourning beliefs and practices have facilitated both the integration of death and the transformations of survivors (Walsh & McGoldrick, 2004). Each culture and religion, in its own ways, offers assistance to the dying and to loved ones who must move forward with life (Rosenblatt, 2013). Most traditions hold a world view and rituals that facilitate acceptance of the inescapable fact of death, including it in the rhythm of life, passage to a spiritual realm, and an abiding faith in a higher power. Most approach loss as an occasion for family and community cohesion and support the expression of grief. Our dominant Anglo-American culture, in contrast, has tended to avoid facing mortality, minimizing the impact of loss and encouraging the bereaved to quickly gain "closure" and move on. With the exception of bereavement specialists, mental health and health care professionals have been slow to deal with loss, reflecting this cultural aversion.

Yet, there has been growing recognition of the importance of facing death and loss. Technology and the media have brought worldwide catastrophic events into greater awareness. Large-scale epidemics such as HIV/AIDS, major disasters, war, and terrorist attacks have heightened attention to the precariousness of life and death in our volatile and uncertain global environment (see Chapter 11).

Amid social, economic, and political upheavals in our times, families are dealing with multiple losses, disruptions, and uncertainties. This chapter focuses on loss through death, yet family adaptational processes apply broadly to loss issues in other experiences, such as physical and mental illness, unemployment, migration, family separations, divorce, foster care and adoption, interpersonal and mass trauma, and community disasters, which are considered in other chapters. In strengthening family resilience to deal with losses, we enable members to deepen their bonds and forge new strengths.

UNDERSTANDING LOSS IN SYSTEMIC PERSPECTIVE

Attention to bereavement in clinical theory, research, and practice has focused primarily on distressed individual grief reactions in the loss of a significant dyadic relationship for a child, parent, spouse, or sibling (Rubin, Malkinson, & Witzum, 2012). Nonsymptomatic family members may be presumed to be functioning normally and not in need of attention. A systemic perspective expands our view to the transactional processes and mutual influences throughout the relational network with any significant loss. Bowen (1978) observed how death or threatened loss can disrupt a family's functional equilibrium. Beyond the grief reactions of the closest members, emotional shock waves can reverberate throughout an entire relational network immediately or long after a death. Unattended grief may precipitate strong and harmful reactions in other relationships—from marital distancing and divorce to precipitous replacement or extramarital affairs (Walsh & McGoldrick, 2004).

As I have seen in my research and practice, how the family handles the loss situation has far-reaching effects, as in the following case:

Marie, a woman in her 50s, came for therapy at the urging of her adult children, who complained, "You've got to stop your overmothering of us—we're grown adults with children of our own!"

In the first session, she said she couldn't help worrying about them. She added that she didn't know how to be a mother of adult children, since she had lost her own mother to cancer when she was 7. As we explored that loss, she recalled feeling abandoned in the months before the death as her father hovered over her mother and tried to shelter her from child care "burdens." She recalled the last night, when many relatives came to the house where her mother lay dying. Marie dressed her younger brother, Jim, and herself in their Sunday best and sat holding his hand, waiting to be called in to say their good-byes. No one came for them, nor were they taken to the funeral.

In the chaotic aftermath, with the father too bereft to care for them, well-intentioned relatives each took in a child, separating them, with uncertainty when or if they would reunite or return home. When she returned home several weeks later, her father, isolated in his unbearable grief, drank heavily and came into her bed at night, abusing her sexually. A year later, his remarriage ended her secret torment. She showed no anger in telling me about this abuse—the first time she had ever revealed it to anyone. When I asked about her feelings, she said she never blamed him because she felt so sorry for his deep sadness and loneliness; it comforted him and eased her fear of losing her only surviving parent. She later married a man who, like her father, was a heavy drinker and endured his physical abuse for many years to keep her family intact for her children. Her close bond with her brother remained her lifeline over the years. It was only at that point in our session that she broke down in tears, revealing that Jim had died recently in the crash of a small plane.

As in this case, some families fall apart with an unbearable loss, with adults unable to care for their children and provide comfort, reassurance, and security through disruptions. Anxieties with secondary losses of separation, unclear communication, and uncertainty about the future increase suffering. Sibling bonds can be vital lifelines through disruption and for years to come. The recent death of Marie's brother was a devastating loss and reactivated her childhood trauma, with reverberations in her relationships with her adult children. Legacies of loss find expression in far-ranging patterns of interaction and mutual influence among the survivors and across the generations. The impact of loss touches survivors' relationships with others, affecting even those who never knew the person who died.

Death or threatened loss can disrupt a family's functional equilibrium. As Bowen (1978) observed, the intensity of the emotional reaction is influenced by the integration in the family at the time of the loss and by the significance of the lost member. The emotional shock wave may ripple throughout an entire family system immediately and long after a significant loss. Therefore, therapists need to assess the family network, the position of the deceased member, and the family dynamics surrounding the loss in order to understand the meaning and context of presenting symptoms.

Loss is a powerful nodal experience that shakes the foundation of family life and leaves no member unaffected. Individual distress stems not only from grief, but also from the realignment of the family emotional field. The meaning of a particular loss event and responses to it are shaped by family belief systems, which in turn are altered by other loss experiences. Loss also modifies the family structure, often requiring major reorganization of the family system.

A death in the family can involve multiple losses: the loss of the particular person, the loss of each member's unique relationship, the loss of role functioning, the loss of the intact family unit, and the loss of hopes and dreams for all that might have been.

Death is more than a discrete event; from a developmental systemic perspective, it can be seen to involve many interwoven processes over time—from the threat and approach of death, through its immediate aftermath, and on into long-term implications. A family life cycle perspective attends to the reciprocal influences of several generations as they move forward over time and as they approach and respond to loss (McGoldrick & Walsh, 2004). Each loss ties in with all other losses and yet is unique in its meaning. We need to be attuned to both the factual circumstances of a death and the meanings it holds for each family in its social and developmental contexts. In family assessment, we explore past, present, and future connections, not with deterministic causal assumptions, but rather in an evolutionary sense. Like the social context, the temporal context of loss holds a matrix of meanings and influences future approaches to loss and to life.

FAMILY ADAPTATION TO LOSS

Contemporary approaches to bereavement, grounded in research, have advanced from early theories of normal grief. There is wide variation in the timing, expression, and intensity of normal grief responses (Wortman & Silver, 1989), and mourning processes have no orderly stage sequence or timetable. Adaptive coping over time involves a dynamic oscillation in attention, alternating between loss and restoration, focused at times on grief and at other times on mastering emerging challenges (Stroebe & Schut, 2010).

Adaptation to loss does not mean resolution, in the sense of some complete, "once-and-for-all" getting over it. Significant losses may never be fully resolved. Similarly, resilience in the response to loss, commonly misconstrued, does not mean quickly getting "closure" on the emotional experience or simply bouncing back and moving on. Rather, mourning and recovery are gradual, fluid processes, usually lessening in intensity over time. Yet various facets of grief may reemerge with unexpected intensity, particularly with anniversaries and other nodal events. Although painful and disruptive, grieving, in its many forms, is a healing process.

Death ends a life but not relationships: mourning processes involve not a detachment from the deceased, but rather a transformation of those relationships from physical presence to continuing bonds through spiritual connections, memories, deeds, and stories that are passed on through kinship networks and to future generations (Stroebe, Schut, & Boerner, 2010; Walsh & McGoldrick, 2004). The ability to accept and integrate loss is at the heart of all healthy processes in family systems (Beavers & Hampson, 2003).

Facilitating Family Adaptational Tasks

Families navigate varied pathways to meet emerging challenges with loss over time. While we must be mindful of the wide variation in individual, family, and cultural modes of dealing with death, families confront basic adaptational challenges. If not addressed, they increase members' vulnerability to dysfunction and the risk of family conflict and dissolution. In developing a systemic approach to loss, grounded in our clinical research, Monica McGoldrick and I delineated four major tasks that facilitate immediate and long-term adaptation for family members and strengthen the family as a functional unit (Walsh & McGoldrick, 2004). We approach these challenges as tasks (as does Worden, 2008, for individual challenges), which families actively engage in and clinicians can facilitate. They involve an interweaving of key processes for family resilience in the three domains of family functioning—belief systems, organizational patterns, and communication/problem solving.

Shared Acknowledgment of the Death and Loss

Family members, each in their own way, need to confront the reality of a death and grapple with its meaning for them and for each other. With the shock of a sudden death, this process may start abruptly. When possible, contact with a dying member facilitates adaptation, including opportunity for children to express their love and say their good-byes. Well-intentioned attempts to protect them from potential upset can isolate them, stir anxious fantasies, and impede their grief process.

Although individuals, families, and cultures vary in their direct expression of information and feelings around death, clear communication is important. Clinicians need to provide support through a climate of trust, empathic responses, and tolerance for diverse reactions. Sharing clear information about the facts and circumstances of the death facilitates mourning processes. A family member who is unable to accept the reality of death may avoid contact with others or become angry with those who are grieving. When death and dying are faced courageously with loved ones, relationships can be enriched. At the death of her partner after a debilitating illness, Bonnie was sad but also at peace:

> "The simple fact is, Jennie's body stopped. There was no unfinished business between us. I had carried a lot of fear about death. Jennie showed me how to feel more alive and more open, even in her last days. She accepted that she was dying, even though she didn't want to go. Acceptance didn't mean feeling jolly or that she liked the situation, just that this was the truth at the moment."

Funeral rites and memorial services provide direct confrontation with the reality of death, the opportunity to pay last respects, and a way for the bereaved to share grief and receive comfort from kin and community (Imber-Black et al., 2012). Families are encouraged to plan ahead for a meaningful service and for burial or cremation, honoring the preferences of the dying or deceased. Increasingly, loved ones take part in the rites—through meaningful eulogies, personal stories, photos, and artistic expression—to remember and celebrate the life passage and the multifaceted personhood and relationships of the deceased. In one especially moving service, a father's son and daughter from his second marriage recounted both poignant and humorous stories from their childhood interactions. Then his son from a previous marriage came forward; saying he was never comfortable with words, he played a stirring flute melody that he had composed in memory of his father.

In the Jewish tradition, as in many others, it is considered even more important to attend a funeral than a wedding, because it both honors a life and marks its loss. Key processes in resilience are movingly expressed in the following Jewish mourners' prayer, read aloud together by those gathered at the shiva after the burial:

> At times, the pain of separation seems more than we can bear; but love and understanding can help us pass through the darkness toward the light. And in truth, grief is a great teacher, when it sends us back to serve and bless the living. . . . Thus, even when they are gone, the departed are with us, moving us to live as, in their higher moments, they themselves wished to live. We remember them now; they live in our hearts; they are an abiding blessing. (Central Conference of American Rabbis, 1992)

Sharing the experience of loss, in accord with family preferences, is crucial in the healing process. I encourage families to urge reluctant members to attend a funeral or memorial gathering. Some may intend to go but say they can't make the time. Others say they'd rather remember the person when alive. Yet, paradoxically, the life and the relationship can be appreciated more fully when the loss is marked.

As it becomes common to announce a death on the Internet to a kin and social network, it can be meaningful if done thoughtfully. One young adult daughter of immigrants invited relatives, friends, and acquaintances from afar to her website, where she had composed a moving tribute to her father at his death. She shared stories of his life journey and a photo album with pictures from his childhood and important milestones in their family life.

It is never too late to hold a memorial service, to lay a headstone at a grave, to hold a ceremony to scatter ashes, or to plant a tree in memory of a loved one. Drawing family members together on an anniversary or at a holiday gathering to "re-member" one who has died can be a profoundly healing and connecting experience. On the 20th anniversary of my mother's death, I wanted to find a meaningful way to celebrate her life with my husband and daughter, who had never known her. My mother's deep love of music as a pianist and organist brought to mind the carillon bells of the Rockefeller Chapel on my campus at the University of Chicago. I arranged a simple concert in her memory, and we were invited to climb to the roof of the bell tower. As the bells pealed harmoniously, we looked out into the evening sky and felt in touch with her spirit among the shining stars.

Shared Experience of the Loss

Open communication is vital for family resilience over the course of loss and recovery processes, especially in the transitional turmoil of the immediate aftermath. We can appreciate the complexity of a family mourning process in light of the many fluctuating and sometimes conflicting reactions of all members in a family system. For instance, sibling differences are common, in part associated with their gender, birth order, age at loss, and family dynamics. Tolerance is needed for members' varied coping styles and timing in grief and recovery processes, as they may be out of sync with one other.

The mourning process involves shared narrative attempts to put the loss into some meaningful perspective that fits coherently into the rest of a family's life experience and belief system. This requires dealing with the ongoing negative implications of the loss, including the loss of hopes and dreams for the future. Nadeau's (1998) qualitative research, based on symbolic interaction theory, explored family meaning-making processes in response to the death of a family member. Nadeau interviewed nonclinical, multigenerational, bereaved families. She found that the story of "what happened" emerged from a process of co-construction, and she identified strategies that families employed in their shared meaning-making process. These included storytelling, dream sharing, comparing the death to other deaths inside and outside the family, "coinciding" (attaching meaning to events that occurred near the time of the death), and characterizing (identifying qualities of the member who died). Families also engaged in "family speak," with an intricate weaving together of individuals' threads of meaning. Communication patterns included agreeing/disagreeing, referencing other members' meanings, and cooperative interrupting by supporting, echoing, finishing sentences, elaborating, and questioning. Family meaning-making was also facilitated by the participation of in-laws, who were less susceptible to family rules and could open discussion of what might be considered taboo subjects. Problem solving at the family level involved finding solutions to instrumental issues. For example, when a family member died, family interactions were aimed at filling the vacant role once held by the lost member. Her study revealed the ongoing interplay of beliefs, organizational patterns, and communication processes.

As a family experiences a loss, members touched in various ways are likely to show a wide range of reactions. Empathy is needed for one another and an ability to respond caringly. Tolerance for different responses and timing is important. Strong emotions may surface at different moments, including complicated and mixed feelings of anger, disappointment, helplessness, relief, guilt, or abandonment, which are present to some extent in most family relationships. In Anglo-American culture, the expression of intense emotions can generate discomfort and distancing in others. Moreover, fears of loss of control in sharing overwhelming feelings can block all communication about the loss experience.

When grieving is blocked, emotions may explode in conflict; some children internalize their grief in symptoms of anxiety or depression, while others externalize their distress in behavioral problems. Adolescents may withdraw from the family and/or engage in risky behavior and drug or alcohol abuse. If a family is unable to tolerate certain feelings, a member who directly expresses the unacceptable may be scapegoated or extruded. Unbearable feelings may be delegated and expressed in a fragmented fashion by various family members. One may carry all the anger for the family, while another is in touch only with sadness; one may show only relief, while another is numb. The shock and pain of a tragic loss can shatter family cohesion, leaving members isolated and unsupported in their grief, as in the following case (see Figure 10.1):

> Mrs. Ramirez sought help for her 11-year-old daughter Teresa's worsening school problems over the past 2 months. In the first session, the therapist and mother focused on Teresa, who seemed at a loss to explain her drop in grades and inattentiveness. As a consultant, I suggested that the therapist explore recent stress events in the family. The oldest son, Ray, age 18, had been caught in the midst of gang crossfire. The shot that killed him had also shattered the family unit. The father withdrew, drinking heavily to ease his pain. The second son, Miguel, carried the family rage into the streets, seeking revenge for the senseless killing. A younger son showed no reaction, quietly keeping out of the way. Mrs. Ramirez, alone in her grief, deflected her attention to Teresa's school problems.
>
> Family sessions provided a context for shared grief work. Family members were encouraged to share their feelings openly and to comfort one another. It was especially important to involve the brother, who had been holding in his own pain so as not to upset or burden their parents further. The therapist helped the parents to obtain legal counsel, gain the necessary information to navigate the court system, and plan and carry out concerted actions, with Miguel's assistance, to seek justice for the murder. They were also encouraged to sort through Ray's possessions, each family member choosing a keepsake—his jacket, a favorite shirt, his prized guitar. Dreading Ray's impending birthday, they were encouraged to plan something they might do together to remember him. The family decided to go to church together—for the first time in a long time—and to light candles in his memory. They

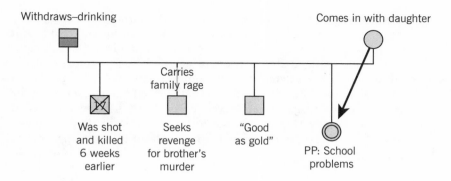

FIGURE 10.1. Genogram highlighting the impact on the family system of the past death of the oldest son.

invited aunts, uncles, and cousins to join them there. Afterward, they spent the whole day together, telling old family stories, as Miguel strummed Ray's guitar.

Such processes repaired the family's fragmentation, promoting a more cohesive network for mutual support and healing. On follow-up, Teresa's school problems and the father's drinking had subsided. The experience of pulling together to deal with their loss had strengthened their resilience, helping them to cope better with other problems in their lives.

Reorganization of the Family System

The death of a family member leaves a hole in the fabric of family life. It can disrupt established patterns of interaction. The process of adaptation involves a realignment of relationships and redistribution of role functions to compensate for the loss, buffer transitional stresses, and carry on with family life. Often, family reorganizational tasks must be addressed before parents are able to deal with their own grief.

One father, an immigrant from Central America, brought his 8-year-old daughter for therapy after the death of the mother. He declined therapy for himself, not wanting to "fall apart" by facing his own grief and guilt. He had contracted HIV/AIDS and had passed it on to her, leading to her death. Moreover, at risk himself, he wanted to keep strong, working, and functional for as long as possible for the sake of his daughter. While respecting his decision not to come to therapy for himself, given his life-threatening condition, the therapist asked if he would come for a consultation concerning his daughter's well-being.

She was careful to express her hopes for his continuing health, while exploring his thoughts and plans for his daughter's custody and care if he were to become too ill or die. He told the therapist he had thought about it: he assumed that a friendly neighbor, with children of her own, would take his daughter in, a common informal arrangement in his home country. But he had not actually asked his neighbor, and he was unaware that legally, in the event of his death, his daughter would become a ward of the state in the foster care system. It was important to work with him and a legal aid consultant to make appropriate arrangements.

Family roles and responsibilities may interfere with mourning. A parent's job demands and breadwinning role may constrain emotional expression in order to keep functioning at work. Children may sacrifice their own needs to bolster a bereaved parent whom everyone depends on, particularly in single-parent families. It is important to help family members structure the time and space for overburdened parents' own grieving, and to rally others' contributions to provide needed respite.

It is crucial to help families pace their reorganization. If a family takes flight from losses by moving precipitously from their homes or communities, further dislocations generate more disruptions and loss of social supports, and children must adjust to a new school and the loss of friends. At the other extreme, others hold on too rigidly to former patterns in family life that are no longer functional, as in the following case:

> After her husband's death, Mrs. Miller vowed to carry on family life and to raise their daughters according to his rules. She took a stressful full-time job, yet continued to keep the house spotless and prepare the father's favorite meals, keeping his empty chair at the head of the table. As the girls reached adolescence, conflict arose because she insisted on continuing his favorite family activities and outings, which they had outgrown. The girls wanted to spend more time with friends and to give up elaborate meals and activities they only pretended to enjoy, yet they didn't want to be disloyal. The mother acknowledged the exhausting strain of trying to be "two parents" and live up to her husband's standards as she idealized him. We worked on finding ways to honor the father's memory, sustain valued continuities, and yet make changes to better fit the daughters' emerging developmental priorities and their structure as a single-parent family.

Family structures can crumble with an overwhelming loss. Leadership and communication may falter, and parents may be unable to nurture and protect children. As we saw in the case of Marie, children can suffer not only from a parental loss and exclusion from family mourning processes, but even more by further separations, confusion, and lack of protection in the aftermath of loss.

With the death of a parent, it is natural for children to worry about losing the surviving parent, so reliable contact is important, especially when living apart. Every effort should be made to keep siblings together, as a vital lifeline. It is important to provide clear information about what will happen and when, and who will take care of them. Extended family members need to help the surviving parent reorganize daily patterns of living and provide appropriate care and protection for children through the disruption. Social supports often dwindle after the first few weeks of a loss, so it is crucial to link those who are bereaved and isolated with kin and community support over the many months that follow.

Reinvestment in Other Relationships and Life Pursuits

As time passes, survivors need to reconfigure their lives and relationships to move forward, reenvisioning their hopes and dreams. Relationships taken for granted often become more valued. New and unforeseen life directions may open up.

In some cases, the formation of other attachments and commitments is blocked by overidealization of the deceased, a sense of disloyalty, or catastrophic fear of another loss. Others may take flight from painful losses through precipitous replacement by a new partner or another child. Well-intentioned friends or relatives may rush the surviving parent unwisely into premature remarriage "for the sake of the children," risking complications if mourning processes were unattended. A bereaved spouse's rapid remarriage may spark upset by children or former in-laws if they view it as disloyal. Often children balk at acceptance of a new stepparent when the loss has not yet been integrated. Therapists can help families to navigate and pace these steps forward.

A resilience-oriented systemic approach to loss requires the same ingenuity and flexibility that families themselves need to respond to various members and subsystems as their issues come to the fore. As changes occur in one part of a system, changes in others will be generated. Decisions to meet with an individual, couple, or family unit at various points are guided by a systemic view of the loss process.

This practice approach encourages active steps that facilitate mourning and recovery processes over time, as illustrated in my continued work with the Miller family (above), whose grief at the father's death had been blocked for several years:

> I encouraged the mother and her daughters to sort through the old sealed boxes stored away in the basement from their past life. They discussed which items to save as keepsakes, sent some to relatives and friends of their father, and gave the remainder to charity. For the approaching anniversary of the death, the mother decided to write a tribute, which she had been asked, but was unable, to do at the time of the death. This prompted one daughter to write a poem and another to make a drawing in memory of their father. With great enthusiasm, they gathered these into a booklet, which they sent to relatives and friends, reviving many valued contacts that had been lost.
>
> This unpacking and reconnection led the mother to request couple sessions with her boyfriend. Soon after her husband's death, Brianna had plunged into this intimate relationship. Lemont was comforting when she had been needy, but now they fought over his controlling nature and her disappointment with his shortcomings. She was uncertain about continuing their relationship. He assured her of his love but said he, too, needed to think it over. The following week, he arrived at the couple session near the end of our time. A large man, out of breath from rushing, he plopped down on the sofa, which cracked down the middle and fell apart. Apologizing, he said maybe the sofa forewarned their breakup. Although they cared deeply about each other, they agreed it was time to go their separate ways.
>
> In the weeks that followed, she was surprised to start dreaming of her deceased husband, waking in tears with a deep yearning for him. We met in individual sessions to address her previously unattended grief. I find it helpful to start by remembering the person and their relationship through reminiscences of their life together as it evolved over time. She recalled how they had met and their courtship, and then traced the milestones, joys, and hard times in their marriage and child rearing over the years. A strong regret she carried was the argument they had had the night before his sudden death in a car crash, and she wished she had made up with him before he left in the morning for work.
>
> In the next session, using the Gestalt "empty chair" technique, I coached her to imagine what she would want to say to him if he were sitting there now. She began by saying how sorry she was for her part in their petty fight. Tears flowed as she conveyed how much she loved him and reminisced about some treasured times: he was the love of her life. We sat in silence for several moments, holding those feelings before ending the session. I asked her if, in the next session, she would like to update him on the developments in the life of the family since

his death. In that session, she related their move to the new city to start a new life, and how hard it had been for her to shoulder all the job and child-rearing responsibilities without him, but how pleased and proud he would be at how smart and beautiful their daughters had become. I added my praise that she had done a remarkable job on her own.

In the following session, we talked about her guilt-tinged feelings of anger and abandonment at how her husband's death had left her with the "heavy load" she had been shouldering alone. She said she now felt it was time to ease up on her unrealistic expectations about providing the "perfect family" for her daughters and to expect more of them, requiring them to share responsibilities around the house to earn their privileges.

At a follow-up session 3 months later, she and her daughters looked more relaxed and happy. Although the girls grumbled at their newly assigned tasks, they enjoyed greater independence and a better relationship with their mom. She had found a new job with better hours and benefits, and began singing in her church choir, which brought her joy and connection. Those new steps bolstered her resolve to stick with a weight-loss program, losing the physical "overload" she had been carrying.

The remarkable resilience and creativity of our clients can emerge through our work. In this case, we flexibly combined family, couple, and individual sessions as priorities emerged. As we had approached her marital grief, Mrs. Miller had asked me if she could tape our sessions. Looking back, she said, "Now that I have it all on tape I don't have to carry it in my head anymore. I can put it on the shelf and listen to it when I want to." She understood what she needed to do to unburden herself—mind and body— regain her spirit, and thrive.

VARIABLES IN FAMILY RISK AND RESILIENCE

The impact of a death is influenced by a number of variables in the loss situation and the surrounding family processes and social context (Walsh & McGoldrick, 2004, 2013), including the nature of the death/loss, the timing of the loss, and the state of relationships and role functions.

Nature and Circumstances of the Loss

The manner of death poses varied challenges for surviving family members and needs to be explored in any clinical assessment. A genogram and timeline are particularly useful in tracking sequences and concurrence of significant events and symptoms over time in the multigenerational family field (McGoldrick et al., 2008).

Sudden Death or Protracted Illness/Dying

With sudden death, family members lack time to prepare for the loss, to deal with unfinished business, or even to say their good-byes. At the other extreme, chronic conditions or protracted dying can deplete family caregiving and financial resources and sideline the needs of other members. Common relief at ending family strain can be guilt-laden (Rolland, 2012). Additionally, families increasingly grapple with agonizing end-of-life decisions about ending treatment or life support efforts (see Chapter 12). These pose profound ethical and religious dilemmas and can generate intense conflict among members (Walsh, 2009c).

Ambiguous Losses

Ambiguity surrounding loss has been found to block mourning processes and to generate anxiety, depression, and conflict (Boss, 1999). Dementias, particularly Alzheimer's disease—called "the long good-bye"—are especially painful for family members as cognitive losses gradually erode personhood, relationships, roles, and even recognition of loved ones (see Chapter 12). Other situations pose ambiguity as to whether a loved one is dead or alive, as in abductions or those missing in a disaster or war. After a plane crash, families commonly report their inability to begin mourning until the body or personal effects are recovered and the death becomes physically real. Families often become consumed by prolonged searches to confirm the fate of missing loved ones. Conflict arises when some want to move on while others do not want to give up hope of return.

Unacknowledged and Stigmatized Losses

Disenfranchised losses—unacknowledged, hidden, or minimized—leave the bereaved unsupported, as commonly occurs with pregnancy losses, the death of a close friend, mentor, or former spouse, or the loss of a cherished companion animal (Doka, 2002; Walsh, 2009b). The bereaved can be isolated, feeling they don't have a right to their grief: that it is inappropriate, excessive, or doesn't fit into socially approved categories. Losses may be hidden when a relationship itself is secret and/or faces family, community, or religious disapproval, such as gay, lesbian, or transgender relationships. The stigma surrounding a suicide or HIV/AIDS foster secrecy, misinformation, and estrangement, impairing family and social support, as well as critical health or mental health care.

Violent Death

Intense grief reactions are felt throughout the family network with violent and traumatic deaths (Walsh, 2007; see Chapter 11). The impact can be devastating, especially for those who have witnessed it, may have contributed to it, or narrowly survived themselves. A senseless tragedy is especially hard to bear, particularly if a result of negligence, as in drunk driving, or deliberate acts of violence, as in neighborhood or school shootings. Murders are committed most often by relatives or close acquaintances and often in cases of domestic violence. Suicides are tormenting deaths for families, particularly when they appear impulsive, senseless, or intended to hurt loved ones. Family members struggle to comprehend these destructive acts, often ruminating over how they might have made a difference.

In cases of suicide, clinicians need to explore possible family influences, such as abuse or abandonment, as well as adolescent peer bullying; career, military, or financial concerns that fuel depression, guilt, or shame; peer drug or drinking cultures; and prescription pain drugs that can lead to self-destructive addictions. The impact of multiple traumatic losses in the families of drug addicts contributes to self-destructive behavior. Major mental illness, particularly bipolar disorder, contributes to heightened risk.

In the aftermath, clinicians need to help family members with their anger or guilt, particularly when they are blamed or blame themselves for the death. Family members' shame and cover-ups distort communication and can isolate them from social support. Clinicians should note family histories of traumatic losses that may heighten the risk of suicide, particularly at an anniversary or birthday.

> Dan, age 14, and his family were at a loss to explain his recent suicide attempt. When asked to describe their family, the parents named Dan and his younger sister but made no mention of an older son, Peter, who had died at age 14. In a session with Dan, he began talking about Peter and revealed that he grew up attempting to take his brother's place in order to relieve his parents' sadness. The father, who could not recall the date or events surrounding the death, wished to remember his first son "as if he were still alive." Dan cultivated his appearance to resemble photos of his brother. When he had reached the age at which his brother died, and his growth spurt at puberty was changing him from the way he was "supposed" to look, he attempted suicide to join his brother in heaven. Family therapy focused on enabling Daniel and his parents to deal with the past loss and relinquish his surrogate position so that he could move forward in his own development.

Therapeutic efforts aim to help families to restore hope to a bleak outlook, assess life options from a clearer perspective, and find meaning and energy to reengage in relationships and life pursuits. Although a therapist or loved ones cannot always prevent a violent death, the risk can be lowered by opening communication, mobilizing the support of family and friends, and fostering a sense of coherence in the meaning of past or ongoing trauma. We can help family members to support one another, integrate painful experiences, and envision a meaningful future beyond disappointments and losses.

The Timing of Loss

The meaning and impact of a death vary depending on the developmental challenges the family and individual members are negotiating (Walsh & McGoldrick, 2004, 2013; see Chapter 9).

Untimely Losses

Deaths that are premature or untimely in terms of chronological or social expectations, particularly early widowhood, early parent loss, or death of a child, tend to be harder to bear for families. Early spousal loss can be a shocking and isolating experience without emotional preparation and can be complicated when others at the same life stage distance to avoid facing their own vulnerability.

A child's death, which reverses the natural order of life, is especially tragic—it seems unjust and dashes shared hopes and dreams. Parents and grandparents often struggle with the question "Why him/her and not me?" Prolonged mourning is common, with heartache often lasting many years and even a lifetime. Because parents are responsible for their children's well-being, they commonly are preoccupied with concerns that they should have prevented a death. With the loss of a child, a parental marriage is at heightened risk for discord, distancing, and divorce, yet spouses who support and sustain each other through the tragedy can forge even stronger relationships than before (Oliver, 1999). The common impetus to have another child can bring solace. Allowing time to experience the loss is encouraged so that the new relationship is not burdened by replacement needs or attachment difficulties.

Pileup of Losses and Other Stressors

The concurrence of loss with other major stressors or losses, incompatible demands, and cumulative strains often overload family functioning and interfere with grief. Complications are more likely when bereavement coincides with other family developmental transitions that require boundary shifts and redefinition of roles and relationships, particularly marriage, birth of a child, or launching of young adults (Walsh, 1983). In multi-stressed families, extended kin and social support are crucial to enable attention both to grief processes and to other challenges.

Past Losses and Intergenerational Legacies

The convergence of developmental and multigenerational strains heightens distress and the risk for dysfunction (Walsh & McGoldrick, 2004, 2013). Inquiry about family experiences of past losses explores how they influence expectations in the present loss situation, from catastrophic fears to a hopeful outlook. Experiences of resilience—in family histories, stories, and role models of adaptive coping and positive growth in response to past adversity—can inspire current efforts.

It is important to note transgenerational anniversary patterns, that is, when symptoms occur at the same point in the life cycle as a significant death or loss in a past generation. Some become preoccupied with their own or their spouse's mortality when they reach the same age or life transition point (e.g., retirement) at which a parent died. Many make abrupt career or relationship changes or start new fitness regimens and feel they must "get through the year," while others may behave self-destructively. Unresolved family patterns, or scenarios, may also be replicated when a child reaches the same age or stage as a parent at the time of a prior death or traumatic loss (Walsh, 1983).

An appreciation of the power of covert family scripts (Byng-Hall, 2004) and family legacies is important to understand the transmission of such patterns in loss. Anniversary reactions are more likely to occur when there has been a physical and emotional cutoff from the past and when family rules block open communication about past traumatic events. This occurred in the case of Martin's breakdown related to his father's past holocaust experience at the same age (see Chapter 1). Interventions aim to open covert patterns and help family members come to terms with the past and differentiate present relationships so that history need not repeat itself.

Family and Social Network

The general level of family functioning and the state of relationships prior to and following the loss should be carefully assessed, including extended family and social networks. Family belief systems, organizational patterns, and communication processes are crucial in mediating adaptation to loss. Particular note should be taken of the following variables.

Meaning-Making

Each family's belief system, rooted in multigenerational, sociocultural, and religious influences, powerfully influences its views toward death and its pathways in adaptation to loss. Meaning-making processes involve family members' attempts to make sense of their loss and put it in perspective to make it more bearable (Nadeau, 1997, 2008). Commonly they grapple with painful questions: Why us? Why my child (or sibling or spouse) and not me? How did this happen? Is someone to blame? Could it have been prevented? What can we do now? Such concerns remain salient when the cause of a death is unclear. Deaths that are sudden and unexpected or seem senseless can shatter core assumptions of normality, security, and predictability.

Clinicians need to explore beliefs that foster blame, shame, and guilt surrounding a death (Rolland, 1994), which can be fueled by Western values of personal responsibility, mastery, and control. Such causal attributions are especially strong when the cause is unclear and questions of responsibility or negligence arise. Family members commonly struggle with thoughts that they or others could have done something to prevent a death. It is important to help them share such concerns and come to terms with any accountability and the limits of control in the situation.

A Positive Outlook: Hope

Hope is most essential in times of deepest despair. Resilience involves mastery of the possible with acceptance of that which is beyond control. Family members may despair that, despite their best efforts, optimism, prayers, and medical care, they can't stop death. The focus of hope must shift from what is beyond their control to the dying process: making the most of precious time, alleviating suffering, and healing relational grievances. Although they cannot bring back a deceased loved one, when death shatters hopes and dreams we can help family members find renewed meaning to go on with life.

Transcendence and Spirituality

Death ends a life, but a relationship transcends death and is sustained through spiritual connection, memories, stories, and deeds. Our own death and that of our loved ones can be faced more openly and courageously through symbolic ways to view ourselves as part of a larger, meaningful whole. Those who believe in a spiritual afterlife or reincarnation find comfort in accepting death as a passage to another realm and, in Eastern and

Native American beliefs, part of a larger evolutionary cycle in the universe (Walsh, 2009d).

Spiritual beliefs and practices foster resilience in the face of death and loss (Walsh, 2009c). Research has documented the positive physiological effects of deep faith, prayer, meditative practices, and congregational support at these times (Koenig et al., 2012). Many find solace in the belief that a tragic death may be beyond human comprehension but part of God's larger plan, or a test of faith.

Religious beliefs can sometimes be a major source of distress. One mother in an interfaith marriage believed that the stillbirth of her second child was God's punishment for not having baptized her first child. In another case, a husband secretly believed the couple's infertility was God's punishment for his past infidelity. Some turn away from their faith. One bereaved father, after the death of his newborn son, who was to be named for him and his father, cried out, "I'm angry at God—how could he take the life of an innocent baby!" It is important for clinicians to include attention to the spiritual dimension in the experience of death, dying, and loss, and to consult with or refer to pastoral counselors as appropriate (Walsh, 2009d).

Suffering can be transcended through creative expression, as in writing, music, or the arts. Many honor the deceased through memorial dedications to benefit others. After the suicide of their young adult daughter, who suffered from bipolar disorder, one family organized public education programs on serious mental illness in her name. Families can transcend their personal loss through social activism or advocacy to prevent the suffering of other families. Healing is fostered by efforts to honor the best aspects of the deceased person and the relationship. As one mother stated after a reckless driver took the life of her daughter, "My daughter wouldn't want me to become consumed by grief or rage; she would want me to honor her life by taking up some meaningful pursuit in her memory." In research by Lietz (2007), resilient families often found new purpose in actions to prevent such tragedy for others.

Family Flexibility and Role Functioning

Family organization—the system of rules, roles, and boundaries—needs to be flexible, yet clearly structured, for reorganization after loss. It is helpful to inquire about what changed and what did not change with a death and how the family can restore or adapt familiar patterns in the wake of loss. A family that becomes disorganized with loss will need help building the authoritative leadership, stability, and continuity necessary to manage the disruptive aftermath. An overly rigid family may need help to modify set patterns and make necessary accommodations to loss.

A loss is greater the more important a person and his or her role function were in family life, such as a parent, grandparent, or sibling who played a major role in child rearing, or an adult child who was the primary caregiver for an elder. The death of an only child, an only son or daughter, or the last of a generation leaves a particular void. Families risk dysfunction if they avoid the pain of loss by seeking an instant replacement. At the other extreme, a family can become frozen in time if surviving members are unable to reallocate role functions or form new attachments.

Family Connectedness

Adaptation to loss is facilitated by strengthening cohesion and mutual support, with tolerance and respect for individual differences in the grief process. In an intensely fused family, any differences may be viewed as disloyal and threatening, leading members to submerge or distort feelings. To avoid the pain of loss, some families may turn to a child, a new partner, or a new baby as an emotional replacement, which can complicate that relationship and pose difficulties for attachment and later separation. Other families may avoid the pain with distancing and emotional cutoffs. When families are fragmented, members are left to fend for themselves, isolated in their grief.

State of Relationships at the Time of Death

All family relationships have occasional conflict, mixed feelings, or shifting alliances. The mourning process is likely to be more complicated if there has been intense and persistent conflict, strong ambivalence, or estrangement. The death of a troubled, abusive, or absent parent is difficult; an adult child may have long grieved for a parent he or she never had. One woman was hospitalized at age 70 with depression following the death of her 94-year-old father. She had vied unsuccessfully with her younger sister throughout her life for her father's favor. On his deathbed, he called for her sister. Even in later life, what pained her most in his death was the loss of future possibility that she might one day win his approval.

In end-of-life care, it is important to encourage family members to reconnect and to repair strained relationships before the opportunity is lost. Often this requires overcoming reluctance to stir up painful emotions or old conflicts. They may fear that confrontations could increase vulnerability and the risk of death. We need to deal sensitively with these concerns, interrupt destructive interactional spirals, and help family members to share feelings constructively with the aim of healing pained relationships, forging new connections, and building mutual support. A facilitated *family life review,* described in Chapter 9, can be a valuable process to integrate varied perspectives, clarify misunderstandings, place hurts and disappointments in the context of life challenges, recover caring aspects of relationships, and update and renew bonds frozen in past conflict. Individuals facing death and their loved ones often become more openhearted, compassionate, and remorseful for past mistakes and hurts, opening possibilities for forgiveness. At life's end, the simple words "I'm truly sorry" and "I love you" mean more than ever.

Extended Family, Social, and Economic Resources

It is crucial to mobilize supportive kin, friendship, and community networks. Internet resources can offer valuable information and support, but it is important to avoid information overload and misinformation. Family recovery is impaired when finances are drained by costly, protracted medical care, inadequate health insurance coverage, or the death of the major breadwinner. It is important to help families discuss such financial issues.

Clear, Open Communication

When a family confronts a loss, open communication facilitates the processes of emotional recovery and reorganization. Clinicians can help members to clarify facts and circumstances of an ambiguous or unacknowledged loss. The cover-up of an alcohol-related accident, a drug overdose, or a suicide carries its own painful legacy for survivors in further blocked communication, cutoffs, and self-destructive behavior. It is important to foster a family climate of mutual trust, empathic response, and tolerance for a wide and fluctuating range of responses to loss over time.

Gender-Related Issues

Although gender roles and relationships have been changing in recent decades, expectations for men and women in families are still influenced strongly by traditional gender-based norms. In bereavement, women have been socialized to assume the major role in handling the social and emotional tasks, from expression of grief to caregiving for the terminally ill and surviving family members, including their spouse's extended family. Men, who have been socialized to manage instrumental tasks, tend to take charge of funeral, financial, and property arrangements. In the dominant U.S. culture, they are more likely to become emotionally constrained and withdrawn around times of loss. Cultural constraints against revealing vulnerability or dependency can block emotional expressiveness and ability to seek and give comfort and contribute to a high risk of serious illness and death for men in the first year of widowhood.

Partners' different responses to loss, especially in the death of a child, can strain couple relationships. Men are more likely to express anger than sorrow and to withdraw, seek refuge in their work, or turn to alcohol, drugs, or an affair. They may be uncomfortable with their wives' expressions of grief, not knowing how to respond and fearful of losing control of their own feelings (culturally framed as "breaking down" and "falling apart"). Grieving individuals may perceive their partners' emotional unavailability as abandonment when they need comfort most, thereby experiencing a double loss (Johnson, 2002).

> Marlene was being seen in individual therapy for inconsolable grief after her only child, 18-year-old Jimmy, had collapsed and died in her arms. Marlene and Matt, a working-class African American couple, had worked very hard to raise Jimmy well and were extremely proud that he had just earned a scholarship to college. Although Matt, too, had lost his only child, he refused therapy for himself, saying he was fine and didn't need any help. Yet he drove Marlene to each session and waited for her in the car. When presented with clinic forms to sign, however, he balked; he did not want to fill out a symptom checklist or to be labeled as needing help. His stoic manner of maintaining control was a source of pride to him. However, he responded to the therapist's encouragement that he could be a helpful resource to his wife by sitting by her side and supporting her in sessions. It wasn't long until he gained trust in the therapist and shared his own deep pain of loss and both spouses found comfort in sharing their grief.

When one spouse has difficulty acknowledging vulnerability and sorrow at a time of tragedy, the other may then carry the emotions for both of them. Resentment may build toward the unavailable partner, who is felt to be insensitive and unsupportive. A couple approach is essential to build empathy, since the relationship is at risk. Interventions can decrease relational polarization so that partners can support each other and share in the full range of human experience in bereavement.

> Doreen and Nick were seen in couple therapy because she felt their "semi-committed" relationship was "deadlocked" and wanted either to get married or to end it. Most nights Nick came for dinner; after her

girls went to bed, he and Doreen would set up a cot next to her bed, where he spent the night, returning to his own apartment each morning. The therapist learned that 6 years earlier, within a few months of the sudden death of her husband, Doreen had accepted an offer by Nick, an old friend, to move with her children to his community to start a new life. Nick found her a job and an apartment—next door to his own. Because they had moved too quickly into this relationship, its status remained ambivalent. Doreen, devastated by the loss of her husband, had initially found support and consolation from Nick and had found the move a welcome escape; yet she became depressed, overweight, and unhappy in her job. Couple sessions revealed Nick's ongoing casual affairs with other women and his refusal ever to commit himself fully again since a bitter divorce and cutoff from his children. Doreen decided to end the relationship and move on with her life. With this loss, she found herself dreaming nightly of her deceased husband and was flooded with intense longings for him, opening up her delayed griefwork in therapy.

It is common for unattended mourning from a past loss to surface at the breakup of a replacement relationship. Individual sessions are valuable at that time to attend to the delayed grief process, review the earlier courtship, marriage, and family life, and explore the many meanings of the loss and subsequent life passages. Issues of loyalty and guilt are crucial to address. With the encouragement of the therapist, Doreen returned to her hometown to visit her husband's grave for the first time since the funeral and spent some time at the gravesite "telling him" all she would have liked him to know about their children's development and budding talents, the memories she would carry on of their life together, and their continuing love for him as they went forward in their lives. This visit and conversation brought her a sense of peace.

Concurrence with Other Losses, Stresses, or Life Changes

The temporal coincidence of a loss with other losses, other major stress events, or developmental milestones may overload a family and pose incompatible tasks and demands. Sketching a timeline can alert clinicians to the concurrence of losses and stressful transitions and their relation to the timing of symptoms. Particular attention should be paid to the concurrence of death with the birth of a child, since the processes of mourning and of parenting an infant are inherently conflictual. Moreover, a child born at the time of a significant loss may assume a special replacement function, which can be the impetus for high achievement or dysfunction. Similarly, a precipitous marriage in the wake of loss is likely to confound the two relationships, interfering with bereavement and with investment in the new relationship in its own right. When stressful events pile up, mobilizing the support of family members is especially important.

Past Traumatic Loss and Unresolved Mourning

Some individuals and families emerge hardier from past traumatic loss experiences, whereas others are left more vulnerable to subsequent losses. When problems with separation, attachment/commitment, or self-destructive behavior are presented in therapy, it is crucial to explore possible connections to earlier traumatic losses in the family system.

HELPING FAMILIES WITH LOSS: THERAPEUTIC CHALLENGES

As we've seen, healing and resilience in the face of loss are not simply matters of individual bereavement, but also involve family mourning processes. Of all human experiences, death poses the most painful and far-reaching adaptational challenges for families. A systemic framework for clinical assessment and intervention with loss is crucial to address the reverberations of a death for all family members, their relationships, and the family as a functional unit.

A family resilience-oriented approach to loss is guided by an understanding of major family adaptational challenges, variables that heighten risk, and key family processes that foster recovery. Given the diversity of family forms, values, and life courses, we must be careful not to confuse common patterns in response to loss with normative standards, or to assume that differences in bereavement are necessarily pathological. Helping family members deal with a loss requires respect for their particular faith beliefs and cultural heritage and encouragement to forge their own pathways through the mourning process.

Individual, couple, and family sessions may be combined flexibly to fit varied adaptive challenges over time. By strengthening key relationships and family functioning, a healing process can reverberate throughout the system to benefit all members. Although open communication and mutual support are emphasized, active processes in dealing with death and loss are also encouraged. The drawing up and discussion of wills, living wills, and directives by all adult family members (not only those most vulnerable) are advised. Planning and participating in meaningful memorial rites are also encouraged, as are visits to the grave—not only at the time of loss, but also on anniversaries, even years later. In cases where mourning has been blocked, we can encourage clients to sort through old photos and memorabilia, which open up memories and trigger the flow of old and new stories. They can share stories and mementos with children, other family members, and friends, setting off a chain of positive mutual influences for recovery and new resilience.

Dying and healing are not incompatible. Finding healing in the face of death involves integrating the fullness of the life and significant relationships. Bereaved families can find strength to surmount heartbreaking loss and go on living a meaningful life by bringing benefit to others from their own tragedy. Clinicians can help clients to find pride, dignity, and purpose in their darkest hours through altruistic actions such as organ donation, memorial contributions to medical research, or taking the initiative in forming support groups for families who have suffered similar losses or community action coalitions.

CHAPTER 11

Traumatic Loss
and Collective Trauma

Strengthening Family and Community Resilience

> Sorrow felt alone leaves a deep crater in the soul; sorrow
> shared yields new life.
> —*Nomathemba* (the Zulu word for hope)[1]

This chapter extends beyond the borders of the family to present a resilience-oriented, multisystemic family and community approach to recovery from traumatic experiences and traumatic loss. Key family and social processes in risk and resilience are outlined. Practice principles, intervention guidelines, and case illustrations are described in situations of community violence, war-related trauma, mass killings, and major disasters to suggest ways to foster family and community resilience.

TRAUMA, SUFFERING, AND RESILIENCE: MULTISYSTEMIC PERSPECTIVES

The word *trauma* comes from the Latin word for wound. Traumatic experiences can wound the body, mind, spirit, and relationships with others (Herman, 1992; van der Kolk, McFarlane, & Weisaeth, 2006). The

---

[1] Musical written by Ntozake Shange, Joseph Shabalala, and Eric Simon that recounts South Africa's turbulent journey from apartheid.

predominant therapeutic models for treating survivors of traumatic events have been individually based and pathology focused, identifying and reducing symptoms of PTSD, categorized as a mental illness. In contrast, a multilevel systemic, resilience-oriented practice approach situates the distress in the extreme trauma experience, attends to its ripple effects throughout relational networks, and strengthens family and community resources for optimal recovery.

The Impact of Traumatic Events on the Family and Community

There is growing attention to the multisystemic impact wrought by catastrophic events, war, and widespread disaster. Family systems approaches grew out of Hill's (1949) groundbreaking study of adjustment in World War II veterans and their families. In the field of trauma studies, Figley and others brought attention to the stressful impact on relational systems of war, catastrophic events, violence, and sexual abuse (Catherall, 2004; Figley & McCubbin, 1983). Families are essential resources in the recovery of a member suffering trauma effects. Yet major trauma affects the closest relationships of survivors and the well-being of loved ones—especially spouses, children, and parents. Secondary traumatization (Figley, 2002) occurs through learning about the trauma experienced, and in ongoing transactions and family life when disruptive symptoms, withdrawal, or harmful behaviors persist.

Families and their communities are intricately intertwined (Betancourt & Kahn, 2007) and can experience shared traumatic effects, as occurs in war, mass killings, and major disasters. Family functioning and vital kin networks can be disrupted, especially with complex, ongoing trauma situations, such as living in conditions of prolonged conflict or blighted communities. Therefore, attention to the family and wider impact of major trauma is essential in any treatment approach. Moreover, family and community networks are essential resources in trauma recovery and rebuilding shattered lives when their strengths and potential are mobilized (Denborough, 2006; Saul, 2013; Webb, 2003).

Resilience and Posttraumatic Growth

Traumatic stress research has brought increasing attention to resilience, with focus primarily on neurobiological and psychological processes in individuals (Southwick & Charney, 2012). Posttraumatic stress symptoms are heightened with greater intensity, frequency, and duration of extreme trauma experiences. But there is wide variation among individuals at the same level of risk. Studies across a wide range of traumatic situations and social contexts find that acute stress symptoms are common in the immediate aftermath, yet most distressed individuals experience recovery and resilience, rebounding over time, gaining strengths, and not suffering long-term disturbance (Litz, 2004; Masten & Narayan, 2012).

Moreover, the struggle to recover often yields remarkable transformation and growth. Studies of posttraumatic growth have found positive individual changes in five areas: (1) emergence of new opportunities and possibilities; (2) deeper relationships and greater compassion for others; (3) feeling strengthened to meet future life challenges; (4) reordered priorities and fuller appreciation of life; and (5) deepening spirituality (Calhoun & Tedeschi, 2013; Tedeschi & Calhoun, 2004; Tedeschi & Kilmer, 2005).

Van der Kolk and colleagues advanced a biopsychosocial understanding of trauma, its treatment, and its prevention, with attention to variables that influence vulnerability, resilience, and the course of posttraumatic reactions (van der Kolk et al., 2006). Although some individuals are more vulnerable to stress, no one is immune to suffering in extreme situations. The effects of trauma and the potential for recovery depend greatly on whether those wounded can seek comfort, reassurance, and safety with others. Strong connections, with trust that others will be there when needed, counteract feelings of insecurity, helplessness, or meaninglessness.

Mental health professionals can best foster trauma recovery by redirecting the predominant pathology focus and individual treatment approaches to address the impact in families and communities and mobilize their capacity for healing and resilience (Walsh, 2007). A multisystemic resilience-oriented approach contextualizes the distress, addresses the collective impact, and strengthens interpersonal and institutional resources for both individual and collective recovery and growth (Saul, 2013).

TRAUMA AND TRAUMATIC LOSS

The experiences of trauma, loss, and grief are intertwined (Figley, 1998; Lattanzi-Licht & Doka, 2003; Litz, 2004; Neimeyer, 2001). Deaths that are untimely, sudden, and/or violent are the most common source of trauma. Trauma situations may involve death; life-threatening bodily harm or disability; abduction, torture, incarceration, or persecution; forced migration/relocation; or relational violence and sexual abuse. Therapeutic attention to trauma recovery has focused mainly on individual survivors of interpersonal/relational violations, especially multiple complex trauma experiences

(Herman, 1992; Courtois, 2004). Serious harm or murder committed by relatives or close acquaintances is so devastating because it is inflicted by loved ones and those who are trusted and depended upon. Posttraumatic difficulties commonly persist for survivors in fears of commitment and intimacy (Johnson, 2002). Systemic approaches have been advanced by Almeida (Almeida & Durkin, 1999); Barrett and Stone Fish (2014); Coulter (2011); and Sheinberg and Fraenkel (2001).

This chapter focuses on shared trauma and loss in extreme situations beyond the family borders, including community violence; widespread atrocities in war and ethnic, religious, or political conflict; and mass trauma in major disasters or catastrophic events.

Various forms of trauma in such situations can involve multiple losses, including:

- Sense of physical or psychological wholeness (e.g., serious bodily harm or torture).
- Significant person, role, and relationships (e.g., family head or community leader).
- Intact family unit, homes, and communities.
- Way of life and economic livelihood.
- Future potential; hopes and dreams for all that might have been.
- Shattered assumptions in core world view (e.g., security, predictability, or trust).

Situations of traumatic loss pose high risk for complicated recovery, as summarized in Table 11.1, and require careful assessment and intervention focus (see also Chapter 10).

In traumatic loss, symptoms such as depression, anxiety, substance abuse, and relational conflict or withdrawal are common. Survivors blocked from healing may perpetuate wider suffering through self-destructive behavior and suicide, or revenge and harm toward others. Massive historical or ongoing trauma, with loss of hope and positive vision, can fuel transmission of negative trangenerational patterns (Danieli, 1985; Pinderhughes, 2004). With brutal atrocities and injustice, the impetus to restore a sense of family or community honor can either fuel cycles of mutual retaliation or spark courageous efforts to rise above the tragedy (see Chapter 14).

When traumatic loss is suffered, most do not experience "resolution" in the sense of completely getting over it. Families may gain partial "closure" on some aspects, such as the certainty or cause of death, but they don't simply bounce back (Walsh & McGoldrick, 2004). Recovery and resilience involve complex, gradual, and fluid processes over time, with various facets

TABLE 11.1. Situations of Traumatic Death and Loss

The meaning and impact of traumatic deaths are influenced by a number of variables in the loss situation that require careful assessment and attention.

- *Violent death.* A violent death is devastating for loved ones and especially for those who witnessed it or narrowly survived. Preoccupation with causal accusations, guilt, or wishes for revenge is common. A senseless tragedy or loss of innocent lives is especially hard to bear, particularly in deliberate acts of violence.

- *Untimely death.* Untimely losses are hardest to bear. The deaths of children and young spouses seem unjust and rob us of future hopes and dreams. The loss of parents with young children requires reorganization of the family system.

- *Sudden death.* With sudden losses, loved ones lack time even to say their good-byes. Like a bolt out of the blue, a sense of normalcy and predictability is shattered. Shock and intense emotions, as well as disorganization and confusion, are expectable in the immediate crisis period. Family members may need help with painful regrets.

- *Prolonged suffering.* With prolonged physical or emotional suffering before death (e.g., assault, torture, or lack of medical assistance), the agony for family members can be great, coupled with guilt, anger, or remorse.

- *Ambiguous loss.* Ambiguity as to whether a missing loved one is alive or dead can immobilize families who may be torn apart, hoping for the best while fearing the worst (Boss, 1999). Mourning may be blocked until bodily remains or personal effects are recovered and the death becomes physically real. Families may need help in pressing for more information and in resuming lives in the face of remaining uncertainty.

- *Unacknowledged, stigmatized losses.* Mourning is complicated when losses or their cause are hidden due to social stigma (e.g., HIV/AIDS). Secrecy, misinformation, and estrangement impede family and social support, as well as critical health care.

- *Pileup of effects.* Families can be overwhelmed by the emotional, relational, and functional impact of multiple deaths, prolonged or recurrent trauma, and other losses (homes, jobs, communities) and disruptive transitions (e.g., separations, migration).

- *Past traumatic experience.* Past trauma and losses can be reactivated in life-threatening or loss situations, intensifying the impact and complicating recovery.

of grief alternating and reemerging with unexpected intensity, particularly around nodal events. Attention commonly oscillates between preoccupation with grief and reengagement in a world forever transformed by the tragedy (Stroebe & Schut, 2010). To foster recovery and resilience in the wake of major traumatic events, we can usefully apply the four tasks in family adaptation to loss (Walsh & McGoldrick, 2004, 2013; see Chapter

10). Pathways in recovery and resilience vary with personal, family, cultural, and spiritual preferences. Family and community forums and interfaith memorial events can help families and communities support, respect, and bridge differences.

Research finds that adaptive mourning involves the transformation of the relationship from physical presence to continuing bonds, rather than the need to gain detachment emphasized in traditional griefwork approaches. This is facilitated through spiritual or symbolic connections, memories, deeds, and stories that are passed on across the generations, bringing forward the best in the lived experience (Stroebe, Schut, & Boerner, 2010; Walsh & McGoldrick, 2004, 2013; also see Chapter 9). Coming to terms with traumatic loss involves finding ways to make meaning of the trauma experience, put it in perspective, and weave the experience of loss and recovery into the fabric of individual and collective identity and life passage.

FAMILY AND SOCIAL PROCESSES
FOR RESILIENCE WITH COLLECTIVE TRAUMA

The family resilience framework presented in this volume (see Chapters 3–8) can help families and communities recover from traumatic experiences and grow stronger. Attention to the following key processes in belief systems, organizational patterns, and communication/problem-solving can reduce vulnerability and risk and foster resilience (see Table 11.2).

Belief Systems

It is crucial to explore family and cultural beliefs that influence members' perceptions and coping responses in traumatic experiences. Clinicians can facilitate the following processes in resilience, which overlap with processes found in posttraumatic growth (PTG) (Calhoun & Tedeschi, 2013).

Making Meaning of Traumatic Experiences

Core beliefs ground and orient people, providing a sense of reality, normalcy, meaning, or purpose in life. Well-being is fostered by expectations that others can be trusted; that communities are safe; that life is orderly and events predictable; that children will outlive their elders; that society is just. When traumatic experiences shatter such assumptions, there is a deep need to restore order, meaning, and purpose (Janoff-Bulman, 1992).

TABLE 11.2. Traumatic Loss: Key Family and Social Processes in Risk and Resilience

Vulnerabilities, risks for maladaptation	Facilitate key processes for resilience
Belief systems	

Vulnerabilities, risks for maladaptation	Facilitate key processes for resilience

• Shattered assumptions; ambiguous or senseless loss
• Sense of failure/fault; blame, shame, guilt
• Hopelessness, despair; bleak outlook
• Powerlessness: helpless, overwhelmed
• Multigenerational legacy: trauma, losses, catastrophic fears
• Spiritual distress; sense of injustice, punishment for sins; cultural/spiritual disconnection, void
	1. Make meaning of traumatic loss experience
	  • Normalize, contextualize distress.
	  • Gain sense of coherence as shared challenge: comprehensible, manageable, meaningful.
	2. Positive outlook: hope, future dreams
	  • Affirm strengths, build on potential.
	  • Master the possible; accept what can't be changed.
	3. Transcendence and spiritual connection
	  • Faith beliefs, practices, community; nature; arts
	  • Purpose, meaningful bonds, pursuits; activism
	  • Learning, transformation, growth

Organizational processes	

Vulnerabilities, risks for maladaptation	Facilitate key processes for resilience

• Rigid, autocratic or unstable—chaotic, unreliable, leaderless
• Enmeshed, highly conflictual, or estranged bonds
• Vital bond or role functioning lost:
• Precipitous replacement, exploitation, or abuse of other
• Inability to reallocate roles or reinvest in relationships
• Socially isolated; unacknowledged or stigmatized loss
• Institutional barriers; economic resources lost, unavailable
	4. Flexibility to adapt and restabilize
	  • Restore structure, routines, predictability
	  • Reorganize; realign role functions
	  • Strong leadership: coordination
	5. Connectedness: family, social, and community
	  • Lifelines; mutual support; social network
	  • Repair estranged relationships
	6. Economic and institutional resources

Communication/problem solving processes	

Vulnerabilities, risks for maladaptation	Facilitate key processes for resilience

• Ambiguous information about death/loss situation
• Secrecy, distortion, denial of loss event
• Blocked emotional sharing or high conflict
• Gender constraints (e.g., "Men don't cry")
• Lack of pleasurable interaction, respite
• Blocked problem solving, decision making
	7. Clear, consistent information, messages
	  • Clarify trauma and loss-related ambiguity.
	8. Open emotional expression, empathic response
	  • Respect individual, cultural differences.
	  • Share pleasure, humor, respite amidst sorrow.
	9. Collaborative decision making, problem solving
	  • Resourcefulness; build on small steps, successes
	  • Proactive planning, preparedness; "Plan B"

Meaning reconstruction in response to trauma and loss is a central process in healing (Neimeyer, 2001). It can reflect a new wisdom from experience and a testament to strengths forged. In our work, we may need to help people envision a new sense of normality, identity, and relatedness to adapt to altered conditions. Our task is not to make meaning for them, but to support their efforts in finding their own meaning out of their experience (Frankl, 1946/1984).

It is important to contextualize family and community members' distress as understandable and common in such traumatic situations. We support their efforts to gain a sense of coherence, rendering their situation more comprehensible, manageable, and meaningful as a shared challenge. When an earthquake destroyed a family's home, the father recounted, "At first we were in a state of shock, disoriented, at a total loss about what to do. Then we dusted ourselves off, took stock of our sorry predicament, and pulled together to clear out the debris and figure out our options. We just kept hugging each other, taking it step by step."

Family members may struggle over a period of time to make sense of what happened, gain perspective, and make it more bearable (Nadeau, 1997, 2008). Commonly, they grapple with painful questions such as "Why us?" "Why my child? Why not me?" "How did this happen?" "Who was at fault?" "Could it have been prevented?" Such concerns persist when, for instance, the cause of a plane crash, fire, or explosion remains unclear. Clinicians can help families gain and share factual information that is helpful. We explore concerns that foster blame, shame, and guilt and help clients come to terms with their regrets, accountability, and limits of control in their situation. Taking lessons from the experience can help to guide future actions.

Hope: A Positive Outlook

In times of deep despair, hope is essential to fuel energies and spirits needed to rebuild lives, revise dreams, and create positive legacies to pass on. We help families direct efforts to "master the possible," gradually coming to terms with what has been lost or cannot be changed. We may need to help some to tolerate prolonged uncertainty and lengthy recovery processes, while holding on to hope in future possibilities with their sustained efforts.

Transcendence and Spirituality

With traumatic loss, transcendent cultural and spiritual values and practices can offer meaning, purpose, and connectedness. Many find solace in believing that catastrophic events beyond human comprehension are a test of faith or part of God's larger plan. Prayer, meditative practices, and/or faith communities can offer solace and support. In human-caused tragedies, faith beliefs can open up a pathway of forgiveness (see Chapter 14). Spiritual connection, memories, stories, and deeds can honor the best aspects of those who died, all that was lost, and the courage and resilience forged. Active involvement in memorial rituals, vigils, anniversary remembrances, rites of passage, and celebration of milestones in recovery all facilitate healing. They also provide opportunities to reaffirm identity, relatedness, and core social values of goodness and compassion (Imber-Black, 2012). Finding ways to celebrate holidays and birthdays, which often go unmarked with turmoil or grief, can boost spirits and reconnect all with the rhythms of life.

Profound suffering can be transcended in creative expression through the arts. Music, such as participation in community or congregational singing, can release sorrow and restore the spirit to carry on. Finding ways to express the experience of trauma *and* survival through writing, drama, music, or artwork can facilitate resilience, especially for children.

Healing is aided through memorial dedications to honor those who were lost. Many find new purpose through community activism or advocacy to benefit others and prevent future suffering (Perry & Rolland, 2009). Learning and growth out of tragedy can spark new priorities and deepened commitments. Recovery is a journey of the heart and spirit, bringing survivors back to the fullness of life.

Organizational Processes

Flexible Structure

For resilience, families and communities must effectively organize to respond to highly disruptive events. Flexibility is needed to adapt to unforeseen challenges and changing conditions. At the same time, it is crucial to restore order, safety, and stability to reduce the sense of chaos and disorientation that comes with transitional upheaval. Children especially find reassurance as daily routines can be resumed or new arrangements put in place. Strong leadership and coordination of response efforts is essential, with collaboration between families and social networks. In major disasters, community groups, agencies, and all government levels involved in rescue, recovery, and reconstruction efforts must have clear plans, lines of authority, coordination, and communication. Clear rules and guidelines are essential, with consistent follow-through. With the loss of basic infrastructure, family and social systems must reorganize, recalibrate, and reallocate roles and functions. Yet, at all levels, they must be nimble enough to readily shift gears as needed.

Connectedness

With traumatic experiences, when helplessness and terror are common, we have an urgent need for connection, to hear the voice of a loved one and to turn to one another for support, comfort, and safety. While high cohesion is essential, tolerance and respect are needed for individual differences in response. Some, especially small children, may show anxious clinging or need constant contact; others may avoid the pain or loss by distancing. In chaotic situations such as evacuations, every effort should be made to keep family members together so they are not left to fend for themselves, isolated in their suffering and worried about loved ones, as occurred in the aftermath of Hurricane Katrina. With separations and ambiguous loss, contact information and communication are essential to ease concerns and facilitate reunion. When trauma has involved a relational violation, trust and security are more difficult to restore. In troubled or estranged relationships, distress may be intensified by unresolved conflicts. Counseling can be helpful to foster healing, reconnection, and reconciliation (see Chapter 14).

Social and Economic Resources and Extended Kin

With collective trauma and loss, it is crucial to mobilize institutional services as well as kin, social, and community networks for emotional and practical support. Social supports might include friends, neighbors, and health care providers; clergy and congregational support; schoolteachers and counselors; employers and coworkers; and community organizations. Multifamily support groups and community forums are valuable for exchanging information, sharing memories and accounts of loss and survival, providing mutual support, and encouraging hope and efforts for recovery. Financial assistance and follow through with expected compensation can be critical with the loss of homes and jobs, medical expenses, or rebuilding costs.

Communication and Problem Solving

Clear, Helpful Information

Families often need help to clarify the facts and circumstances of traumatic events and the steps they can take to improve their situation. Practical guidelines can assist them in rebuilding their lives. To avert confusion and frustration, those in charge of emergency and recovery plans should provide consistent and accurate information, correcting errors and updating changes swiftly. After the failed response to Hurricane Katrina, one resident in the stricken area remarked, "If FedEx can track packages worldwide why can't the government even track the delivery of ice?" (which melted in trucks awaiting communication on their destination).

Emotional Sharing and Support

Traumatic events can trigger a wide range and fluctuation of intense feelings among survivors, with ripple effects throughout the kin and social network. One boy said the emotional upheaval was like "a roller-coaster ride that wouldn't stop." When painful or unacceptable feelings can't be expressed, or are seen as disloyal or threatening, it is important to foster a climate of mutual trust, empathic response, and tolerance for differences over time.

Collaborative Problem Solving/Proaction

Practical assistance with immediate needs is a first priority. Goals should be approached concretely with practical, realistic steps, tasks, and projects. Over time, with the slow pace of recovery and rebuilding of lives, it is important to rally family and community efforts to experience small gains and mark progress. Above all, it's crucial to shift from a crisis-reactive mode to a proactive stance, learning lessons for preparedness planning to lower future risks and meet new threats with greater resilience.

WHEN FAMILIES SUFFER
FROM VIOLENCE IN THE COMMUNITY

Every day, violence takes a terrible toll in communities worldwide (Aisenberg & Herrenkohl, 2008). As Kaethe Weingarten (2004) notes, it can become a common shock, affecting us yet barely arousing us until our lives or the lives of those we know are directly affected. Each violent incident is a tragedy for the families it touches.

Collaborative actions by families and communities, facilitated by helping professionals, can promote healing and resilience, as in the following case. A tragic shooting death, in a neighborhood near my home, began on a warm summer evening with an escalation of taunts between white and Latino youth, which turned lethal. With the catalyzing engagement of a parish priest and his congregation, and the courageous efforts of the parents of the boy who was killed, a remarkable journey of recovery, transcendence, and transformation was forged over the following year (Shefsky, 2000; Terkel, 2000, 2002).

When Mario Ramos, an 18-year-old Latino gang member, was charged with the shooting death of another boy in the community, his family's parish priest, Father Oldershaw, told his congregation, "He is a son of our parish; we must reach out to him and his family and offer our prayers and assistance." He visited Mario's loving parents, hardworking immigrants, who were in deep pain and struggling to comprehend their son's violent act. The priest visited Mario in detention, ministered to him, and encouraged parishioners to write to him and also to pray for the Young family, whose son he had killed. Although the Youngs were not members of his parish, Father Oldershaw extended himself, going to their home to offer his condolences and to let them know he was there for them if he could ever be of assistance. Mr. Young was at first angered by the visit: "This was his kid who killed our son!" But a few nights later, unable to sleep, he called the priest after midnight and they talked for over an hour. The priest's outreach and compassion led the parents to visit his parish, where they found solace in the caring community.

Over several months, the faith community's outreach to Mario fostered a genuine transformation in Mario; he left the gang, affiliated with a Christian group for support, and wrote a letter to Mrs. Young to express his deep remorse for the killing and to ask for her forgiveness.

Mrs. Young's own deep faith from her childhood led her to write to Mario to offer compassion and forgiveness. Their letters crossed in the mail. As she later explained, she came to this decision in order to heal from the tragedy and be better able to help her family in their unbearable suffering. Her husband hadn't been able to work for months, her surviving children were devastated, and the youngest son had run into traffic hoping to be hit so he could join his big brother in heaven. She understood her husband's deep anger, and the common impulse for revenge, but she spoke out against any retaliation. She said she felt she would lose her mind if she didn't try to draw something positive out of the tragedy. She found inspiration from her religious upbringing, recalling from the Bible that unforgiveness corrodes the body, the mind, and the spirit. In offering forgiveness, she clearly held Mario accountable for the killing and its devastating impact on her entire family. She continued contact with him and urged him to take responsibility for making something good of his life, investing herself in his rehabilitation. As she later said, "He came into our life through an act of violence, but now he's in my heart. . . . There's no way to bring back my son, but here's a life with potential that I don't want to waste."

Although her husband did not take her path of forgiveness, it was crucial for their relationships that he respected her way of healing. Mr. Young forged his own transcendent pathway, channeling his anger and sorrow through community activism. He took leadership in an organization to stop gun violence and worked tirelessly on behalf of the many families in the larger community who had lost a child. His wife joined him in that effort, both finding that their efforts furthered their healing and yielded more energy to devote to their children's recovery.

At Mario's sentencing hearing, Father Oldershaw accompanied his mother, saying, "I want to sit at your side to give you courage." When Mr. Young arrived, the priest introduced them. Although Mrs. Ramos spoke no English, Mr. Young saw the sorrow in her eyes for his loss and tearfully embraced her, realizing that they both had lost their sons: his to a grave and hers to prison.

Key processes in resilience are evident in this remarkable case. Gradually, over many months, the Youngs and Mario became determined to "master the possible," directing their energies to forge some good out of the tragedy and to prevent future violence. Most significant was the power in tapping relational connections and spiritual resources—through faith beliefs, the involvement of the clergy and congregation, and new purpose in community activism. These resources, long neglected in the mental health field, can be vital pathways in resilience.

Families of victims—and those of offenders—need ongoing support and advocacy. Most are better able to go on with their lives when they feel that justice has been served. Yet many experience further trauma in lengthy, convoluted processes in the criminal justice system. Families of offenders often face social condemnation, isolation, and neglect with presumptions of blame. In the case above, the priest's bridging of the two families transcended barriers and fostered mutual compassion. On the first anniversary of the tragedy, he invited both families to join him for dinner and prayers. With the efforts of the two families, the parish community, and a pro bono attorney, Mario's sentence was significantly reduced and he continued on a positive path. Their efforts were grounded in a deep conviction in the worth and potential of the offending youth. Movements for restorative justice emphasize such actions to repair harm and restore the humanity of the offender. When families and community members join efforts, the results, as in this case, can be transformational.

Mass Killings

The fatal shooting of 26 small children and staff at Sandy Hook Elementary School in a peaceful New England town underscored the vulnerability of all children and families to unthinkable tragedy. Under the glare of the national media, each family struggled to find its own path in healing. The families recognize that they will never be "over" their grief, and will likely carry their sorrow though their lives, yet for most, it gets easier to bear over time. Many forge resilience through efforts to honor the memory of their child. Here is just one story, excerpted from a local newspaper report (Dobbs, 2014):

> In the 14 months since 6-year-old Catherine was killed, her immediate family and distant relatives have channeled their memories of her into building a living tribute: an animal sanctuary that will bear her name. They've kept youngsters involved throughout the whole process, organizing bake sales and selling T-shirts to help spread the message. Catherine's 10-year-old cousin, Jack, wanting to pitch in, created a fundraising group called Catherine's Peace Team and spread the word on the Internet, gaining Facebook followers and donations from around the world. Several teenagers involved in Catherine's Peace Team held a fundraising dance and a Peace Party. When Jack thinks of his cousin, he recalls a time when they were playing tag in the yard—how Catherine lost interest quickly and went off to chase butterflies instead. When family members were thinking of a way to honor her legacy, her love of animals led them to the sanctuary. "It's definitely an outlet for us to do what we know Catherine would want," said her mother.
>
> Yet, as the rest of the world has moved on, her relatives carry a sadness that few others can comprehend. Her uncle says, "The pain is still there. . . . Nothing can replace her. But you figure out a way to cope with it every day." Her mother adds, "It's hard to see Freddy (her brother) sledding by himself. Last year, it was too painful to even talk about the times when she and Freddy went sledding. But that's becoming more doable, and we can cherish those memories." Now, when Freddie has a dream about Catherine, it becomes a happy topic of conversation, rather than a painful reminder of her death. Increasingly, they push past her death and think about her life: how she'd catch bugs and frogs and whisper to them; how she'd try and help the old family dog to its feet, though it was twice her size. About how much she would've loved the sanctuary that they're building. "We have a lifetime of healing. It will never be the same," her mother says. "But we're starting to put down roots for what will be Catherine's legacy. What we're doing is building something beautiful." She adds, "Her hand is in everything that we do."

Ongoing Community Violence

An entire community suffers with complex, ongoing trauma in blighted neighborhoods affected by chronic stresses of poverty and discrimination. Daily life for children and families is much like living in a war zone (Garbarino, 1997). With the proliferation of guns in the United State, lethal violence takes a tragic toll on young lives, too often in poor minority communities. It is frequently the result of personal grievances, domestic violence, or suicide, or is associated with gang and drug activity, At times, it is the result of misguided law enforcement and racial profiling, shattering the community's trust in those who should be protecting it and fueling outrage at injustices. Tensions and violence are often sparked by repeated experiences of racial or ethnic profiling and disrespect toward those who live on the margins of society and who lack social acceptance, resources, and opportunities for educational and economic advancement. Catastrophic fears and destructive behavior patterns often emanate from multiple traumas and losses across family generations. With a brother in prison and a son recently killed in a drive-by shooting, one mother sadly observed, "We never know who will be with us or lost tomorrow." Some individuals try to numb the recurrent pain, terror, and helplessness with alcohol or drugs, or by shutting off emotions and concern about themselves or others, in the belief that "If I don't care, then it won't hurt."

Yet when we think of community violence, we need to be careful not to blame and write off the community or assume the worst of its residents. In the face of such conditions, most families show remarkable resilience in carrying on their lives each day, striving to raise their children well, toward a better future. However, in many housing projects and dangerous neighborhoods, families are often isolated from one another, lacking supportive connections. Ongoing parent groups, with easy access, offer a context for sharing concerns and strategies for overcoming obstacles (see Chapter 13). In many programs (see Chapter 8), older men form mentoring relationships with gang members and youth at risk in efforts to stem the tide of violence and encourage school and job pursuits toward a better life. Neighborhood-based programs, such as Take Back the Streets, build family and community resilience, as they combat violent crime by bringing together residents, police, and social agencies to work collaboratively and build a sense of pride and empowerment.

MAJOR DISASTERS:
COLLECTIVE TRAUMA AND HEALING

Major disasters produce widespread disruption and loss. The distinction of natural versus human-made disasters has blurred, with recognition of multiple factors in many situations, as in climate change and environmental calamities such as earthquakes, extreme drought, and the widespread destruction wrought by Hurricane Sandy along the U.S. East Coast. In many cases, human actions, or inactions, compound the effects of natural events, as in the breach of faulty levees that flooded the city of New Orleans with Hurricane Katrina.

Each survivor's experience is unique in sources of suffering and pathways in resilience. Helping professionals can assist in healing emotional wounds by understanding the particular impact and meaning of a trauma situation and by reknitting fractured relationships, as in the following case:

> In Southeast Asia, many months after floodwaters inundated a coastal community, a teacher in a nearby town found a 12-year-old boy sleeping in the streets, suffering deeply. When asked what had happened, he told her that the day of the flood, he had been arriving home with his father when they saw his mother carried off in the surge. His father yelled at him to swim out and save her, but he stood frozen in place as his father berated him. Afterward he ran away and had not seen his family since. He was too ashamed to tell his father he didn't know how to swim. He couldn't forgive himself for not saving his mother's life. Still reluctant to visit his father, he agreed to go with a counselor to see his uncle. Upon hearing the account, his uncle reassured him that the floodwaters that day were too strong for even a good swimmer to save the lives of the many who were lost. He added that he knew that the father himself could not swim, which was why, in his own helplessness, he had turned to his son with such desperation. The uncle took the boy in and arranged a reunion of father and son, beginning their healing from that tragic day.

The pileup effect of multiple losses, dislocations, and adaptational challenges can be overwhelming. The sadness is compounded when former lives can't be restored; as one parent put it, "It's a cascade of sorrows." Meaning-making and recovery involve a struggle to understand what has been shattered, how to build new lives, and how to prevent future tragedy. As in an earthquake, we need to learn what weaknesses in structures contributed to their collapse—but we can learn even more from the strengths of those that withstood such damage.

Even small scraps of family life salvaged from the wreckage of a disaster can hold special meaning. When a recent tornado slashed through a town near Chicago, residents emerged from basements and community shelters to find their homes ripped from the foundations, with furniture and possessions scattered widely. Residents in surrounding communities set up a website, posting photos of found items—a page of a love letter, a child's doll, framed photos. One family found great comfort in retrieving a vase—cracked but not shattered—that had blown over a hundred miles away. It stands on the new mantelpiece in the home they are building on a more solid foundation.

As attention goes to bereaved families, those who survived a disaster can face a lonely road ahead. After a school fire killed nearly 100 children, one girl who survived became depressed when everyone kept telling her how brave and lucky she was. No one asked about her terrifying experience, and she never revealed her deep shame: how in panic she had clawed her way through the smoke-filled classroom, stepping over fallen classmates, to reach the window to jump. Another girl, who suffered spinal injuries when she jumped, was welcomed home from the hospital as a hero by friends and neighbors; yet many later avoided contact with her, too uncomfortable at seeing her injuries and being reminded of the tragedy. Another surviving child had lasting self-doubt from the inadvertent meaning she had taken from the message of her pastor, who consoled the bereaved families by saying that God had taken his special angels: "What did it mean that God didn't choose me?"

PATHWAYS IN RECOVERY AND RESILIENCE

Early intervention is important for those who have suffered trauma and traumatic loss (Litz, 2004). Relieving acute distress and mobilizing resources for recovery can be crucial to prevent more serious and chronic PTSD. Yet we should be wary of a "quick fix." Crisis intervention can be immensely helpful in providing initial information and support. However, some debriefing programs designed for crisis workers (e.g., Critical Incident Stress Debriefing) have been found to be unhelpful and in many cases increased distress when applied in a one-session format with survivors of collective trauma immediately after the event (Emmerik, Kamphuis, Hulsbosch, & Emmelkamp, 2002). Suffering was exacerbated by a narrow focus on individual trauma symptoms; by increasing worry that common trauma reactions could be an early sign of PTSD, a psychiatric disorder; and by opening up intense, overwhelming, and painful memories and feelings, including helplessness and rage, and then sending individuals home without follow-up.

Multifamily groups can provide a supportive context for those who went through a harrowing experience. Early interventions are most helpful when they (1) normalize and contextualize distress; (2) draw out strengths and active coping strategies for empowerment; (3) mobilize family and social support for ongoing recovery; and (4) offer follow-up sessions, as well as mental health services for those in severe and persisting distress.

The following facilitator guidelines are useful in multifamily group sessions:

- Start with grounding in members' personal, family, community, cultural, and spiritual identity and connections.
- Invite them to share a few aspects of their crisis experience that stood out for them. Offer acknowledgment and compassionate witnessing of recent and ongoing crises, losses, hardships, or injustices that they have suffered.
- Draw out and affirm their strengths and the potential shown by their endurance and coping efforts—their own and those shown in stories of others' positive responses demonstrating courage, ingenuity, or generosity.
- Facilitate shared meaning-making and mastery over several sessions. Refocus sensitively from what has happened to them to what they can do about their situation—from helplessness or victimization to active initiative and empowerment. Shift from a global sense of despair and immobilization to a more hopeful outlook and manageable step-by-step progress.
- Identify resources for resilience in important connections in their lives (link to those noted above in initial grounding) as lifelines in their recovery process, such as their extended kin network, ethnic or religious community, or personal faith in contemplative practices.
- Identify personal, relational, and spiritual resources that their families drew on in past times of adversity, such as pride in their "can-do" spirit," and stories of resilience that might inspire current efforts.

Families, teachers, counselors, and other workers find journals, music, and artwork especially helpful with children and adolescents. One program designed for use in many disaster situations to facilitate meaning-making, emotional expression, and active coping uses activity books to help children express their experience of both suffering and resilience (Kliman, Oklan, Wolfe, & Kliman, 2005). Drawing, coloring, and word activities help children to remember, document, and integrate not only the sad, bad, and scary parts, but also the helpful, brave, and good things people did. In journal format, older children are invited to describe what they learned; what would be helpful now; and things that they, their families, and their community could do to rebuild and to be more prepared in the future.

We attend to family processes in recovery over time. As one study of family resilience following Hurricane Katrina documented, all directly affected families had an initial drop in functioning, one parent saying they "hit rock bottom." Over the following months, most families experienced a roller-coaster course with the recovery efforts, facing a pileup of ongoing disaster-related stressors and other family crises, such as the death of a caregiving grandmother (Knowles, Sasser, & Garrison, 2010). Yet many rose above past baselines, achieving higher levels of family functioning and positive growth, and evidencing key processes in the family resilience framework presented in this volume (and in Walsh, 2003). In particular, families gained resilience through spiritual resources, efforts in meaning-making, open emotional expression, and collaborative problem solving. The study also found that families who experienced long-term lowered functioning lacked social supports, job opportunities, and economic resources. Many were stuck in overcrowded government-supplied trailers, without job opportunities or progress in the rebuilding of their homes.

I've served for many years as a consultant to the Porter-Cason Institute at Tulane University in New Orleans, founded to provide strengths-based family-centered training and community services. On one visit, 5 years post-Katrina, at a community mental health agency in St. Bernard parish—which had lost nearly 100% of its housing—families were still facing persistent obstacles beyond their control. Community residents who demonstrated resilience in their own recovery efforts were involved as peer counselors in a collaborative program to serve families that were struggling. One mother, still in a temporary FEMA trailer with her five children, summed it up: "We're alive but we're not yet living."

Nearby, in Plaquemines Parish, three-generation fishing families, many of whom were refugees from Southeast Asia after the Vietnam War, were struggling to recover from the major oil spill that devastated the coastal region. Meaning-making efforts and future planning were confused and frustrated by repeated unclear and inconsistent information over many months by government and industry officials about future expectations: Will fish be safe to eat and will the fishing industry survive or be destroyed? Should the younger generation rebuild the family business or disperse to find new livelihoods elsewhere, breaking up the strong family networks that supported their resilience with migration? In such widespread disasters, professionals are urged to work not only with families in distress but also with the larger systems affecting their recovery, especially government authorities, to clarify and support future prospects for recovery, post updated website information and resource contacts, and hold community forums to facilitate communication and collaborative efforts.

The revitalization of New Orleans as a vibrant community has been remarkable. The annual Mardi Gras was held amidst the devastation just 6 months after Katrina. Musicians and floats in the parade expressed a mix of sorrow, pride, hope, humor, satire, and surrealism—some came in costume as mold, mocking the failures of public officials and FEMA. Leading jazz musicians were concerned that many local musicians had lived in inadequate housing prior to the catastrophe and remained displaced. They rallied support to create a new housing development, Musicians' Village, which became a cornerstone of the New Orleans Area Habitat for Humanity post-Katrina rebuilding effort (*www.nolamusiciansvillage.org*). The core idea behind Musicians' Village was the establishment of a community for the city's several generations of musicians and other families. A central part of this vision was the Ellis Marsalis Center for Music, a focal point for teaching and performance, sharing and preserving the rich musical tradition of a city and reaching out to involve low-income youth and families.

The long and varied paths in healing emotionally and rebuilding lives require a longitudinal approach to take into account emerging stressors and adaptational processes over time (e.g., Litz, 2004), with the flexible availability of professionals and the support of kin and social networks over many months, and often much longer. Survivors frequently note that there were times when they suffered so deeply they didn't know if they could face another day, or felt that life no longer had meaning—but then they rallied to carry on. With the press of immediate practical demands, family members may suppress emotional needs. They may not seek counseling until months later, after initial social support wanes and the full impact of losses and emerging challenges is felt or distress intensifies. This will require pacing of interventions attuned to each family at various nodal points, weaving back and forth in attention to grief, emerging challenges, and future directions, and allowing time for respite and replenishing of energies.

As studies of resilience amply document, in struggling through hardship, reaching out to others, and making active coping efforts, people tap resources they may not have drawn on otherwise and gain new abilities and perspectives on life. Each survivor's experience is unique, yet the human compassion and generosity that emerge are remarkable. In the widespread Ebola outbreak in West Africa, one physician noted that amid the horrible deaths in the isolation wards, there were moments of grace. Mothers whose babies had died would feed and care for children who were orphaned.

It can be devastating for those who could not save loved ones in a disaster. One man was distraught that he had been unable to hold on to his wife, who was severely disabled, as they tried to escape their burning apartment building. Still, her last words kept him going: "Take care of the kids." He said, "It's hard every day; I've never had to do this before. I didn't know how—but I'm finding I can do it. Her voice and her spirit give me the strength and determination."

Another disaster can reactivate past trauma but also offer opportunities for further healing. Families of the victims of a terrorist-caused plane crash over Lockerbie, Scotland, found their pain revived by another plane crash 8 years later—one father described it as being "like a scab torn off a deep wound." Yet many of those families came forward and offered support to the recently bereaved families, finding that their assistance furthered their own long-term recovery as well.

Multisystemic Approaches to Recovery and Resilience

In humanitarian crises, multisystemic resilience-oriented approaches draw on and expand individual, family, and community resources that have a recursive synergy and are the critical components of healing from widespread trauma and loss (Miller, 2012; Mollica, 2006; Saul, 2013; Weine, 2011). Landau's LINC framework, grounded in disaster recovery experience in many parts of the world, identifies and links with these natural resources to create a matrix of healing (Landau, 2007; Landau, Mittal, & Wieling, 2008). Professionals take a consultative role, encouraging natural leaders and change agents within the community. Family and community members with diverse skills, talents, and ages can contribute in different ways to the resilience of the community. The elderly can bring memories and lessons of coping with previous adversity, while the young renew the capacity for play and creativity. This approach is highly effective in ensuring long-term viability and hope for the future.

With massive psychosocial trauma in major disasters, Landau and Saul (2004) have found that community resilience encompasses the following four themes:

1. Building community and enhancing social connectedness as a foundation for recovery by strengthening social support systems, coalition building, and sharing information and resources.
2. Collective storytelling and validation of the trauma experience and response, with the emerging story broad enough to encompass the many varying experiences.
3. Reestablishing the rhythms and routines of life and engaging in collective healing rituals.
4. Arriving at a positive vision of the future with renewed hope.

These themes fit closely with the key processes in resilience described above in belief systems, organizational resources, and communication processes. Widespread disasters that disrupt structures and services may lead to family and community fragmentation, conflict, and destabilization when larger systems are unresponsive. The failure of government rescue and recovery efforts compounds the trauma, suffering, and chaotic displacement of residents. As too often occurs in a disaster (Boyd-Franklin, 2010; Norris & Alegria, 2005), those most affected—and most neglected—are those most vulnerable and marginalized, especially people of color, those with limited means, the elderly, and those with serious health problems. For disaster preparedness and recovery, the utmost importance of local and national emergency planning, coordination, communication, and follow-through should be emphasized (Norris, Stevens, Pfefferbaum, Wyche, & Pfefferbaum, 2008). As Knowles and colleagues (Knowles, Sasser, & Garrison, 2010) concluded, families are often called the bedrock of a society, yet when disaster strikes, the lack of resources renders them vulnerable. Therefore, the commitment to post-disaster planning for sustainable communities must prioritize policies and practices for resilient families.

MILITARY FAMILIES AND COMBAT-RELATED TRAUMA

The predominant treatment models for war-related trauma have been individually based and focused on reducing symptoms of PTSD and related disorders. Military families suffer the impact of physical, psychological, and relational wounds with prolonged service in war, repeated deployments, highly stressful reentry transitions, and shifting roles and relationships for spouses, parents, and children (McDermid et al., 2008). Rising rates of PTSD, disabilities, traumatic brain injuries, substance abuse, suicide, violence, and divorce ripple through the entire family, affecting all members.

Families are also affected by moral injuries of service members or veterans (Nash & Litz, 2013). Military chaplains and family life educators can be especially sensitive to these issues. The recent concept of *moral injury* concerns the damage to moral belief systems through participation in events in war zones that violate one's deepest moral values, producing deep shame, guilt, and self-loathing. Such incidents might involve betrayals of trust in actions or failure to act; extreme or disproportionate violence or mistreatment; harm or loss of life of civilians, especially women and children; and within-ranks violence, "friendly fire," or sexual abuse. Profound shame and guilt involving acts of inhumanity leave service members feeling morally unfit to reenter the human community, receive praise and awards for their valor, or accept the love of spouses and family members. Morally injurious events cannot be undone, but healing involves a journey of forgiveness, with attempts to make symbolic reparations. As one military chaplain advised a serviceman unable to forgive himself for mistakenly opening fire on a family and killing five children: "Go out and find five children you can rescue."

Abundant research has documented the psychological and relational effects of trauma on military spouses and children related to the service member's war-zone deployments, combat exposure, and postdeployment disturbances and the influence of family processes as crucial moderators of this effect (MacDermid, 2010).

A family resilience framework situates the many varied facets of trauma—including the spiritual (moral) dimension—in the extreme experience of war and contextualizes intense distress as a normal reaction to the abnormal conditions. Interestingly, the Vietnamese term for PTSD translates as "spiritual sadness." Interventions address family stresses, strengthen bonds, and facilitate family support of a returning service member's resilient adaptation to life. Consultation with a pastoral counselor may be helpful.

The framework presented in this volume has been applied in military family resilience research (MacDermid, Sampler, Schwartz, Nishida, & Nyarong, 2008), in training family life educators, chaplains, and therapists, and in services for military personnel and their family members. Family resilience-based programs, utilizing workshop and weekend retreat formats, have been designed to help families navigate pre- and postdeployment challenges and to foster healing from injuries, trauma, and losses as they revitalize family relationships and re-vision future possibilities.

In a major initiative, Saltzman and colleagues at UCLA and Harvard designed FOCUS, a widely used brief intervention for military families dealing with wartime deployments and parental injury (Saltzman et al., 2011, 2013; also see timeline activities, Chapter 6). The program aims to improve child and family functioning and adaptation during and after highly stressful times by enhancing key family resilience processes. It combines family psychoeducation and developmental guidance; structured communication and narrative sharing experiences; and specific family-level skills targeting family resilience processes drawn from the Walsh (2003, 2007) family resilience framework. Intervention aims include:

- Developing shared family narratives.
- Enhancing family awareness and understanding.
- Improving family empathy and communication.
- Fostering confidence and hope.

- Supporting open and effective communication.
- Enhancing selected family resilience skills (stress management and emotion regulation, collaborative goal setting and problem solving, and managing trauma and loss reminders).

The program was adapted and refined to fit broadly diverse multicultural families and military cultures, and was found to be effective for children and families from diverse backgrounds. Improvements in specific aspects of family functioning—including communication, affective responsiveness and involvement, role clarity, and problem solving, all linked to the core family resilience processes—were associated with reductions in parent and child distress and improvements in their adaptive functioning overall. The program has also been effectively used with families contending with a range of trauma situations, illness, and loss.

TRAUMA SUFFERED IN WAR-TORN REGIONS AND THE REFUGEE EXPERIENCE

We've seen the vast human toll and the devastation wrought by war, violent ethnic, tribal, religious, and political conflicts, and genocide or ethnic cleansing campaigns in many parts of the world. Family members are forcibly separated, kidnapped, or made to witness the brutal killing and abuse of loved ones. Young boys and girls are pressed into combat, enslaved, or sold in sex trafficking. Efforts to reconnect survivors with their families and communities, or welcome them in asylum settings, are vital to their resilience.

The comfort and security provided by warm, caring relationships is critical in withstanding trauma for populations affected by war, including social and personal uprooting, family disruption, separation and loss, mental and physical suffering, and vast social change (Weine, 2006). The security provided by families in war zones buffers such stresses as bombings, air raids, and the horrors of witnessing violent death (Masten & Narayan, 2012). With evacuation, children fare best when they are able to stay together or in close contact with parents and siblings.

Refugee families face a myriad of challenges: overcoming the experience of physical and psychosocial trauma and loss, and further privation, separations, and relocations in migration. Many are forced to leave their homeland and seek asylum to escape persecution. Others are displaced by harsh environmental conditions. Often they must move from place to place or are trapped in refugee or IDP (internally displaced persons) camps for years or even decades. Abduction, starvation, torture, rape, imprisonment, and dehumanizing treatment are all too common. Many have suffered multiple traumatic losses of loved ones, homes, and communities and have witnessed brutal atrocities (Weine, 2006). For a description of the resilience-based multifamily groups for Bosnian and Kosovar refugees developed by the Chicago Center for Family Health, see Chapter 8.

From his extensive work with refugees, Mollica (2006) believes that there is an intricate relationship between connections to the environment and the healing of mind and body; in experiencing beauty or social connection, neurochemical processes are activated that literally begin to heal psychic wounds. Beauty in the wake of disaster can be experienced through exposure to nature and the arts, while social connectivity comes from family, friends, colleagues, and community groups.

When family members take flight, they are often separated from one another, with loved ones missing or their fate uncertain, as in the tragic ongoing war in Syria, which has displaced over half the population. With heightened stress and anxiety concerning ambiguous losses, family members have a critical need to gain information, to learn if others are alive and safe, and to restore contact whenever possible. One innovative program, Refugees United (*www.REFUNITE.org*), was founded by two brothers to respond to this urgent situation worldwide. Their nonprofit directly reconnects refugee families through technology, partnering with public and private organizations. Specially designed, secure Internet and mobile search tools enable family members to search for, locate, and then communicate directly with their loved ones.

Resilience–Oriented Family and Community Services in War-Torn Regions

The success of our resilience-based multifamily groups for Bosnian and Kosovar refugees led to a multiyear project in Kosovo to develop community-based, resilience-oriented, family-centered training and services (see Chapter 8). The Kosovar Family Professional Educational Collaborative (KFPEC), a partnership between mental health professionals in Kosovo and a team of American family therapists, aimed to enhance local capacities to address the overwhelming service needs in the war-torn region. Growing out of that program, other collaborative projects have been developed, addressing treatment and prevention of substance abuse, HIV/AIDS, and serious mental illness, as well as adolescent developmental challenges in the context of the economic, social, and systemic upheaval common in war-torn regions. The spirit of resilience persists in creative efforts to build a new community-based family-focused mental health care system for Kosovo.

Ongoing Complex Trauma

In some troubled regions, such as Colombia and Sudan, war and conflict have been ongoing across decades and generations, producing complex trauma and suffering for all directly affected. As Barrett and Stone-Fish (2014) have found, essential ingredients for resilience include: the importance of a meaningful vision of the future; the experience of being valued and valuing others; hope of a better world and life worth living; feeling empowered (versus helpless); and collaborative efforts to create workable solutions. One particularly meaningful experience for me was a 2006 brief training conducted on trauma, loss, and family resilience for the Community Mental Health Programme of the United Nations Relief and Works Agency (UNRWA), serving the Palestinian refugee communities in Gaza and the West Bank. The multiday training group experience in Ramallah fostered more open sharing by counselors and their supervisors of their professional challenges and strengths, as they brainstormed effective strategies and planned team meetings for greater collaboration and mutual support in their work.

I had tremendous admiration for the courage and dedication of the Palestinian counselors, who work with children and families suffering from ongoing complex trauma as they and their families experience these same conditions and shattering losses. In our discussion, they found most helpful our application of the keys to family resilience to their own resilience as counselors, especially the power of positive belief systems. They highlighted the importance of sustaining/restoring hope, as distinguished from optimism: faith that their positive efforts have the potential to make a difference for children's future despite pessimism about immediate prospects for an end to their occupation, degrading treatment, and reactive cycles of violence. With the larger political stalemate beyond their control, the key to resilience that most resonated with them was "mastering the art of the possible" and the quote "Do all you can, with what you have, in the time you have, in the place you are." Spirituality, experienced in the deep and abiding Islamic faith of the Palestinian people, is their deepest wellspring for resilience, nourishing their unwavering efforts to counsel those in distress.

Due to the closing of the Gaza border, training with the Gaza UNRWA counselors was arranged via videoconferencing from the United Nations offices in Jerusalem. My deep appreciation of the counselors' tireless efforts to alleviate the suffering of families in Gaza led to continued contact with them through e-mail exchanges and a writing collaboration on spiritual sources of resilience (Wolin, Muller, Taylor, Wolin, Ranganathan, et al., 2009). This online connection became a link to the outside world for several counselors later, when they contacted me during an Israeli military incursion into Gaza to relate their experience of the atrocities, the terror felt by children, and the widespread destruction. The profound suffering and the ongoing challenges faced by families and communities experiencing trauma and loss are not problems for brief solution focus, a cheerful optimistic mindset, or therapist techniques for change. I was humbled by how little I could offer, but I could bear witness. That was important to them, and it sparked me to do more in raising awareness and advocacy for a just resolution.

Such experiences have taught me that in our training and practice from a resilience orientation, it is our relationships with those we serve that matters most of all. Our connectedness, even in brief or long-distance contact, can nourish their resilience, from our compassionate witnessing of experiences of suffering and struggle to our belief in the human capacity for resilience.

MASS CASUALTIES IN TERRORIST ATTACKS

In this age of widespread terrorist attacks, we are all living in a more volatile and insecure world. With the attacks of September 11, 2001, trauma for Americans was intensified by the utter shock at such unimaginable events happening out of the blue, shattering illusions of invulnerability (Walsh, 2002b). Yet that was not the first attack in the United States. Valuable lessons can be learned from the experience of the Oklahoma City bombing.

Lessons from the Oklahoma City Bombing: Community Response and Resilience

A remarkable demonstration of community resilience emerged after the 1995 Oklahoma City bombing of the Murrah Federal Building, which killed 168 people and injured 842, including children in day care (Sitterle & Gurwitch, 1999). Although foreign terrorists were immediately suspected, it shocked the nation to learn that the bomber was a young, white Christian American, who plotted the attack with his friend. Amid the immediate chaos and suffering, local people came together in recovery efforts, collaborating in outreach and organizational efforts to aid and support those severely impacted. Thousands of professionals, volunteers, and rescue workers joined forces in providing effective crisis intervention for those in need and a strong support system for responders.

One notable program was the Compassion Center created in a local church, where hundreds of families gathered for information about their loved ones. Overcoming initial chaos, a multiagency effort was quickly organized to provide accurate information about rescue progress, facilitate identification of victims, and offer emotional support. The center coordinated the response of multiple emergency and community organizations to meet the many needs of survivors. Mental health services had three core aims (similar to the organizational and communication keys to resilience described above): (1) to provide a safe and protective environment for families to share their suffering; (2) to help families regain a sense of order, predictability, and structure; and (3) to provide information respectfully to the families.

Rituals were important in fostering unity and healing for survivors, families of the deceased, and the wider community. They channeled grief and terror into meaningful and life-affirming activities and instilled faith in the long healing process. Informal memorials and offerings were created at the bombing site and around the lone "survivor tree," which had been damaged but not destroyed by the blast. An official memorial and later remembrance events paid tribute to all those whose lives were lost and all who contributed to the recovery.

Case studies of group recovery (Zinner & Williams, 1999) have found that the grief experiences may become either a developmental crisis or a growthful opportunity for that community. Catastrophic events, traumatic loss, and suffering can lead to a breakdown in community morale and the stagnation of future development. In Oklahoma City, it strengthened resolve to rebound and propelled the community into new areas of growth. Learned resourcefulness—rather than helplessness—marked their recovery. Community members stepped forward, volunteering to fill many roles and provided mutual benefits by helping others in need and gaining an empowering sense of efficacy. It was this process of collaboration, making meaning and mastering at least *some* part of the traumatic experience, that promoted their resilience.

Resilience in the Wake of the 9/11 Attacks

The terrorist attacks on September 11, 2001, had widespread ripple effects for families and communities near and far. A few notable illustrations, offered here, reveal the resilience possible when families and their communities rally in the wake of tragedy.

In New York City, thousands of people gathered at the site of the World Trade Center attacks to organize support services, aid in the recovery of bodies and cleanup of the site, or simply to lend a helping hand wherever needed. Rituals were vitally important in sharing grief and in healing. Numerous remembrance events took place, at candlelight vigils, community gatherings, and places of worship. Again, a community showed that it could endure and surmount the worst. Caring responses poured in from strangers around the nation and the world. Notably the Oklahoma City community offered assistance to grieving families and sent a huge shipment of teddy bears to comfort those awaiting news of missing loved ones.

Sparks of this resilience kindled many positive developments (Walsh, 2002b). Two months later, a plane crashed after takeoff in a neighborhood of Queens, a working-class Irish and Italian American community that had lost many firefighters at the World Trade Center. On that flight to the Dominican Republic, most casualties were from the Dominican community in Washington Heights, a poor neighborhood in upper Manhattan at the other end of the subway line. As all New Yorkers reeled from yet another plane crash and fear of more terror strikes, a Dominican community leader and the city mayor were moved by the intertwined suffering of these two communities and together seized the moment to plan a joint memorial service, bridging a long-standing racial divide and bringing together communities that rarely had contact. Family members remarked that they had always assumed they were so different and had nothing in common. In coming together in sorrow, they discovered their shared values of strong families, hard work, and deep faith.

Yet the greater challenge lies in sustaining the strong spirit and connection that emerge in times of crisis after people return to their everyday lives. Over time, bereaved families organized into advocacy groups, such as the "Jersey Moms" and "Voices of September 11" to provide resources and support. They spoke out in public arenas to press for an independent commission to understand how the attacks came about and might have been prevented, and drew up recommendations to avert and prepare for any future threat. Their concerted efforts to clarify and make meaning of the crisis event, draw lessons from it, and take proactive steps are core processes in family and community resilience.

As Landau and Saul (2004) note, community members, who make up the natural support system, have many advantages over outside providers in effecting change after a crisis. They have greater access to local knowledge of existing resources and to vulnerable populations and have relationship networks that have developed over time. They are often already engaged in positive social processes that build solidarity, such as community association meetings and volunteer work. Because these efforts are driven by their experience and priorities, they can be more successful than programs imported by outsiders. Community members, with greater investment in the development of their neighborhoods, are more likely to maintain activities long after the funding for a recent crisis dries up or attention shifts elsewhere.

The Lower Manhattan Community Recovery Project

In neighborhoods directly affected by the terrorist attack, schools were closed and families displaced from their homes for several months. Mental health professionals initially focused on potential pathology in children, with little place for families to discuss their concerns. Parents became distressed on reentry, when children returned to their schools, where they had witnessed the horror. Saul and colleagues organized a neighborhood-based program involving local agencies and residents to facilitate child, family, and community resilience (Landau & Saul, 2004; Saul, 2013). Multifamily groups and networks of parents, teachers, counselors, and school staff were set up as a resource to share experiences, respond to children's concerns, provide mutual support, and mobilize concerted action in recovery efforts.

These support groups developed into a series of community forums, expanding the notion of healing beyond a focus on individual stress reactions to community-wide recovery. In this context, varied reactions were normalized and a framework was offered identifying common phases in disaster recovery:

1. "United we stand": Initially, people experienced shock and then came together, sharing and letting down their guard.
2. "Molasses and minefields": With growing fatigue and irritability, stresses accumulated, tempers flared, and people retreated into groups where they felt safer. At this stage, the focus was on ways to reduce stress and tensions in the community.
3. "A positive vision of recovery": At this stage, the community came together to build hope for the future, gaining understanding that recovery is not a passive process, but an active collaboration for a common purpose.

Through this process, community connectedness provided a matrix of healing and support along with sound information and feedback. A videotape of the forums was available to parents.

A community needs assessment led to the creation of a neighborhood resource center, a public space to gather and share ideas and creativity. The center formed a disaster preparedness initiative and developed such projects as a video narrative archive, a theater of witness project, a community website, a computer education program for seniors, art projects, and even a samba school. These programs have had long-lasting positive effects.

Family Meetings as Community Intervention for Ambiguous Loss

Another team of systems-oriented therapists, co-led by Pauline Boss (Boss, Beaulieu, Weiling, Turner, & LaCruz, 2003), worked with families of World Trade Center labor union workers who were missing after the attacks. Multifamily group meetings were held in the union hall, where families felt more comfortable than in a mental health setting. Additional counseling services were available. To be sensitive to the culturally diverse families, mostly immigrants, intervention teams were multilingual, multiracial, and attuned to the cultural diversity of the families. Group leaders helped families share anguishing experiences and communicated their basic premise: When a loved one remains missing, it is the traumatic situation of ambiguous loss that is abnormal, not the reactions of the distressed family members.

The group interactions and mutual support were empowering and healing. One daughter, devastated by the loss of her father, was helped enormously when a surviving coworker spoke up. He informed her that he had seen her father in one of the towers and that he had saved 1,000 lives before he perished. He told her that when she goes to football games and sees all the people in the stands, she can be proud of her father's courage in saving so many lives. The families voted to extend the sessions over many months; several widows took on leadership roles, and they prepared a memorial tribute on the first anniversary.

Challenges and Missed Opportunities

In the wake of those terrorist attacks, national surveys found that most Americans found strength, comfort, and solace by turning to their families and loved ones and to their faith. With the likelihood of continuing terrorist threats worldwide, we had to redefine normality and carry on with our lives in the face of fear and uncertainty. The rush to demonize enemies and seek revenge tragically led to two wars and their unintended consequences, as it has all too many times throughout history. It also fueled the profiling of suspected terrorists and outright racism, discrimination, and mistreatment. The greatest challenge is to better understand the many roots of terrorism and seek to address inequities and injustices that contribute to it. We must question old assumptions, learn more about our world, gain understanding of the suffering of others, and engage in shared reflection and positive actions for meaning-making, healing, and transformation.

We can do better as a society. As the response to the bombing at the 2013 Boston Marathon revealed, times of great tragedy can bring out the best in the human spirit: ordinary people and local officials showed extraordinary courage, compassion, and generosity in helping kin, neighbors, and strangers receive urgent care, undergo arduous healing journeys, and rebuild their lives. The Boston community emerged stronger with enhanced pride and resourcefulness.

FORGING RESILIENCE IN THE WAKE OF TRAGEDY

Traumatic losses reverberate throughout families and their communities; in turn, their collective response can help or hinder recovery. Catastrophic events can awaken us to what really matters in life and inspire us to reorder our priorities and take initiative in caring actions to benefit others. Communities have shown that they could endure the worst forms of suffering and grief and yet, with time and great effort, rebuild and grow stronger. After a fire destroyed the city of Chicago in 1871, forward-looking community leaders gathered the world's greatest city planners and architects to rebuild it, literally out of the ashes. That resilient response to tragedy made possible the transformation of the skyline and lakefront with innovative skyscrapers and vast public parks. In our times, we will need strong leadership, investment, and collaborative efforts to rebuild devastated communities and the lives of families that sustain them.

As helping professionals, we cannot heal all the wounds suffered in major trauma and humanitarian crises. We can create a safe haven where family and community members are able to share deep pain and renewed strivings. Of value is our compassionate witnessing of their suffering and struggle and our admiration for their courage and endurance. When we shift focus from symptoms to strengths and potential, people find they have, and can build, many unexpected competencies and resources. We can rekindle their hopes and dreams for a better future and support their best efforts. We can encourage their mutual support and active strategies to overcome their challenges. Multisystemic, resilience-oriented practice approaches help families and communities expand their vision of what is possible through collaboration, not only to survive trauma and loss but also to regain their spirit to thrive.

Thus recovery becomes a creative process arising from the synergy of members coming together to work toward a common purpose. The goal of courageous engagement with life guides our work as helping professionals, accompanying our clients on their journey in rebuilding and transforming their lives. The courageous people I have met and worked with—families, therapists, and others in humanitarian efforts—have taught me the power of *vicarious resilience*. This concept, developed from studies by Hernandez and colleagues (2002, 2010), refers to the benefits to helping professionals of working from a resilience perspective. In bringing forth accounts of resilience by those who have suffered traumatic experiences, we ourselves are inspired and reinvigorated in our work and in our lives, often in transformative ways (see Chapter 8).

In the wake of tragic events, remarkable resilience emerges in the many stories of recovery, heroism, and courage. Through crisis, trauma, and suffering, extraordinary compassion, generosity, and wisdom are forged. Over time, with shared reflection, we strive to integrate the fullness of our experience with traumatic events into the fabric of our individual and collective identity. Our response to tragedy can embody the humanity that binds us all together. We are, despite our differences, one human family.

CHAPTER 12

Serious Illness and Disabilities

Family Challenges and Resilience

All the world is full of suffering; it is also full
of overcoming it.
—HELEN KELLER, *Midstream: My Later Life*

Serious illness and disability pose a myriad of challenges for families, requiring considerable resilience in coping and adaptation. A health crisis can also be experienced as a wake-up call about our lives. It can heighten and alter our sense of priorities, which are too often lost in the helter-skelter demands of daily living. Persistent and recurring conditions can require changes in our patterns of living and reorient our hopes and dreams. This chapter highlights salient issues for a family resilience approach with serious health and mental health challenges.

LEARNING THE ART OF THE POSSIBLE: LESSONS FROM LIFE

Over the life course, serious illness strikes us all; therapists are not immune. Our own experiences with illness and caregiving challenges can teach us many things about resilience. It can also deepen our work with individuals and families who are striving to live as well as possible with chronic, debilitating, and life-threatening conditions.

Some years ago, I was hospitalized with viral meningitis on my return home from a consultation in Morocco. I was informed of the diagnosis but

265

received no information about what I might expect. The first few nights, nurses woke me repeatedly but never told me why, so I presumed that it was to make sure I was still alive. After a week, I was informed that the crisis period was over, my EEG appeared normal, and I could go home and resume "normal activity." When I asked for guidelines, I was told only to "avoid stress for a while." My husband was told I might be "a little irritable." That weekend, I hosted a dinner party for visiting friends—for me, a "normal activity," celebratory and fun, and not what I considered stressful. I collapsed before the end of the evening. At my follow-up appointment with the neurologist, I was angry. I asked for clearer guidelines: "How should I know what's too stressful?" I'll never forget his reply: "If you walk to the corner and need an ambulance to get home, then that was too much." This was not helpful. If I only found out *after* I required an ambulance, I had no guidelines to protect myself and avert a health crisis.

The year that followed was a long nightmare as I struggled to meet the demands of a flourishing career and of parenting an active 3-year-old child. I could pull myself out of bed to get my daughter off to nursery school and then teach a 3-hour seminar, only to collapse with piercing headaches, dizziness, and exhaustion for the rest of the day. I had no memory of what I had said in class. I tried to work on a book draft, only to have excruciating difficulty finding words and forming coherent sentences. My doctor was amiable but patronizing, each time telling me simply to "take it easy" and I'd soon feel better, as if I were exaggerating my difficulties to gain sympathy. I felt helpless and despairing. My resilient self was not bouncing back.

After a year of "taking it easy," I was still not much better. I consulted another neurologist, whose further tests found that I had suffered neurological damage, especially to the vestibular system. Despite the bad news, this physician was more helpful and hopeful. His approach was closer to a healing and resilience philosophy than to the traditional treatment paradigm. Its core assumption: the human brain has considerable plasticity. It is able to repair itself and modify its wiring to compensate for injury and loss *if* we actively mobilize our resources for recovery. Working collaboratively, he took time to listen to my concerns and answer my questions, gave me informational brochures, drew diagrams of the brain injury, and helped me to comprehend my illness experience. Medication controlled the pain and dizziness. Convinced that the brain, like other parts of the body, needs exercise to function well ("use it or lose it"), this physician recommended a program of strengthening exercises to reduce my vulnerabilities and restore my mental energy and functioning. He encouraged me to persist in my teaching and writing efforts, but in an incremental way to regain my proficiency gradually. He helped me to not become discouraged when symptoms worsened at times of high stress, to anticipate such times in the future, and to restructure my life to buffer stress more effectively. Months later, much improved, I asked him how he and my first neurologist could have approached the same patient so differently. He laughed and said, "I've known Dr. X for years; we play tennis together. When he has an injury, he stops playing for months and takes it easy. When I have an injury, I get physical therapy and get back on the court as soon as I can. It's all in our world view."

Indeed it was. Yet I was also fortunate, as some serious conditions cannot be improved. Looking back, I can see that the successful approach to my case embodied many of the key processes in resilience and was based in a collaborative therapeutic partnership. Unfortunately, one link was missing: inclusion of the family. Although I came through the worst of the ordeal personally strengthened and able to care well for my child, my marriage, already strained, didn't survive. Yet the many months of quiet contemplation enabled me to gain a new perspective on my life. My friends were my mainstay. I learned to reduce my work overload, focus on the things that really mattered, set aside petty grievances, and find more joy in life. Over time, I had to come to grips with the long-term sequelae of the brain injury. I learned to compensate for losses: Left-handed, I lost strength and coordination in my left hand, so I had to build my right-handed abilities—and one-handed keyboard agility. I had to overcome impaired vision and dizziness. I chuckled at one specialist's remark: "Your eyes really don't work together, do they?" In mastering the ongoing challenges, I was grateful for the deeper wisdom and bonds forged by the experience. I learned to practice the art of the possible.

THE ILLNESS EXPERIENCE:
A SYSTEMIC PERSPECTIVE

A family resilience approach to serious illness is grounded in a systemic orientation; it involves language and concepts that humanize the challenges of illness and encourage optimal functioning, personal well-being, and relational connection.

Biopsychosocial Orientation

An integrated biopsychosocial orientation to psychiatric and medical disorders is widely advocated but not readily put into practice. Emotional, interpersonal, situational, and environmental stresses all contribute to a wide range of symptoms, lower physiological immunity and neurological functioning, increase the risk, course, and severity of health problems, and can hasten death. Medical training and practice increasingly aim toward treating the whole person, yet integrated care is primarily symptom focused, and family and social influences receive insufficient attention (McDaniel, Doherty, & Hepworth, 2013; see also the website of the Collaborative Family Healthcare Association at *www.ccfh.net*).

It is well documented that physical illness significantly impacts family functioning and that family beliefs and practices can influence the physical and mental health of members (Campbell, 2003; Carr & Springer, 2010). When living with a serious condition—from diabetes, cancer, or multiple sclerosis, to traumatic brain or spinal cord injury, to major mental illness—individuals and their families need to cope with crises and navigate a challenging terrain over time.

Although most studies of family influences have focused on the negative, family systems approaches reveal the positive impact of family strengths on the course of illness and quality of life for all family members (Weihs, Fisher, & Baird, 2001; Rolland, 2012). Efforts to strengthen family resilience can buffer stress, bolster neurophysiological immune processes, and contribute to enhanced functioning and well-being. A family resilience framework connects individuals with their families, communities, and cultural and spiritual resources. This holistic approach increasingly integrates Eastern medicine and such teachings and practices as mindfulness meditation and yoga, along with Western models of care (Walsh, 2009c).

Addressing the Cultural and Spiritual Dimension of Illness, Suffering, and Resilience

Illness and suffering involve cultural and spiritual matters, opening questions about the human condition, our physical, mental, and emotional vulnerability, and our mortality (Wright, 2009; Wright & Bell, 2009). In a multicultural society, our clients' varying ethnic traditions, spiritual beliefs, and healing practices must be understood, respected, and integrated in practice (Falicov, 2009; Walsh, 2010). For instance, many ancient cultures have understood mental disturbances as forms of possession by spirits. Many immigrant families turn to indigenous healing approaches alongside Western medicine and may not mention their beliefs and practices if not asked. Kirmayer, Dandeneau, Marshall, Phillips, and Williamson (2011) found that the cultural and spiritual traditions of immigrants, refugees, and indigenous peoples in Canada are powerful sources of resilience in coping with serious health and mental health challenges. Their extensive research informs their call for an integrative orientation in all mental health services, particularly for oppressed and marginalized groups, to draw on resilience-enhancing family and tribal traditions and the power of connectedness with communities, the environment, and the spiritual realm beyond.

The Illness Experience in Families

The term *illness experience* best captures the essence of living with symptoms and suffering (Kleinman, 1988). It refers to how impaired persons and members of their family and social network perceive, cope with, and master the physical and psychosocial challenges associated with painful symptoms, disability, and treatments. Life-threatening or life-shortening conditions pose the challenge of carrying on with life in the face of an uncertain prognosis and anticipation of death and loss (Rolland, 2012). When illness strikes a loved one, the entire family requires attention for optimal coping and adaptation.

In practice, for instance, the therapeutic discussion of a woman's experience of breast cancer, mastectomy, and radiation and chemotherapy treatments would broaden to include how it affects her sense of identity, body image, and sexuality; her mental functioning ("chemo brain" symptoms); bonds with intimate partners and children; family and job responsibilities; and life priorities in the face of possible recurrence. With all medical conditions, we explore such questions as:

- How are family, work, and social functioning affected?
- What is the illness experience for the spouse? For children?
- How can a couple shelter their relationship to weather strains over time?
- How can parents approach their children's concerns about loss? About the threat of the same condition for themselves?
- How can helpful extended kin and social resources be mobilized?

With advances in genomic science and technology, clinicians increasingly will need to help individuals and their families grapple with decisions about genetic testing, sharing results with others, and informing children, siblings, or other family members who may be at risk for heritable disorders (Rolland & Williams, 2005). Yet genetic predisposition does not determine fate. Recent epigenetic research reveals the potential family and environmental influences in the expression and course of most genetic conditions (Spotts, 2012), underscoring the need to strengthen family processes.

As helping professionals, our approach to illness can facilitate coping and adaptation. Our images and language need to convey respect and humanize an illness experience, for example, referring to a "person with a disabling condition." Caution is needed to keep the diagnosis of a chronic disorder from reinforcing pessimistic views of limited lives or hopelessness. At the other extreme, unrealistic images of superstars who defeat all odds, while inspiring, can inflame feelings of failure for those unable to forestall or reverse a devastating condition. With medical advances, more people are living longer with chronic conditions that vary widely in their course, severity, and degree of functional impairment. Although they may not (yet) be curable, most can be managed well through individual and family efforts, with collaborative health care systems and community resources (Rolland, 1994, 2012).

The needs of "well" spouses, caregivers, siblings, or other family members also require attention. Those who are consumed by caregiving demands are at risk for depression, illness, and premature death. Yet, if not overloaded or lacking in support, most do well and many find their relationships enriched through meaningful involvement and mutual support of family members through the challenges.

Family Systems Approaches to Health Care

In comprehensive systems-based health care, the family is the central unit of care in the integrated treatment of health problems and the accompanying psychosocial challenges (Heru, 2013; Kazak, 2006; McDaniel et al., 2013; Rolland & Walsh, 2005). Family interventions with serious illness address the ongoing mutual interactions of biological vulnerability and environmental stresses and supports. Interventions aim to help clients cope with and master illness challenges, to reduce stress, and to strengthen individual and family functioning and positive adaptation. We engage families as indispensable partners in a team approach. Enhancing their potential for resilience increases both patient and family quality of life.

Meeting Varied Psychosocial Challenges over Time

The particular challenges of specific illnesses vary; yet there are many commonalities, depending on the psychosocial demands and the timing of an illness. The family systems–illness model developed by Rolland (1994, 2012) provides a useful framework for evaluation and resilience-oriented intervention. The model casts the illness in systemic terms according to its pattern of practical, emotional, and interpersonal demands over time. The progression of a chronic condition involves the intertwining of the illness phases with individual and family life cycle patterns (see Chapter 9). How we help families think about success or mastery will vary with their challenges, their resources, and their values. The model addresses three dimensions: (1) psychosocial types of illnesses; (2) phases in their course; and (3) core family system variables.

On the first dimension, illnesses are grouped by key biological similarities and differences that pose distinct psychosocial demands on the individual and family. Illness patterning can vary in terms of onset (acute vs. gradual), course (progressive, constant, relapsing, or episodic), outcome (fatal, shortened life span with possible sudden death, or no effect on longevity), incapacitation (none, mild, moderate, or severe), and the level of uncertainty about the trajectory. Each psychosocial type of condition poses a pattern of practical and emotional demands that can be addressed in relation to the style, strengths, and vulnerabilities of a family.

On a second dimension, the concept of time phases provides a way for clinicians to think longitudinally about chronic illness and disability as an ongoing process that families navigate with landmarks, transitions, and changing demands. Crisis, chronic, and terminal phases have salient psychosocial challenges, each requiring particular family strengths or changes. For instance, the crisis phase involves the initial period of socialization to chronic illness. Family developmental tasks include (1) creating a meaning for the disorder that preserves a sense of mastery, (2) grieving the loss of the pre-illness family identity, (3) undergoing short-term crisis reorganization, and (4) developing family flexibility in the face of uncertainty and possible threatened loss. Gradually, families need to come to accept the persistence or permanence of a chronic condition, learn to live well with illness-related symptoms and treatments, and forge ongoing collaboration with professionals and health care systems. In the chronic phase, families must also pace themselves to avoid burnout, rebalance relationship skews (e.g., caregiving), and juggle the competing needs and priorities of all family members. They need to find ways to conserve or revise individual and family goals, accounting for constraints of the illness, and to sustain intimacy in the face of threatened loss. With a life-threatening or fatal condition, families do best when they shift their views of mastery and control over the illness to making the most of precious time.

The psychosocial demands of a condition are addressed in relation to each phase of the disorder. The model informs an assessment of ways the illness interfaces with individual and family dynamics and development; the family's multigenerational history of coping with illness, loss, and other adversity; and the meaning of the illness experience for family members. Key processes in family resilience, involving belief systems, organizational patterns, and communication processes, can be targeted as they fit the evolving situation. The Rolland framework can guide periodic family consultations, or "psychosocial checkups," as salient issues surface or change over time. Family psychoeducational groups and support networks can provide useful illness-related information, management guidelines, and support for family members in meeting caregiving challenges, coping with the myriad of stresses, and making the most of their lives.

As therapists, we need to be flexible in helping families to meet emerging challenges over the uncertain course of a serious, life-threatening illness.

I worked with Kate, a vivacious woman, periodically at various phases and transitions over 8 years of her journey with breast cancer. She and her husband, Wayne, showed remarkable courage and resilience through two recurrences, with active initiative in searching out the best treatment options and keeping informed of medical advances. I coached them to listen and respond sensitively to their children's concerns as they emerged, and to keep channels of communication open. Wayne was supportive of Kate and flexible in shifting his work schedule to be more available in parenting their three children during difficult periods. A few couple sessions were held at a time when Wayne became remote, to explore his unexpressed fears of loss and of inability to manage parenting responsibilities on his own. Kate decided to maintain her part-time clerical job, which she experienced as "an island of normality," taking her mind off her own condition as she tackled mountains of paperwork and enjoyed socializing and light banter with coworkers. She was open in informing colleagues of major changes in her status or treatments, and took time off when needed. Otherwise, she preferred not to discuss her illness at work, keeping a boundary to preserve non-illness-focused aspects of her life. She took "long vacations" from therapy during periods of remission and stable plateaus, wanting to "just smell the roses." Yet, she called proactively when new complications loomed on the horizon. Sometimes she came in when, as she put it, she lost her compass and needed to reorient herself on her journey.

A year ago, when the cancer spread to her lower spine, Kate underwent an experimental bone marrow transplant, once again beating the odds and doing well over the critical months. However, in the midst of her recovery, her 70-year-old mother was diagnosed with untreatable colon cancer, which progressed rapidly to death. A month later Kate called, concerned about Mollie, her 12-year-old daughter. She had found a letter that Mollie had written to a friend saying that she was desperately unhappy and wanted to run away. We held a family session, where at first Mollie railed against her teachers, wanting to go away to boarding school because "life sucks!" When I asked how the grandmother's recent death had affected family members, Mollie's eyes filled with tears. Her parents' receptiveness helped her to share her fear: "Grandma's death scared me so much. She had cancer, and Mom has had cancer three times. If *she* could die, so could Mom. Sometimes I have nightmares that the cancer hasn't all gone away. Then I just want to run away." Both parents held her, soothing her as she sobbed. Mollie's siblings were encouraged to share their feelings and concerns as well. I supported the parents' efforts to talk about the dilemmas in living with uncertainty and their wish that they could just make the cancer go away once and for all. Both parents reassured the children that Mom indeed was continuing to do well and vowed to be honest with them if the situation changed. The discussion turned to ways they could make the most of family time together.

This case illustrates how systemic therapists may combine individual, couple, and family sessions, holding a resilience-oriented systemic map to guide intervention priorities over time. Even when parents handle an illness experience as well as possible at one crisis point, others will arise later that require further conversations. Here, the death of the grandmother shattered the shared optimism (positive illusions) that the mother would always continue to beat the odds. Also, developmental transitions are nodal points when new concerns often surface. As Mollie approached adolescence, she had greater comprehension of her mother's condition and all it would mean to lose her. She also began to worry about her own risk of breast cancer. The time had come to talk more openly about those issues.

Coming to terms with an illness and its ramifications is never a once-and-for-all matter, but a process worked on periodically over time. Kate's long-term goal was to be there for her daughters until they were independent, which she first defined as getting their drivers' licenses. At that milestone, she set a new goal: until they were launched and off to college. When that transition occurred, she met with me, saying, "Well, I guess I'd better come up with a new reason to keep on thriving!" We talked about meaningful pursuits for her and travel she and her husband would enjoy together. Such life-cycle transitions can be valuable touch points for consultation.

Keeping the Illness in Its Place

With a serious and chronic condition, families can't simply "bounce back" to the old normal life, but must navigate a new terrain, which some describe as "leaving the normal world and entering the illness world." It is crucial for families to gain a perspective on the illness so it doesn't define individual identity or rule family life. The challenge is to recognize the influence of the condition, master what is possible, accept what is beyond control, and come to terms with living with it well. To do this successfully, families need to find ways to "put the illness in its place" (Gonzalez & Steinglass, 2002). Setting boundaries as to when, where, and with whom illness concerns are discussed can be helpful, just as Kate (above) kept boundaries in her work life to preserve what she called her "island of normality."

Over time a chronic condition can skew a couple relationship between the impaired partner and the caregiving or "well" spouse (Rolland, 1994). The persistent intrusion of an illness into all aspects of family life can fuel despair.

> Mike and Delores, a working-class couple in their mid-40s, came for therapy as growing conflict threatened the survival of their marriage. In the first session, they argued over money, sex, and Mike's whereabouts on weekend nights. Neither partner mentioned that Delores had been suffering for many years from multiple sclerosis, despite her evident difficulty in walking with a cane. When asked about her condition, both minimized it as "nothing new" and resumed fighting over petty grievances.
>
> Separate individual sessions were held to hear more about the illness experience for both partners, affording each the opportunity to express concerns more freely. Mike revealed that he was alternately depressed and furious at Delores because of her increasing disability and dependence. They had traditional breadwinner–homemaker roles in their marriage. As her illness progressed, she was less able to keep the house clean or to manage cooking, shopping, and errands, and had lost all interest in sex. It bothered Mike to come home and find her "lying around" while he worked an exhausting construction job plus overtime to keep up with her medical bills. He harbored fantasies of leaving her, became irritated with her over small things, felt ashamed, and then drowned his frustration in bouts of heavy drinking at a neighborhood bar on weekends. As for Delores, the less she felt in control of her body, the more controlling of Mike she became. She alternated between feeling guilty for being such a burden on him and then irritated and resentful that he wasn't more attentive to her needs.
>
> In the next couple session, it was important to reframe the relational distress as not attributable to his failings or hers, but rather as a shared dilemma arising from the burdens imposed on their lives by a progressively debilitating illness. Appreciation of the impact of the illness enabled the spouses to hear and comfort each other as they shared the ways each had been affected and how it had ravaged their relationship, their financial security, and their future hopes and dreams. Strains also concerned the uncertainty about the future progression of Delores's condition and the possibility of early death. Their marriage was strengthened as they pulled together to find ways of reducing the intrusion of the illness in their lives and to find pleasure together. Delores, reassured that Mike's night out with the boys was not an

extramarital affair, encouraged him to go out to sports games he enjoyed when she couldn't; in turn, he agreed not to drink to excess. Feeling less trapped, he was kinder toward Delores and supported her need for outlets and visits with friends. Knowing her love of nature, on his days off he took her to nearby parks and the Botanic Garden to brighten her spirits. They decided to set aside a little money each week toward a trip for their upcoming anniversary.

When the cumulative effects of a chronic illness loom increasingly large—imposing heavy physical, emotional, relational, and financial burdens, and diminishing future hopes and dreams—it is crucial to help clients regain a view of each person and their relationship as defined by more than the illness. Similar to White's (White & Epston, 1990) technique of externalizing the problem, the illness is framed as an unwelcome intruder; by joining forces family members can regain control of their lives. Couple therapy can help each partner gain empathy for the other's position, address such issues as guilt and blame, and rebalance their relationship, enabling them to live and love as fully as possible.

Key Family Resilience Processes: Navigating the Challenges of Chronic Illness

Recent studies have identified an array of ways that key family processes can be helpful in chronic illness, particularly with childhood illness and physical, mental, and developmental disabilities (Beavers & Hampson, 2010; Greeff & Nolting, 2013; Greeff, Vansteenwegen, & Gillard, 2012; Greeff & van der Walt, 2010; Knestricht & Kuchey, 2009; Levine, 2009; McCubbin, Balling, Possin, Friedrich, & Byrne, 2002; Retzlaff, Hornig, Müller, Gitta, & Pietz, 2006; Shapiro, 2012).

Belief Systems

The belief systems of the affected person, the family, their cultural and spiritual traditions, and their health care providers intersect in the illness experience and in all healing transactions. We may need to work with distressing causal attributions of how and why health problems have occurred or persist, as well as beliefs about the role of helping professionals and the family in the treatment process. For instance, several studies above find that a shared sense of coherence and a larger family vision or sacred beliefs contribute to family resilience.

Epidemiological research points to the importance of hope in the face of uncertainty with life-threatening conditions. Taylor (1989) found that cancer patients were better able to rally when they held "positive illusions" in their potential to overcome a poor prognosis. Unlike denial, this involves a choice to maintain a strong focus on healing and well-being while clearly understanding the grim situation. It fuels active initiative and perseverance in steps (such as stress reduction, social support, healthy diet, and exercise) to maximize the likelihood of a positive outcome. Even when patients did not live longer than expected, their quality of life and relationships were significantly more satisfying and meaningful as they made the most of precious time.

In helping families initially face elevated risks of death and loss with a health condition, it is important not to undermine their hope and to encourage their best efforts for optimal well-being and quality of life. If an illness progresses, sensitivity is needed in helping families to reconstruct the meaning of realistic or reasonable hope (Weingarten, 2010) as they confront the greater *probability* of a poor outcome, such as a limited recovery or death. In the event of a terminal condition, and the *certainty* of death, they can be encouraged to redirect their hope, prayers, and efforts to the amelioration of pain and suffering, enhanced comfort, emotional and relational well-being, and spiritual peace of mind. Even then, the length of time they have to live may be uncertain, depending on such variables as the slow or rapid progression of a condition, as in amyotrophic lateral sclerosis (ALS). Feelings of hopelessness are common when a condition becomes incurable, suffering unbearable, or treatment overwhelming. In families, members may be divided between holding on to hope or giving up (Flaskas, 2007). Therapists need to allow space in the therapeutic conversation to discuss feelings of hopelessness, what hope means to various members, and, where possible, to support clients in reorienting to a new vision of hope and mastery of what is possible.

Making meaning of the condition and prognosis is crucial. It is useful to ask families what illness information they have received and what each member believes about the future course, exploring their best hopes and worst fears. When these beliefs are polarized among family members, it can generate strong conflict, particularly if decisions must be made about whether to pursue or forgo further treatment options. We can help families obtain clearer information about the medical prognosis, treatments, and management issues to guide collaborative decision making. As the course of a condition worsens, we can help families reevaluate their options and chances, and encourage their efforts to master the possible and accept what may be beyond their control. Although their best efforts may not result in the hoped-for outcome, they can greatly impact the quality of life and enhance their relationships. Activism and advocacy for prevention and treatment are a valuable pathway in resilience for families. One father, afflicted with multiple sclerosis, maintained a positive outlook despite a poor prognosis:

"I'm not happy I have it, but I'm a happy man living with it." Taking part in research gave his life greater meaning. "If I can help others it gives me satisfaction. My glass is half full—and I have hope for future generations."

Organizational Processes

With severe disabilities, studies find that establishing rhythms in family life, such as consistent rules, rituals, and routines, fosters child and family resilience. Family organizational patterns may need to shift with various adaptational demands over the course of an illness. For instance, in a family with teenagers, a father's heart attack generates a crisis, drawing family members together in high cohesion. Family life is disrupted by the initial anxiety and turmoil. Over the following weeks, as the father recovers, the family restabilizes, regaining household order, resuming daily routines, such as shared mealtimes, and expanding attention to others' priorities, such as schoolwork and activities. Several months later, family functioning may remain closer and more structured. Members may be vigilant and cautious not to upset the father, out of fears of recurrence. An adolescent may be constrained from leaving home for college under pressure to support parents. Although all families change in response to a crisis, some need help in readjusting roles and interactional patterns to maximize their resources and coping skills, especially if a crisis recurs or a condition becomes chronic.

Communication

Positive patterns of communication facilitate family resilience in dealing with serious health challenges. Open communication in families and with health care providers is vital to clarify an illness diagnosis, prognosis, treatment options, and management guidelines. Framing events, such as receiving a diagnosis, cast meaning on a serious condition and may help or hinder in dealing with it (Rolland, 1994). Health care professionals may unwittingly contribute to blocked communication and isolation among family members by telling only a spouse or parent about a life-threatening prognosis. Some might presume that it is unwise to talk openly about it together or harmful with the patient. When clinicians sensitively help family members to share information and clarify an illness situation and options, they are better able to support each other in mastering their challenges.

Clinicians also need to explore cultural differences and each family's preferences. In traditional Japanese culture, the family may be told that their loved one is dying but the patient is not told, for fear that it could hasten death. Yet we should not assume that all families would want to follow their traditional norm. Often, patients are aware of their condition but don't talk with loved ones about it, wishing to spare them upset. Care needs to be taken not to contribute to a "conspiracy of silence," which can rob them of opportunities for important conversations.

Studies have shown the importance of good communication in the adaptation and competence of families with a child with serious physical and mental disabilities. Countering assumptions that families inevitably suffer chronic sorrow and dysfunction, those families who dealt openly with their feelings adapted well, increasing their mutual support with members able to express a wide range of feelings, including joy. As one critically ill young girl said: "We have to live and love it up!"

Collaborative Caregiving Team

A family resilience approach expands our society's narrow, individualistic focus on a designated primary caregiver to involve all family members as a caregiving team. Family intervention priorities include (1) stress reduction; (2) information about the impaired member's medical condition, functional abilities, limitations, and prognosis; (3) concrete guidelines for sustaining care, problem solving, and optimal functioning; (4) linkages to supplementary services to support family efforts; and (5) focus on ways for family and friends to share meaningful and enjoyable contact. To meet caregiving challenges, communities must support families through a range of services from day programs to assisted and communal living and commitment to full participation of individuals with disabilities in community life.

Illness and Caregiving in Later Life

With the aging of societies and medical advances, more elders are living longer with chronic health conditions (Qualls & Zarit, 2009). In the United States, health problems and their severity vary greatly with disparities associated with income, race, and adequate, affordable health care. While more people are healthy through their 60s than in the past, for those over 75—and especially for frail elders over 85—progressive, degenerative physical and mental conditions and chronic pain are increasingly common and require long-term care.

Family caregiving for elders can be demanding and strain intergenerational relations. Issues of autonomy and shame-laden dependence also come to the fore as aging parents lose functioning and control over their bodies and their lives (see Chapter 9). As family size decreases and childbearing occurs later, those at midlife—the so-called "sandwich generation"—face multiple pressures: meeting job demands, raising children, and caring for aging parents, grandparents, and other relatives. Caregiving has burdened women disproportionately in their roles as daughters and daughters-in-law. In our mobile society, adult children often live at a distance; shuttling back and forth further strains the ability to provide support in times of need. Adult children past retirement age, facing their own declining health and resources, increasingly assume responsibilities for infirm parents in their 80s and 90s.

Family and friends are the front lines of support. Growing numbers of elders with chronic conditions receive home-based care for daily functioning and require costly medications and periodic hospitalizations. Prolonged caregiving can take a heavy toll in depression, anxiety, and health decline. Some aspects of elders' chronic conditions are especially disruptive for families, such as sleep disturbance, incontinence, delusional ideas, and aggressive behavior. Useful management guidelines, support groups, home health aides, and day care programs can reduce exhaustion and revive spirits.

Progressive Dementias: The "Long Good-bye"

Progressive dementias, affecting over 40% of elders over 85, are especially challenging for families (see also Chapter 9). Alzheimer's disease, accounting for most dementias, is one of the most devastating illnesses of our times. Dementia gradually strips away mental and physical capacities, with gradual memory loss, disorientation, impaired judgment, and loss of control over bodily functions. The irreversible disease course, called "the long good-bye," can persist for 10 to 20 years. Families need help in dealing with the many ambiguous losses (Boss, 1999), including gradual loss of identity, family roles, relationships, and even recognition of loved ones, who are confused with others, even those long deceased. Finding humor can lighten spirits.

> Danny, who was devoted to his parents, found his father's worsening dementia heartbreaking and lamented the frustration and sadness it caused his mother, who tended to him despite her own medical ailments. Danny had dinner with them frequently to help out. One night, as his mother cleared the table, his father leaned over to him and said, "See that woman over there—she's a darn good cook and good-looking, too. If I wasn't a married man, I could really go for her!" Danny hugged his father and replied, "Pop, you're a lucky man—because you ARE married to her! She's your wife!" They all had a good laugh, his mother was pleased by the compliment, and they retold the story many times.

Bonds with companion animals are found to facilitate resilience for elders with declining health (Walsh, 2009a, 2009b). One grandfather with dementia could no longer follow family conversations but found contentment petting the family dog, snuggled close to him on the sofa. He took great delight in sneaking sausages under the dinner table to his attentive companion. Service dogs, trained to assist persons who are functionally impaired or have life-threatening conditions such as diabetes or seizures, provide vital companionship and enable them to live independently.

We would be mistaken to view later life only as a time of decline and loss. This period also holds potential for personal and relational change and growth (Walsh, 2012b). One father's cognitive decline was accompanied by a softening of his prickly defenses and mellowing of his affect from his former gruff demeanor, enabling his adult children to engage more warmly with him. The challenges of caregiving also present opportunities for greater intimacy and for healing relationship wounds.

Difficult Family Dynamics

Intergenerational tensions often arise over dependency issues (Walsh, 2016b). It's helpful for family members to appreciate that meeting increasing parental needs is a normative filial responsibility, not a parent–child "role reversal." An aged parent deserves respect as a family elder, with declines in functioning not demeaned as "childlike." Family therapists can open conversations about dependency issues with sensitivity and a realistic appraisal of strengths and limitations. An elderly father driving with serious impairment may be unwilling to admit dangers or give up his autonomy. Adult children can be encouraged to intervene respectfully while supporting their elders' desire to be as fully engaged in life as possible.

When past grievances have ruptured family relationships, caregiving and life-and-death decisions often become more complicated. If one adult child steps in and becomes overburdened, resentment can brew toward others on the sidelines. Yet a medical crisis can become an opportunity for family members to heal strained relationships and collaborate as a caregiving team.

> Joellen, a 38-year-old single parent, came to therapy with an agonizing dilemma. Her father, hospitalized for complications of chronic alcohol abuse, had asked her to donate a kidney to save his life. She felt enraged to be asked to give up something so important when he had not been there for her as a father. He had been a mean drunk, often absent and many times violent. She was also angry that he had brought on his deteriorating condition by drinking and had refused

to heed his family's repeated pleas to stop. Yet, as a dutiful daughter and a compassionate woman, she also felt a sense of obligation and guilt: She did not want her father to die because she had denied him her kidney.

I broadened the dilemma to include Joellen's siblings, suggesting that she discuss it with them. But she dismissed that idea, saying that they had been estranged for many years and were rarely in contact. So I encouraged Joellen to talk with her mother—who informed her that her father had also asked her siblings for the kidney donation. She was furious that old rivalries were stirred up as to who would be seen as the good, caring child or the bad, selfish ones. Fired up, she now took the initiative to get her siblings together. When the meeting proved hard to schedule, I encouraged her to keep trying. When they met, old rivalries melted as they began to grapple with the shared dilemma.

I refocused the discussion with questions about the future, wondering if they had considered that other challenges would likely arise in caring for both aging parents, or the surviving parent, if widowed. They had avoided looking ahead, but I encouraged them to begin thinking about ways to collaborate as a team in meeting future challenges—and the immediate crisis. With this conversation, the oldest brother, Vick, volunteered to donate his kidney for their father. He said he felt less conflicted remembering good times with him in earlier years before the problem drinking. The others then stepped up, agreeing to support him through the surgery. As the beginning of a new solidarity was forged, all agreed to keep in contact and come together around their parents' future needs. Over time, Vick shared stories of their father's life struggles, expanding his younger siblings' understanding and compassion for him.

Family members commonly distance out of sheer exhaustion and depleted resources. Recurrent crises can fuel helplessness, hopelessness, frustration, and escalating conflict. Some distance from painful past experiences, failed rescue attempts, anger over destructive behavior, or the fear that they will be pulled into a bottomless pit of selfless caregiving and the sacrifices extracted by an illness. Loss issues and survival guilt are common as well: "How can I be successful and enjoy life when my loved one's life has been devastated by illness?" Yet the relief of a cutoff is sometimes overshadowed by worry about the parents' well-being and later sorrow or guilt at abandoning them in their time of need.

My experience has taught me never to give up on relational recovery even—and especially—when physical recovery is not possible. My work with many in this position—parents, siblings, and adult children of frail elders—has heightened my appreciation of their many struggles and has strengthened my conviction that it is rarely too late to repair frayed bonds (see Chapter 14).

Placement Decisions

When declining health requires consideration of extended-care placement, it can be a crisis for the whole family. Placement is usually turned to only as a last resort—when family resources are stretched to the limit and in later stages of mental or physical deterioration or high risk of harm to oneself or others. Yet feelings of guilt and notions about institutionalization can make a placement decision highly stressful for families, especially when it is seen as abandonment in their family or cultural context.

> Mrs. Gupta called for help with her teenage son, stating that she "felt helpless to control" him and feared that he "needed to be institutionalized." A family assessment revealed an escalating cycle—his defiance of her attempts to control his every activity—over the past several months—since Mrs. Gupta's mother had been brought to live in their home. She wept as she described her mother's deteriorating Parkinson's condition, feeling unable to provide round-the-clock care. She couldn't sleep at night after finding her mother on the floor. Control struggles with her son deflected her heightened concern: that her mother's condition was beyond her control but "institutionalizing" her was out of the question. At her father's deathbed, a year earlier, he had asked her to promise that she would always care for her mother. She had also heard stories that in regions of India widowed women were banished from their homes and communities. She could not bear to abandon her mother. She felt alone with her dilemma, as her husband had distanced, preoccupied by his work. In a couples session, he acknowledged that he was avoiding his own guilt over having left the care of his dying mother to his sisters. The family crisis now became an opportunity for him to support his wife and mother-in-law's well-being. The couple's bond was strengthened as they explored together how to provide the best care, with in-home nursing assistance or in a nearby care facility, without abandoning their loved one—or each other.
>
> Family sessions can help members to assess needs and resources, weigh the options of in-home and placement options, and share feelings and concerns before reaching a decision. Often through discussion new solutions emerge that can support the elder's remaining in the community without undue burden. Home-based health care services and community backup resources are vital for the respite and well-being of family caregivers. When placement is needed, we can help families see it as the most viable way to provide good care and help them navigate the maze of options.

Terminal Illness

Families face many painful challenges with terminal illness. Dilemmas may include whether and how long to pursue more treatments with little or no chance of prolonging life, toxic side effects, and lowered quality of life for the remaining time. When the dying process has been prolonged, family caregiving and financial resources depleted, and the needs of other members long on hold, relief at ending the strain on the family can be guilt-laden for survivors. Clinicians need to attend to unmet needs for pain control and palliative care, and to worries about financial and emotional burdens on loved ones. Family collaboration is essential to reduce suffering and make the best arrangements to keep the seriously ill person comfortable and comforted while balancing the needs of other family members.

Families need wise counsel as they approach life's end and grapple with personal, cultural, and spiritual matters (Walsh, 2009d). Gawande (2014) encourages health care professionals to have vital conversations with patients and their loved ones, exploring four basic questions: What is their understanding of their health or condition? What are their goals if their health worsens? What are their fears? What are the trade-offs they are willing to make and not willing to make? Most important are conversations about their priorities as they approach death and loss. Some prioritize living long enough for a project completion or a special event, such as a child's graduation; others might prefer to end pain and suffering and forgo further treatments.

Advanced planning of end-of-life wishes is advised. Clinicians can help family members discuss living wills, share feelings about complicated situations, weigh various options, and come to terms with decisions taken. Over time, such decisions should be reviewed and flexibly revised to fit changes in health status, as people's priorities commonly shift over the course of a disabling condition. In some cultures it is taboo to plan for death or discuss it openly, so clinicians must be sensitive to family beliefs. Increasingly, families face agonizing end-of-life dilemmas. There is growing public support in the United States for physician-assisted dying when requested by someone who is terminally ill to enhance dignity, peace of mind, and control over the dying process. Decisions to maintain or withhold life support efforts for a loved one raise fundamental questions of when life ends and who should determine that end, involving medical ethics, religious beliefs, patient/family rights, and even the possibility of criminal prosecution. Families can be torn apart by opposing views and decisions.

A terminal illness may hold unexpected gifts, particularly at life's end, when family members fully engage with loved ones and make the most of precious time.

James, age 52, came to talk with me about his unbearable sorrow at his mother's terminal illness. We explored his complex feelings. A devout Catholic, she had done all she could to keep her family intact while enduring an abusive marriage and many relocations that uprooted the family due to his father's alcoholism and repeated job loss. After the father's recent death, James had bought a new home for his mother in high hopes that, at last, she could enjoy her later years in peace and comfort. He was devastated that her illness so quickly shattered these dreams. "It's just not fair! She deserved some good years."

He and his sisters had scattered around the country in adulthood and maintained little contact. Since their mother's cancer diagnosis, she had uncharacteristically asked them to make several trips to visit her. Now she had just called them together, he feared, for their last good-byes. He was tormented as he left for the visit.

When I saw him after his return, he seemed transformed: his inner turmoil had subsided, although his mother, indeed, had died during the visit. He told me, "I knew my mother was a strong woman, but she was most amazing as she faced her own death—she deliberately brought me and my sisters in to care for her, time and again, to knit us back together. Her final request made sure that we'll continue our bonds. She told us she didn't want to be buried where she lived, so far from her children and her roots. Instead, she asked to be cremated and that we take the urn with her ashes and travel together to each town where our family had lived and scatter some of her ashes in a beautiful place we had enjoyed. Her courage inspired us to go even further in honoring her wishes. We told her we would save a portion of the ashes and make a trip to Ireland together to scatter the last remains in the town of her grandparents, which she had always wanted to visit. She was so pleased and died peacefully a few hours later as we sat around her singing Irish ballads she had loved.

This potential for transformation, forged in the midst of suffering, dying, and loss, distinguishes the concept of resilience from coping well. As we've seen, resilience entails more than shouldering a caregiving burden, bearing the sadness of loss, or adjusting dreams downward. This moving story reveals the core of relational resilience: Family members rallied together to practice the art of the possible. They made the most of limited time together and transcended the immediate death and loss, inspired by their mother to carry out her wishes, thereby honoring and sustaining her memory and spirit. In the process, they and their bonds were transformed. In resilience-oriented practice, we can facilitate such processes.

FAMILIES COPING WITH MENTAL ILLNESS

We now have ample evidence of the complicated mutual influences between biogenetic vulnerability and family and social environmental factors in the expression and course of major mental disorders (e.g., Tienari et al., 2004). Yet, a biopsychosocial orientation is not well integrated into most treatment, currently prioritizing psychopharmacological and cognitive-behavioral approaches. I was fortunate that my first year of clinical training in 1968 was on a model psychiatric inpatient unit (T-1) at Yale Medical Center, combining individual, group, family, and multifamily therapy approaches with newly developed psychotropic medications. My very first family therapy experience taught me the value of this multilevel approach:

> Emmy Lou was admitted to the psychiatric unit during an intense psychotic episode. She had been suffering from bipolar disorder for over 20 years. Walt, her devoted husband, took her to the best treatment centers; stood by her through recurrent breakdowns, hospitalizations, and brief recoveries; and never stopped hoping for an effective treatment.
>
> As Emmy Lou began taking lithium, a newly experimental drug at that time, she and her family were also referred for family therapy. A first-year psychiatry resident and I eagerly worked with our first family, and as Emmy Lou made an astounding recovery, we jokingly credited our skillful family interventions.

Even when a condition is biologically based and responds to psychotropic drugs, family involvement in treatment is crucial for optimal patient and family adaptation. The family didn't *cause* her disorder, but they too suffered its impact. The family members didn't *need* Emmy Lou to be ill; nor did her symptoms serve a function for them (mistaken beliefs by some early family therapists). However, they had structured their family life around her dysfunction over the years. Any recovery, while everyone's greatest wish, involves a disruptive transition. Although medication can reduce florid symptoms, loved ones must reorient their relationships and patterns of living. And, as with a serious condition and drug treatments, the path forward may not be smooth.

> It was important to help Walt and their two teenage sons relate to Emmy Lou not as a chronic patient, but as a beloved wife and mother recovering from a devastating condition. To enhance her functioning and worth, they needed to alter patterns of family functioning set in place over the years to compensate for her deficits and diminished

sense of self. Walt had increasingly taken over parenting and house-hold responsibilities, with Emmy Lou assigned to menial tasks such as walking the dog. To restore her competence and confidence, the paren-tal partnership needed to be rebalanced. Walt and their sons needed to shift their expectations. They were nervous and uncertain about how to relate without the illness defining their roles and relationships.

Discharge planning and posthospitalization reentry sessions—critical components of the treatment unit—enabled Mary Lou and her family members to share their hopes and concerns and to reorganize family life. We scheduled a follow-up family session for early spring, the time they anticipated a recurrence. This offered an opportunity to discuss fears of a setback, to adjust medication, and to sustain the family's gains.

To optimize functioning and reduce the risk of serious relapse, it is crucial to engage family members as partners from a hospital admission through discharge, with planned follow-up and referral for outpatient sus-taining care. The first few weeks and months postdischarge can be the most challenging. Relational tensions commonly mount as difficulties arise. It is helpful to support realistic expectations and offer useful guideline, reorga-nizing stressful interactional patterns and building communication skills to strengthen both individual and family resilience.

From Deficit-Based to Resource-Based Therapeutic Approaches

A focus on deficits, reinforced by psychiatric nomenclature, exerts a pow-erful influence in clinical practice. When those with recurrent emotional distress seek help, they often carry pathology-loaded baggage from previ-ous treatment experience. A resilience-based approach aims to transform this experience.

Jessie and Ted, a recently married couple in their late 20s, sought help for Jessie's phobic anxiety, which prevented her from leaving their apartment without a panic attack. She was evaluated for psy-chotropic medication, which lowered the intensity of her anxiety; yet she remained alone in the apartment all day, becoming increas-ingly depressed and ruminating about the emptiness of her life and the hopelessness of her emotional problems. The couple had recently moved from Jessie's hometown for Ted's new job. In the first few ses-sions, Jessie talked at great length about her "dysfunctional family," her mother's chronic drinking and depression, and her own recurrent episodes of panic, which had led to three brief psychiatric hospitaliza-tions. She had spent the last 6 years in psychoanalysis, with sessions several times a week until their move to Chicago. Now fearing she was coming "unglued" again, she was making crisis calls to her former therapist. Ted was attentive and caring toward Jessie, yet frightened by her agitated state and catastrophic fears.

A deficit-oriented therapy might have continued to focus on past family damage and Jessie's resulting limitations and emotional fragility. Some therapists might have felt sympathy for the "normal" spouse stuck with a "damaged" partner. Or they might have assumed both partners in a marriage to be equally dysfunctional, and searched for underlying pathology in Ted as well. A family resilience approach identified and encouraged their strengths and potential. Ted was solid, stable, and caring. His attraction to Jessie was understandable: she was a lovely woman, warm, affectionate, attractive, and smart. Ted's fears from a past failed marriage also played a part. Recently divorced by a woman who had left him to pursue her career, he was reassured by Jessie's dependency and devoted loyalty. However, he neither anticipated her intense suffering nor "needed" her helplessness.

As our sessions became dominated by Jessie's accounts of how her "messed up" family and her long history of emotional problems "explained" her current plight, I shifted focus to the recent transitional crisis in the couple's life—the disruption wrought by their relocation. I asked how the decision had come about. The partners had shared their feelings, concluded that on balance it would be a good move, and arrived at the decision jointly. Still, there was a skew in the experience of the transition, generating more stress for the more vulnerable partner. The move furthered Ted's career advancement and gave him a sense of pride. It also brought welcome contact with his family, who lived nearby. Jessie, who wanted to assume a homemaker role and hoped to start a family soon, had lost her community network, a satisfying job, and her therapist. She felt isolated in long, empty days in their apartment in an unfamiliar city. The loss of structure and support fueled her anxiety, rumination, and self-doubts.

Helping the couple to make meaning of the recent symptoms in the context of this major transition was pivotal to Jessie's adaptation and the couple's resilience. I expressed my conviction that a major relocation is very stressful for a relationship as well as for individuals, and that by strengthening their resilience as a couple, they would both more likely make the best adjustment. To help them begin forming a new support network and to anchor them in their new community, I explored their interest in joining a church that fit their beliefs and lifestyle, encouraging them to make several visits. Within weeks they found a new "spiritual home" and a congregation of "kindred souls." Jessie met several women through the church who took her under their wing, helped her get oriented, recommended good neighborhood resources, and accompanied her on errands. These small concrete supports eased her insecurities and helped her gain a sense of mastery over the "foreign" environment. As her comfort increased, we talked about the library job she had left behind and her love and knowledge of books. Ted encouraged her to volunteer in the church's fund-raising book sale. Her success in that endeavor led to a volunteer position with the neighborhood library. In turn, that experience led within a few months to a part-time job in a bookstore, a short bus ride away. With Ted's confidence in her, she overcame her "fear of becoming panicky" and excelled in the job, which she found to be a rewarding challenge.

It was vital to our work that Jessie stop defining herself as damaged, but rather broaden her identity as a likable and interesting person, with many assets as well as vulnerabilities. It was also crucial that she experience therapy not as a place to nurse old wounds endlessly (as in her past therapy), but as a place to develop latent talents and abilities. Jessie came to look back on her prior therapy as an addiction. Over the years, her vulnerability and overdependence on her therapist had increased to the point where she doubted her ability to survive on her own.

Our therapy ended successfully after 5 months. Jessie's medication was tapered off gradually. A year later, I received a birth announcement with a very cute baby picture and a note of appreciation for helping the couple launch their new life. Yet life doesn't follow an orderly course. Six months later Jessie called in a panic: Ted's company had been bought out, and he might be downsized out of a job. Over several sessions, the couple proactively considered possible options if a "worst-case scenario" required another move. When the ax fell a few months later, the couple was prepared and Jessie didn't panic. Ted had already begun a job search, landing a good position in a desirable community where Jessie planned to return to college. We met for a few sessions before the move, and I linked them to a trusted colleague there if the need arose. Jessie's physician recommended that she resume her antianxiety medication if needed during the expectable turmoil of the move. We scheduled a follow-up phone contact, and they sent a card at holiday time expressing their pride at how smoothly the new transition had gone. With all they had learned from their previous move, they now considered themselves experts on relocation. Jessie even thought about writing an article for a magazine on the subject.

Respectful Collaboration

Clinicians and investigators have long sought to understand and effectively treat the most debilitating mental disorders but have too readily pathologized families. For decades, the concept of the "schizophrenogenic mother" blamed the purported character and parenting deficiencies of mothers for causing schizophrenia; "refrigerator mothers" were thought to cause autism. The family systems paradigm countered linear, deterministic assumptions to recognize the multiple, ongoing recursive transactions in the family unit. Still, some early family therapists focused on dysfunctional family processes in so-called "schizophrenic families" that were thought to maintain symptoms, approaching families adversarially as dangerous "barracudas" and calling their interactions "dirty games" (Anderson, 1986). However, strengths-oriented family therapists eschewed such pejorative approaches and emerging research confirmed a biological base in schizophrenia and found a wide range of functioning in patients' families (Walsh & Anderson, 1988).

Studies have examined the role of family processes in the future *course* of mental illness. For instance, high "expressed emotion" (i.e., critical comments and emotional overinvolvement) predicted later symptom relapse for highly vulnerable individuals. In studies of adopted-away identical twins with high genetic risk for schizophrenia, those growing up in families with communication deviance were significantly more likely to develop the disorder (Tienari et al., 2004). Notably, those studies also documented the importance of family protective factors: adoptive families with healthy communication patterns protected children at high risk from developing the disorder. By identifying such process elements, we can target interventions to lower stressful interaction patterns and enhance communication to strengthen both individual and family functioning.

Family Intervention and Psychoeducational Approaches

Research and practice developments have informed helpful family interventions with a range of serious and persistent mental disorders and developmental disabilities. Success depends on mobilizing family and community resources through collaborative relationships. Assessment and intervention engage family members as caring and vital resources for an impaired loved one's long-term adaptation. Interventions aim to reduce stress and strengthen a supportive network.

Clinicians need to counter the stigmatizing experiences of families who have felt blamed and shamed for their loved one's symptoms or failed treatment efforts. The family may be coping as well as can be reasonably expected in the face of recurrent psychotic or destructive episodes. Referral for family therapy should be disengaged from causal assumptions and based on the value of family involvement in strengthening effective coping and mastery with the stressful challenges of living with a persistent mental health condition.

Brief family therapy, providing structured, focused interventions, can be useful for strengthening individual and family functioning and reducing stress and conflict. It is crucial to set concrete, realistic objectives that can be tracked and tweaked, achieving small successes and a more solid base. On reaching a higher level of functioning and stabilization, gains can be sustained and setbacks averted with periodic family consultations or in multifamily groups.

Family psychoeducational approaches provide useful information, management guidelines, and social support. Combined treatment strategies that include family psychoeducation have been most effective in treating schizophrenia, bipolar disorder, major depression, and other serious disorders (Anderson, Reiss, & Hogarty, 1986; Lucksted, McFarlane, Downing, Dixon, & Adams, 2012; Miklowitz, 2010). Numerous studies have demonstrated the effectiveness of this approach in preventing relapse, improving recovery, and increasing family well-being. Drug maintenance may be needed to control the severity of symptoms and to prevent destructive behavior or repeated hospitalizations. Additionally, involvement in a social skills group and productive activity boost functioning and decrease isolation.

In the Anderson et al. (1986) model, a connecting phase established an empathic alliance, with the therapist attending noncritically to family needs and experiences and specific areas of stress in their lives. A daylong survival skills workshop providing information and management guidelines is followed by brief family therapy to support taking concrete steps toward stable functioning in the community. Monthly multifamily groups sustain gains. The basic principles of psychoeducation have been adapted for brief focused family consultation and effective prevention and early intervention programs (McFarlane, 2002). Family consumer groups critical of more traditional treatment have responded positively to these developments.

Psychoeducational multifamily groups are valuable with both mental and physical conditions (Gonzalez & Steinglass, 2002; McFarlane, 2002; Steinglass, 1998). They prevent or delay relapse, increase medication and treatment compliance, reduce stress, and improve individual and family functioning. Professionally led groups, typically with four or more families or couples, focus on ways to manage situational stress, loss, and transition while strengthening relationships and problem-solving abilities. The group context provides a social support network and opportunities for family members to learn from one another's experiences, to gain perspective on their own situation, and to reduce isolation and stigma, as well as guilt and blame. Group interventions may have a short-term or modular structure, typically as a daylong workshop, or 4–6 weekly sessions. Monthly meetings sustain gains, avert crises and setbacks, and address ongoing challenges and new or recurrent strains. Multifamily self-help groups are also useful in sustaining care and support over the long haul of a chronic condition.

Other family-based approaches have been developed in situations of maternal depression. Riley, Valdez, and colleagues designed Keeping Families Strong, using a multifamily group format to promote child and family resilience (Riley et al., 2008). Fortalezas Familiares (Family Strengths) is a 12-week community-based prevention program designed to address relational family processes and promote well-being in immigrant Latino families when a mother has depression (Valdez, Abegglen, & Hauser, 2012; Valdez, Padilla, Moore, & Magana, 2013).

Mobilizing Community Connections

Despite vital service needs, social policies and funding cuts have drastically reduced hospital stays, limiting them to treatment with medication and rapid stabilization, with inadequate outpatient services and community supports to sustain independent living. We see the failure of these policies in the tragic numbers of seriously troubled persons locked up in prisons or living precariously in the streets and shelters. The expectation for families to assume the primary caregiving burden over the chronic course of a mental illness, often with combined substance use issues, and the unresponsiveness to their concerns have led families to mobilize (Lefley, 2009). Consumer advocacy groups such as the National Alliance on Mental Illness (NAMI) provide valuable networks and information for families and lobby for more research and support. The Balanced Mind Parent Network (recently merged with the Depression and Bipolar Support Alliance) evolved out of efforts by families struggling with their youths' serious and volatile mood disturbances. Forming a virtual kitchen table community—a network of allies accessible anywhere, anytime—their web-based connections and programs share understanding and resources for educating, empowering, and ending isolation (*www.thebalancedmind.org*). As one mother said, "It's a beacon in our storm."

HELPING FAMILIES LIVE WELL
WITH CHRONIC CONDITIONS

General Clinical Priorities

With serious physical and mental conditions, it is vital to build family strengths, resources, and successful coping strategies. Families are better

able to handle stresses and to be more proactive to prevent and ameliorate future crises when we (1) identify and address common illness and
treatment challenges; and (2) offer problem-solving assistance through predictably stressful periods. Flexibility is needed to tailor interventions and
respond to family members as needs arise over the course of the illness and
with changing life challenges. Priorities include the following:

1. Reduce the stressful impact of the illness/disability experience on
   the family.
2. Share information about:
   • The illness/disability, treatment approaches, and expectable
     course
   • Individual vulnerabilities, abilities, and potential
   • Importance of compliance with medication, treatment, or diet
     regimens, and physical therapy/rehabilitation to reduce vulner-
     ability and enhance functioning
   • Expectable psychosocial challenges for the individual and family
     over time
   • Interaction with individual and family life cycle priorities
3. Offer practical guidelines through various phases of a chronic con-
   dition for:
   • Ongoing stress reduction
   • Managing symptoms, treatments, and complications
   • Problem solving and crisis prevention
   • Building strengths for optimal functioning and well-being
   • Respite and attention to other family members and life priorities
4. Provide links to services that support functioning in the community
   and the family's caregiving efforts, for example:
   • Home health care support
   • Day care, structured work programs, and social contact
   • Assisted living and group homes
   • National and local consumer groups; useful Internet resources
   • Faith-based communities and services

   Family members facing the demands of a serious illness are often
unsure whether they are doing too much or too little and how to navigate
unfamiliar and challenging situations. They value information, management guidelines, and help in setting realistic expectations. A neglected family issue is the need for respite—time and space from illness and caregiving
concerns for family members to meet their own needs, enjoy pleasurable
shared experiences, replenish their energies, and revitalize their spirits.

Attention is also needed to the many losses that often accompany a chronic condition—loss of functioning or cognitive capacity, loss of limbs or disfigurement, loss of a sense of intactness and "normality," loss of valued roles and functions in the family, loss of employment and status, and loss of personal and shared hopes and dreams for the future.

> Mick, a construction worker left permanently disabled and wheelchair bound by the collapse of a building, began to drink heavily. One night Peg, his wife, found him passed out on the floor with his hunting gun ready to be fired. In individual and conjoint sessions, we explored the multiple losses he had experienced: his family role as breadwinner, his "tough guy" image, and the active life he had prized. In family sessions, he realized how much he was loved, valued, and needed by his wife and children, which was most crucial to his inner healing and resilience. Their support and encouragement recharged his will to go on living and make the most of his life, seeking new ways to be productive and active. As Peg increased her job from part-time to full-time, he took over cooking and helping with his children's homework, which provided new satisfactions and closer family bonds. Over time, he set up a web-based small business and began coaching his daughter's soccer team. He told Peg that although he never would have wished for his disability, his life and loved ones now meant more to him than ever before.

Crisis Intervention/Crisis Prevention

Crisis intervention is urgently needed by families in times of acute distress, since most chronic disorders involve periodic exacerbation of symptoms. Without such help, many individuals and their families veer from one crisis to the next, achieve few gains over time, and risk emotional exhaustion, serious conflict, and relationship cutoff. Therapists must be active and provide enough structure to help temporarily overwhelmed families reorganize and gain control of threatening situations. Because individuals with cognitive impairment may lack motivation, use poor judgment, or not take needed medication, family collaboration is crucial to sustain involvement in treatment and to reduce stress. Periodic "psychosocial checkups" and prevention-oriented consultations can be timed around major changes in a condition or disruptive life transitions to help families "bounce forward" with resilience.

Community-Oriented Family-Centered Health Care

Both family and community resilience can be nurtured if all helping professionals reach out to persons with disabling conditions and their families, respect their dignity, and work to forge viable extended kin and social supports. In many cases, basic needs for human connection and productive functioning can be met through such programs as structured group living arrangements and sheltered workshops, tailored to the vulnerabilities and potential strengths of residents. Families are essential resources in treating serious and persistent illness and disability. We can encourage collaboration, understand their challenges, and support their best efforts. Yet families cannot carry the burden alone. Despite rhetoric supporting strong families, family-centered prevention and intervention services are lacking, despite evidence of their effectiveness. Families and helping professionals must complete burdensome paperwork and navigate confusing and frustrating compliance and reimbursement bureaucracies. Families living in impoverished conditions, especially ethnic and racial minorities, are most vulnerable to the risks of serious illness and disabilities, caregiver strains, and inadequate health care and mental health services. A system of care—a spectrum of integrated family-focused services, medical, personal, social, and rehabilitative—is required. A continuum of care and community services is essential to meet changing needs over time and to sustain independent living, optimal functioning, and well-being.

Seeing Differences as More Than Disabilities

A resilience orientation embraces the whole person, supporting families' loving abilities to see beyond disabilities to cherish their loved one and encourage positive interests, abilities, talents, and potential. Moreover, many parents raising a child with autism or other developmental disabilities are quite resilient (Bayat, 2007) and view the family experience as a gain, not a loss (Dura-Vila, Dein, & Hodes, 2010). This is especially important in countering the stigma of mental disorders. Many individuals with difficult lifelong challenges forge satisfying and productive lives and find meaningful expression in music, the arts, and other arenas. Some have special gifts that can be nurtured by families. Temple Grandin, a remarkable woman with autism, credits her mother's love and dedication with helping her make the most of her life. She achieved an advanced academic degree and channeled her hyperfocus and sensory differences into an extraordinary ability to relate to animals and take in the world as they do, recognizing their cognitive and emotional abilities (Grandin & Johnson, 2004). Her sensitivity to animal suffering led to the design of systems for more humane treatment of livestock. She has also been an inspiration to so many who have been labeled with severe deficits by viewing many autistic symptoms, such as hyperspecificity, as strengths rather than weaknesses. Her visual thinking allows her to find solutions that others might not see. She notes that whooping cranes can memorize long migratory routes they've flown only once by using a brain capacity similar to that shown by some individuals with autism in making complex drawings with perfect perspective. We need to see physical and cognitive differences in terms of *assets*, not only in terms of liabilities. By appreciating and enhancing each family member's interests and abilities, families can bring out their best and share joy in their bonds.

CHAPTER 13

Nurturing Resilience in Vulnerable, Multi-Stressed Families

Hope has never trickled down; it has always sprung up
—STUDS TERKEL, *Hope Dies Last*

Many families, especially those in poor and disadvantaged communities, are buffeted by frequent crises and chronic stresses that overwhelm their functioning. A family resilience approach is most needed and beneficial when families feel beaten down and defeated by repeated frustration and failure. This chapter offers a conceptual base and practice guidelines for strengthening highly vulnerable families—supporting their best efforts to manage their stress-laden lives and overcome the odds of high-risk conditions. By focusing on their positive aims and potential, families gain a sense of hope and confidence that they can rise above persistent adversity.

UNDERSTANDING MULTI-STRESSED FAMILIES

Multi-stressed families struggle with serious problems cutting across many dimensions of their lives. They can become overloaded and destabilized by a pileup of internal and external stresses over time. Couples are at high risk for conflict and breakup; single parents become depleted; and children or other family members may suffer from serious medical, behavior, or emotional problems, substance abuse, violence, or sexual abuse. Too often in mental health, social service, and juvenile justice systems, highly vulnerable families have been defined by their deficits. The label of "severely dysfunctional family" reinforced the view of a pathological family, prejudged as hopeless and untreatable. A narrow focus on the interior of the family and the label "multiproblem family" often blame families for their problems, many of which are beyond their control and not of their making. Seeing these families as "multi-stressed" (Madsen, 2009) better contextualizes family difficulties, recognizing their precarious life conditions and overwhelming challenges.

It is important to understand how multi-stressed families become overloaded and undersupported, rendered vulnerable by many past and ongoing challenges and unmet needs. Crisis situations are often embedded in their environmental conditions or trigger reactivation of past trauma. While many vulnerable youth and families are at high risk for serious problems, Swadener and Lubeck (1995) urge us to see them as children and families "at promise," with conviction about their potential and investment in helping them surmount barriers to positive development.

Family Challenges of Poverty and Discrimination

In a cruel paradox, crisis and disruption may be a constant in the lives of disadvantaged families. In the United States and other countries with vast economic, social, and racial disparities, low-income families confront relentless stress from unemployment, substandard housing, discrimination, and inadequate medical care. Parents struggle to provide their children with the basic essentials of food, clothing, shelter, and education. Life prospects are bleak for those with limited job opportunities and access to resources. When families live close to the edge, a job loss or medical crisis may plunge them into a financial abyss. Prolonged unemployment and temporary or part-time work without benefits make it hard to break the cycle of poverty and despair. Such problems present mammoth challenges to even the healthiest families.

The combined psychological, social, and economic burdens of poverty and discrimination place poor minority children and families at greater risk for multiple problems. Recent immigrants face the additional barriers of cultural and language differences. When surrounded by neighborhood blight, crime, violence, and drugs, parents worry constantly about their children's safety (Garbarino, 1997). Intertwined family and environmental stresses contribute to school difficulties and dropout, gang and criminal activity, and teen pregnancy—all of which worsen family strains. Interventions to reduce family vulnerability must address the environmental forces that pose such threats to family survival and positive child development.

Pileup of Stressors and Family Developmental Challenges

Family vulnerability is heightened by the cumulative impact of multiple stressors over time. Recurrent crises, trauma, losses, and dislocations can overwhelm coping efforts and disrupt family life. The demands of persistent challenges drain resources. Chronic distress can carry over from year to years and from one generation to the next. Overstressed and depleted family members are more likely to stumble or make poor choices, compounding their difficulties. Interventions for stress reduction and mutual support are imperative to break the cycle.

A single crisis event can have cascading effects (Masten, 2014). For instance, a catastrophic injury and disability may result in a job loss, loss of the family's housing, and relocation, triggering losses and adaptive challenges for children in a new neighborhood and school, with new peer relationships. Therapeutic response to a child's emotional or behavioral problems must be attuned to cumulative stresses. We can help families to gain perspective and to pace and buffer disruptive changes.

In multi-stressed families, a systemic assessment with genogram and timeline construction can reveal past and ongoing trauma, disruptions, and loss. Without trying to address each specific incident, which would overwhelm therapeutic efforts, it is important to identify major crises and attend to recurrent patterns. Even in brief counseling focused on current problems, it is crucial to understand how symptoms and catastrophic fears may be fueled by past trauma or the cumulative impact of experiences over time. In work with one couple in crisis, a partner's fears of commitment, withdrawal, and drinking are better comprehended when he recounts the many separations and losses he experienced throughout childhood in his family of origin and the foster care system. His drinking stirs his wife's catastrophic fears stemming from painful memories of a previous marriage shattered by alcohol abuse. An understanding of where families are coming from increases their ability to make meaning of their current dilemma, informing and empowering their actions and future directions.

STRENGTH-BASED, FAMILY-CENTERED SERVICES

Core Principles

Families that present multiple, complex, and severe problems and recurrent crises make up a disproportionately large segment of human services caseloads. Unfortunately, they are more likely to be ill served and to fall between the cracks (Kaplan & Girard, 1994). Traditional services have tended to be deficit based, individually focused, fragmented, crisis reactive, inaccessible, and defined for clients by "expert" professionals.

In contrast, strengths-oriented services stress the following core principles:

- Identify and build on family strengths and resources that empower families.
- Take a family-centered approach to individual problems.
- Provide flexible, holistic services.
- Emphasize prevention and early intervention.
- Build community-based, collaborative partnerships.

From Deficit-Based to Resource-Based Model

Uri Bronfenbrenner (1979), a champion of families, decried deficit-based public policies and services requiring recipients to document their families' inadequacies to qualify for help. Categorizing an individual or family with a pathological label is a dehumanizing and stigmatizing experience: negative stereotypes of parents as destructive, hostile, and uncaring; preconceptions of them as unreachable, unmotivated, and untreatable; and thick files of past problems and failed interventions—all create adverse expectations for any therapeutic contact.

It is crucial not to underestimate the ability of vulnerable families to understand and tackle their problems. Most show remarkable strengths alongside their difficulties (Orthner, Jones-Sanpei, & Williamson, 2004). Many are resilient simply in making it through each day of unrelenting hardship; many are resourceful in the inventive ways they manage on meager earnings. Most parents care deeply about their children and want a better life for them, although the crush of difficulties may block their ability to act consistently on their best intentions. They often know what they need to change in their lives, and can take positive steps if we value their input, listen well, and support their best efforts (Madsen, 2009).

When therapy with multi-stressed families is overly problem focused, it grimly replicates the problem-saturated experience of family life. A resilience-based perspective empowers them to navigate the challenges in their stress-laden lives. Interventions facilitate positive interactions, support coping efforts, and build resources to reduce stress, enhance pride and competence, and strengthen family functioning and bonds.

From Individually Based to Family-Centered Approaches

Compartmentalized services tend to categorize clients narrowly by presenting symptoms, inattentive to the whole person, the family, and the social context. Often agencies avow, in principle, the importance of strengthening families yet in practice usually see an individual child or adult, occasionally meeting with a primary caregiver. With heavy caseloads and complicated family situations, workers may doubt whether they can be helpful. A failed experience may reinforce their beliefs that multi-stressed families are beyond repair.

One of my students, eager to work with families in the juvenile justice system, found that despite her agency's stated mission to work with incarcerated youth and their families, in practice no families were seen. She was told that over the years, agency staff had found it too difficult "to get such dysfunctional families motivated for treatment" and no longer "wasted their resources." They met individually with the youth offenders, even though most youths maintained close contact with family members and returned home. In our experience, it is crucial to involve families in order to (1) enlist family support for incarcerated youths' transition back into the community, counter gang involvement, and encourage educational and job training pursuits; and (2) reduce family stresses and encourage their best efforts (Walsh, 2013a). When the family foundation is strengthened, the home becomes a more solid base for at-risk youths. If parents are unable to provide this structure, we recruit positive models and encourage mentoring relationships in the kin network (Ungar, 2004; see Chapter 8).

When any family member seeks help—a parent or caregiver, a child, a spouse—we broaden attention to the relational network. Maintaining a family focus doesn't require seeing the whole family together in ongoing sessions, which may not be feasible in overstressed or fragmented families. What matters most is maintaining a systemic perspective to address the important connections between family members, their problems, and potential resources for change and growth.

From Fragmented to Holistic Services

Human service systems intensify family confusion and frustration—and hamper workers' efforts—when they lack coordination, handle problems in a disorganized, piecemeal way, and require families to navigate a bureaucratic maze of agencies. In a family, one child may be seen by a school-based professional, a sibling by a juvenile justice counselor, and another member in a drug treatment program; a grandparent in the home may need extensive medical care, while an overloaded single parent suffers with depression. With fragmented services, no one is addressing interrelated concerns or building concerted efforts.

A family-centered resilience-oriented approach strengthens collaborative service delivery across systems. A broad, comprehensive approach aims to coordinate and integrate services and pool resources. Services are viewed holistically, tailored to each family's challenges and drawing on community, cultural, and spiritual resources.

From Crisis-Reactive to Prevention-Oriented Services

Mental health, human services, and school contacts with families tend to be crisis reactive. At such times, brief interventions cannot sufficiently address more complex or entrenched problems, or prepare families to meet future challenges. A limited focus may not foster relationship building or restructuring of family life to consolidate gains. Flexibility and responsiveness over time are needed to address persistent or recurrent problems and prevent future crises.

Prevention-oriented services—seriously underfunded—are far more effective and less costly than most treatment programs. By investing in families "up front," we increase their coping ability and resourcefulness, preventing problem escalation and chronicity (Harris, 1996). A preventive approach can identify highly vulnerable families—those in precarious situations, underresourced and beset by numerous problems. Through outreach, early intervention to strengthen family functioning can prevent more serious and chronic problems.

Building a Collaborative, Family-Centered, Community-Based Partnership

The early movement advocating family support and preservation programs for at-risk children and families, linked with the child development field, was founded on the belief that families are our best resource (e.g., Dunst & Trivette, 2009; Kagan & Weissbourd, 1994). Head Start's successful preschool program was designed to empower families and improve young children's life chances, encouraging family involvement in all aspects of the program. Parents collaborate in program decision making and serve as volunteers, observers, and paid support staff. By working closely with professional staff they gain the skills to help their children and improve their own lives.

Family support programs have tended to focus on early mother–child bonds, although many have expanded to involve the family caregiving network. Consumer oriented, they operate at the grassroots level, concentrating on prevention and early intervention for capacity building. Local, accessible family resource centers provide a range of information and services to support and strengthen vulnerable families. Professionals and neighborhood paraprofessionals assist families with stressful life cycle transitions, such as parenting education and support, particularly for single teen parents. They link families with formal and informal services and support networks, pooling efforts by communities, school systems, hospitals, and corporations.

Family preservation programs have a dual commitment to protect vulnerable children and to strengthen their families. Based on the conviction that the best place for children is with their families as long as safety is assured, these programs aim to support and strengthen troubled families instead of replacing them. To prevent out-of-home placement, they provide immediate, home-based intervention to defuse a crisis, stabilize the family, and teach problem-solving skills to avoid future crises. Trained staff work intensively with families in their homes, addressing areas of concern. With accountability for any future neglect or abuse, family members are actively involved in assessing risks, reducing stress, and strengthening leadership, nurturance, and protection. Additional support is available as needed. Placement is necessary when children are at high risk of serious neglect or abuse and family interventions are unworkable. Efforts are made to link residential and foster care rather than sever family ties, with family reunification when possible (Kaplan & Girard, 1994).

Multilevel Systemic Approaches

Programs based on a strengths-oriented multisystemic approach build family and community partnerships, fortifying the collective capacity to surmount adverse conditions (Saul, 2013). Services are designed to be accessible, affordable, and offered through home-based and neighborhood programs (Madsen & Gillespie, 2014). Multilevel approaches address individual issues, such as a child's school or behavior problems in a challenging social context, through family and larger systems interventions, such as family–school partnerships. SAFE Children, a model program in Chicago, builds on Head Start to help parents in violent neighborhoods get children off to a good start in first grade. Efforts are made to connect families and build a strong sense of community, overcoming isolation and mistrust through informal contact, shared projects, and activities. Families participate actively in setting priorities and seeking solutions, building networks and structural supports.

Fraenkel (2006; Fraenkel, Hameline, & Shannon, 2009) developed an effective collaborative program for homeless families residing in shelters, in transition from welfare to work. He stressed that to truly collaborate with families in building programs, professional program developers must view families as experts on the life situations that challenge them and as the best informants on what they would find most useful in a program to support their coping and resilience. This approach is particularly appropriate in working with families marginalized by class, race, ethnicity, or other dimensions of difference and discrimination, who often receive programs created with little or no consultation from them. As a result, families may not find the programs engaging or relevant, may elect not to attend them, and are then viewed as "resistant" or "unmotivated." However, families will eagerly engage in programs when they have some control over the processes used to create the program; when they have contributed to the program's content and structure through their wisdom, experiences, and desires; and when the relationship between professional program developers and recipients is collaborative and mutually respectful.

A multisystemic perspective integrates various program efforts involving families and communities, from preventive approaches, such as family life education and psychoeducational support groups, to more intensive interventions for crises and entrenched problems. A family life cycle orientation can guide services to foster healthy pregnancy and early child rearing; child and adolescent development; stable family units; and elder care (see Chapter 9). Workers with vulnerable youth and families can increase their effectiveness and reduce burnout through training in strengths-oriented systemic assessment and family intervention skills (e.g., Berg, 1997; Madsen & Gillespie, 2014; Minuchin, Colapinto, & Minuchin, 2007). Madsen's (2011) Collaborative Helping maps are a valuable tool to guide efforts, by focusing on clients' positive vision, identifying and mobilizing potential supports, overcoming obstacles, and taking active steps toward aims.

Several evidence-based, family-centered, multisystemic intervention models have been effective with high-risk and troubled youth, their families, and larger community systems (Henggeler, Cunningham, Schoenwald, & Borduin, 2009; Liddle, 2013; Sexton, 2011). These approaches, used with youth conduct disorder and substance abuse, yield improvements in family functioning, including increased cohesion and communication and improved parenting practices that are significantly linked to more positive youth behavioral outcomes than those achieved with standard services. With varied formats, family therapists may involve school counselors, teachers, coaches, and peer groups, and work with police, probation officers, and judges to address legal issues. They might help a youth and family access vocational services, youth development organizations, social support networks, and religious resources. All contacts draw out strengths and competencies for change.

ASSESSMENT AND INTERVENTION PRIORITIES

A family resilience orientation is grounded in the conviction that even the most troubled families want to be healthy and have the potential for change and growth. However, environmental obstacles, depleted resources, or self-defeating survival strategies may block efforts and ability to see positive options in their situation. Engaging family members collaboratively, therapists help them develop a shared sense of hope, active agency, and empowerment. Efforts are made to identify and overcome barriers to success in the therapeutic, family, and social contexts.

Assessing Family Stress, Vulnerabilities, Strengths, and Potential

A resilience-based refocus begins in the first contacts with a family. In assessment, we need to be explicit that our intentions in gathering information are to understand family stresses and their impact, as well as family objectives and pathways for moving forward. Past experience with judgmental, deficit-based evaluation may lead family members to hear even neutral questions as blame laden. In resilience-oriented practice, we assess families within a positive framework, searching for resources and potential as well as vulnerabilities and constraints, all in relation to their challenges and their aims.

Most often, help seeking centers on an immediate crisis focused on one family member. On contact, a number of problems often become evident and other members may be in distress. When we understand how a son's vandalism, a father's disappearance, financial hardship, and a mother's depression are all connected, we can better focus on common concerns and aims. When presenting problems are reactive to family stress—and exacerbate that stress—we mobilize family teamwork to make things better. This collaborative approach alleviates distress and instills hope and confidence that other challenges can be mastered.

Information gathering lays the groundwork for identifying strengths and prioritizing areas of concern. What are the significant family and community connections? How do family members view their adverse situation? How have they attempted to deal with it? What patterns of interaction escalate or reduce anxiety or conflict? Increase or reduce vulnerability and risk? Which members are helpful in strengthening the family? How do they do that? What hidden resources might be tapped to manage stresses and overcome barriers to success? How can change in the core family unit have a positive ripple effect for each member? When a family is in perpetual crisis and members' attention is scattered, it's important to understand major stresses in early sessions and identify patterns connected with members' distress.

Genograms (McGoldrick et al., 2008) are essential tools for diagramming very complex family systems—for instance, those extending across households in binuclear, stepfamily, and foster or extended families; those where a parent has had multiple partners and children have different fathers; and those with members in and out of various living arrangements (see Chapter 6). Drawing a large genogram interactively with a family readily engages family members. Children are often very interested to see how people are connected and where each one fits in the relational network. Seeing everyone on the same page facilitates a sense of coherence for fragmented families that have experienced many losses, dislocations, and reconfigurations. Visualizing systemic patterns helps both therapist and family to feel less confused and orients intervention planning.

Drawing a family timeline fosters a developmental perspective, as family members recall key events and their impact over time (see Chapter 6). How did a family attempt to handle traumatic events? What organizational shifts occurred with major transitions? In a multi-stressed family, a timeline helps to order the jumble of events and changes in family life over time. For instance, family members can better comprehend a parent's withdrawal into alcohol when seen in its stress-laden context. The genogram and timeline are valuable in assembling many disconnected fragments of experience into a fuller, more coherent family narrative.

When family life has been saturated with problems, it's essential to identify particular relationships, events, and periods of time that have offered islands of calm, satisfaction, connection, and hope in the midst of the turbulence. These positive experiences, often invisible when assessment and therapy are problem focused, offer resources to be drawn upon and enlarged. A teenager abused by her mother's boyfriend may have found shelter in a nurturing relationship with a grandmother. Even if that person is no longer nearby or alive, identifying the positive qualities in the relationship can provide a template for forming new, healthier relationships.

Diagnostic assessment can be essential in identifying serious mental illness and substance abuse, determining risk for destructive behavior, and evaluating the need for psychotropic medication. However, labels that locate the problem in a person's character structure tend to reinforce a sense of permanent damage and defect. It's more helpful and hopeful to identify problematic behavioral and interactional patterns that people can take steps to change. We should also be careful not to label a family by a member's problems (e.g., "an alcoholic family") and should put nothing in a case report that disrespects clients. By encouraging them to read and offer input in letters to agencies or courts we value them as active partners in therapy.

Key Processes in Family Resilience: Framework for Assessment and Intervention

The three-domain framework of key family resilience processes presented in Chapters 3–5 was initially developed for effective intervention with families presenting many serious and chronic problems. It facilitated my own shift from labeling families as "severely dysfunctional" to identifying particular vulnerabilities and resources that could be strengthened. Multi-stressed families and clinicians can be flooded by intense emotions and chaos in the midst of crises. The framework keeps me mindful to search for strengths and not become overwhelmed by a myriad of problems. Even when information emerges helter-skelter in the course of interviews, we can map it in a way that allows us to keep a systemic perspective and target key processes in interventions aiming to strengthen family resilience.

Belief Systems

When families experience recurrent crises, disappointments, and frustrations they are more likely to believe that things will turn out badly. This expectation generates pessimism, skewing perceptions of future possibilities. The inability to see viable alternatives or solutions further erodes confidence and blocks initiative. All-or-none global generalizations are common, in extremes of always or never, all-powerful or powerless, victim or villain. Catastrophic fears and destructive behavior patterns often radiate from constant exposure to community violence and a socially toxic environment (Garbarino, 1997) or can ripple down from multiple traumas in family history.

When families struggle with severe and persistent conditions that are largely beyond their control, professionals need to help them counter a pervasive sense of helplessness and hopelessness. It is crucial not to give up on families that seem at first to resist our help. Listening to their prior experiences can shed light on their pessimism and mistrust: they expect that their efforts will be futile or that we will let them down, as others have. By steadily conveying our belief in their worth and potential, despite missteps or setbacks, we can help families to believe in themselves, fostering pride, courage, and hope for the future, which fuel positive action and perseverance.

Cultural and spiritual resources can be wellsprings for resilience in poor and marginalized communities, where grim life chances breed a foreshortened sense of future for youth. With a high proportion of young men lost to violence, drugs, or prison, families and communities must be all the more determined to raise their youth to overcome these challenges, drawing on their cultural heritage, as in the wisdom of an Ashanti proverb, "You must act as if it is impossible to fail."

Strong faith beliefs, practices, and congregational involvement counter despair and sustain a spirit of love, courage, and endurance for most families in poor communities (Walsh, 2009d, 2012d). They facilitate positive parenting and, when shared with at-risk youth, protect youth from delinquency (Mahoney, 2010). Harry Aponte's (2009) work with poor minority inner-city families led him to recognize their spiritual as well as their physical needs. A pervasive sense of injustice, helplessness, and rage is rooted in being denied access to opportunity, power, and privilege in society. Aponte urges therapists not to limit our work to pragmatic solutions but also attend to spiritual needs to counter the despair that robs lives of meaning, purpose, and hope. He also calls on therapists to work as catalysts for community activism, to mobilize the spirit of hope to transform oppressive conditions.

Organizational Processes

Most multi-stressed families seen in human service agencies live in single-parent households and have complex family structures. Research shows that families of varied forms can function and raise their children well. However, unremitting stresses and scarce resources wear down family functioning and stability, deplete parental energies, and heighten risks for child maladaptation. Multiple parental repartnering, repeated losses, and dislocations compound the difficulties. The family organization, role functioning, interaction patterns, and relationships can become fragmented and chaotic. Therapeutic priorities are to strengthen the stability and cohesion of the family unit and draw on extended family and community resources.

Building Structure, Stability, Leadership, and Collaboration. Strengthening family organization is a high priority. With chronic stresses, roles and rules can become blurred, impairing the collaboration needed to structure daily life and resolve problems that accumulate. A lack of security, stability, and consistency can ensue with multiple repartnering, separations, and shifting household membership. Amid chaos is a deep longing for order, security, and stability.

Some families fluctuate between extreme rigidity and disorder. With upheaval they may hold on tightly to what is familiar. An unspoken rule might be "Don't rock the boat," with the fear of "capsizing" again. When families are overwhelmed, the therapeutic setting must provide a safe haven and solid structure with reassuring calm, order, predictability, and stability. Pushing too quickly for "therapeutic change" may fuel fears of more upheaval and loss of control. It is more helpful to start with small, grounded incremental steps to build on. Although we cannot control our clients' lives—nor should we—therapists should take charge of sessions and interrupt runaway processes or destructive escalations so families feel in control of the helping process and their lives.

Interventions aim to strengthen authoritative parenting. Family leadership, worn down by stress, may become erratic and ineffective, with inconsistent limit setting, monitoring, and follow-through until a parent reaches a boiling point and explodes. When a parent is unsure how to provide both nurturance and discipline, it can be helpful to frame discipline as setting caring limits and loving consequences.

When overwhelmed parents are unable to control unruly children, it can reinforce a sense of helplessness and incompetence if a professional helper simply takes over. It's important to put parents in charge and support them in setting rules and limits. We empower parents by joining forces with them and backing them up to bolster their authority and leadership. We may need to take charge initially in sessions, yet aim to increase parental competence and confidence to provide leadership.

In multi-stressed families, especially single-parent households, teamwork among all members is essential. Clear and age-appropriate expectations for older children to pitch in with delegated tasks can build their competencies and support family functioning. Skews of overfunctioning–underfunctioning members need to be rebalanced, with parents clearly in charge, and no child overburdened, or siblings simply free to roam. Concrete guidelines, such as posting a chart of weekly chores fairly allocated, can reinforce structure and follow-through. Positive reinforcement, grounded in social learning models, is especially needed in multi-stressed families to counter the barrage of problems and the focus on misdeeds and punishment. Praise and privileges reward efforts and build a sense of personal responsibility and a sense of value and belonging.

Assessing whether overwhelmed families are motivated poses the wrong question; rather, we need to ask how we can support their best efforts to manage the myriad of stresses and reduce frustrations. We should take care not to pile still more demands on already overloaded parents. Inability to follow through only reinforces their sense of deficiency.

It's important to acknowledge and contextualize difficulties in their position. After just an hour of pandemonium in a session, or hearing about the many problems during the week, we can use our own feeling of being overwhelmed to identify with parental challenges and applaud their efforts and perseverance.

Building Connection and Mutual Support. When overwhelmed families become fragmented and disengaged, members are left to fend for themselves and lack caring and enjoyable contact. Frustrations can boil over into intense conflict or disruptive behavior, further splintering family bonds. Families in blighted and marginalized living conditions, who often experience uncaring, denigrating mistreatment, may become socially isolated and alienated and feel unsupported, all of which contributes to abuse and neglect. Depleted parents may be unaware of children's whereabouts, sexual activity, or drug or alcohol use. Some parents take flight from responsibility or seek escape themselves in substance use. A sense of desperation may fuel threats to send a misbehaving child away. Youth who have a sense of belonging and of being nurtured and valued by their families and communities are at lower risk of conduct disorder, early pregnancy, and gang involvement (see Chapter 8). Intervention efforts focus on facilitating family connection, teamwork, mutual support, and links to extended kin and community resources.

In more disturbed families, vulnerable and highly anxious members become enmeshed: clinging to each other, boundaries blurred, and thoughts, feelings, and needs fused or distorted. Unclear boundaries contribute to violation in sexual abuse. Parents may entangle children in their marital strife. Jenny, age 17, was seen for self-destructive behavior after carving small crosses in her arms. Embroiled in her parents' intense conflict, she said she felt "caught in the crossfire." Other siblings may cut off all contact or oscillate between distancing and falling back into helpless dependence— a pattern common in drug and alcohol abuse. Jenny's brother "took the geographical cure" (as he put it)—abruptly leaving home and driving 500 miles to a remote area and a cabin off a dirt road. Yet he returned, curious to "check out" the family therapy, and sat quietly near the door throughout a session with a bemused smile. Later he told me he had been high on drugs in order to keep "a safe distance." Such intense, ambivalent attachments and loyalties often aren't simply resolved by physical separation. Family therapy, combined with individual work, can untangle members and help them achieve a more differentiated connection.

In some instances, family life has spun frighteningly out of control, as in the following case:

The Washingtons were referred for family therapy after two brothers, ages 13 and 15, were arrested for vandalism. Most recently, they had set their mother's bed on fire. It was learned that the mother had given her bedroom to her oldest son, age 17, and appointed him "man of the house," after evicting the father because of recurrent drunken, assaultive behavior. The mother's family-of-origin relations were also complicated by alcohol abuse and violence. Her sister, a single parent living in poverty, had "lost all control" and beaten her small child to death.

The therapist, understandably overwhelmed by the history, was unsure of where to begin. It was important to identify and alter interactional patterns that reinforced vulnerability. When clear structure is lacking, things get out of control; catastrophic fears takes hold: anything can happen, from violence to murder to sexual violations. Although the household was safer from violence with the father gone, the mother had relied on his "law and order" authority and felt unable to take charge. Further, a demanding factory job and long commute left her exhausted when she got home. Their apartment was in disarray. The mother slept on the living room sofa, while the 12-year-old daughter was sharing a room with her two "wild" brothers. Their living structure heightened risks and reinforced their sense of chaos.

It was crucial to shore up family stability, leadership, and boundaries. The therapist framed these objectives normatively, affirming the mother's position of respect and authority as head of the household and the healthy needs of all family members. He strongly encouraged the mother, as a hardworking sole parent with "two shifts" of job and family demands, to reclaim her own room, where she could close the door for needed respite. The family members were encouraged to be creative and come up with ways to rearrange their apartment so that everyone could claim a space of their own. In the next session, they sketched the floor plan with magic markers and cut out drawings of furniture to arrange. They enjoyed this fun task and it gave them a sense of control in planning their living space. The therapist affirmed the mother's suggestion that a small storage room could be cleared out for the daughter. He framed this good idea normatively, in terms of teenage girls' need for privacy from their brothers. The mother had the eldest move back in with his brothers, helping to calm them down and assist them with homework. The therapist supported their eagerness to decorate their own personal space around their beds with photos and posters. As in this case, we can facilitate structural changes in families by encouraging their inventive solutions in everyday life.

Nonresidential Parents and Extended Family and Social Networks. While the household functioning is most crucial, it is also important to increase the reliability of commitments to children by nonresidential parents. It's important to ask about the amount and dependability of contact and financial support, especially where children have different fathers, or a parent has dropped out of the picture. Even where custodial parents and their extended family are pessimistic about partners who were unreliable in the past, we should not reflexively write them off without exploring their current status (e.g., they may be gainfully employed or in stable recovery from substance abuse). More often than expected, uninvolved fathers care deeply about their children and have a strong desire for contact. With the custodial parent's agreement, we can contact the nonresidential parent to explore his or her situation, potential involvement, and any risk concerns. If the response is favorable, then facilitating cooperative coparenting arrangements will benefit the children (Waller, 2012). A clearly structured stepwise process can knit together frayed bonds. Demonstrating reliability and trust are paramount. To ensure children's protection in cases of past risk, carefully monitored visits can be arranged, often involving the extended family. In my experience, it is never too late for uninvolved parents to become more supportive of their children's positive growth.

Extended family networks are vital lifelines for multi-stressed families, including aunts, uncles, godparents, and informal kin. Co-residence can ease financial concerns. Grandmothers often fill a crucial caregiving role in overstressed and fragmented families. We should also explore the potential contribution of grandfathers and stepgrandfathers, often overlooked. Many who were uninvolved with their own children or made serious missteps earlier in life have deep regret and welcome the opportunity to step forward for the next generation. In one urban neighborhood plagued by street crime, drugs, and violence, a grandfathers' watch group was formed to protect children walking to and from school, a dangerous daily passage.

Communication Processes

Clarity. Pervasive unclear communication processes heighten family vulnerability. Parents may need help being more consistent in words and deeds. Messages may become distorted or family members may think they can—or should—read minds, further confusing their thoughts and expectations. Important information remains murky, increasing anxieties. Helping families clarify their problematic situations, options, and aims should be a priority.

We need to be clear and consistent in defining our therapeutic partnership: our role and commitment to family members, what they can expect of us, and what we will expect of them. It's important to keep our contacts on a regular, predictable schedule as much as possible, and to make every effort to follow through on expectations. In sessions, setting and maintaining communication rules brings order and focus to chaotic family interactions. For instance, a rule about turn taking can be helpful when members talk at once, interrupt, and don't listen to others, or go off on tangents. "Only one person talks at a time. That way, when it's your turn, everyone will be able to listen to you." Framing the rule in terms of the positive benefits is more effective than criticizing offenders for interrupting others. A toy microphone or "talking stick," like those used in tribal meetings, can facilitate communication.

Emotional Expression. A pileup of family stresses can shut down emotional sharing or heighten reactivity as tensions reverberate. It's important to help family members tolerate a range and fluidity of difficult emotions—sadness, anger, frustration, helplessness, repeated disappointment, or fears—while helping them to modulate their intensity and respond empathically to each other (Johnson, 2002). Therapists must actively interrupt destructive cycles and help family members feel safe and handle negative feelings in constructive and respectful ways. Repeated negative interactions corrode relationships and block mutual understanding as family members stop listening, counterattack, or withdraw. Some families suppress upsetting feelings and avoid conflict, fearing it will escalate into violence or family dissolution, as it may have in the past. Yet when tensions mount and emotional needs go unmet, risk is heightened for periodic explosions of pent-up feelings (again, in an all-or-none pattern). It's important to understand catastrophic fears, shore up mutual support, and help family members express emotional needs and hurts in ways that foster understanding and healing. We can help them gain skill in managing and repairing conflicts. By setting and maintaining facilitative ground rules in our sessions, we help family members feel safer to express concerns. When highly sensitive issues can be discussed more calmly, anxieties lessen and problems are tackled more effectively.

It's even more important to facilitate positive interactions in problem-saturated families. Most needed is the genuine expression of love, appreciation, and gratitude toward each other. Shared humor, laughter, fun, and pleasurable activities revitalize family life, counteracting exhaustion and burnout from constant demands. We need to be mindful that parents, as well as children, need nourishment. They urgently need appreciation for their efforts and respite from the storms of life in order to replenish their energy and spirits. I recently observed a session with a struggling family at a clinic in Hong Kong. Before the session, the director and therapist, Wei Yung Lee, and I thought it might be an interesting idea to serve tea to all family members. Since she didn't have tea handy, she filled a large pot with hot water, taking it in on a tray with cups for everyone. The mother, who had been quite discouraged and slumping in her chair, sat up and eagerly drank cup after cup, becoming more lively and engaged with every sip.

Collaborative Problem Solving. Action-oriented, concrete problem solving is essential in work with multi-stressed families, also helping them to reduce the negative impact of problems that can't be solved. A first priority may be addressing a family's immediate needs, such as housing, employment, day care, or job training. Clear, attainable objectives should be defined, with small, manageable steps toward them. Each success builds more confidence in the ability to deal with more complicated issues. It also builds trust in the therapeutic relationship and in family teamwork. Tasks should be designed to reduce stress and to strengthen family structure. We need to help family members prioritize and focus their attention. When we normalize and anticipate possible setbacks or upheaval if a new crisis hits, they are less discouraged by inevitable bumps in the road. Failure is not falling down, but staying down. Although we and our clients can't control everything, what matters is the determination to rebound and redouble our efforts.

Therapy empowers families by helping them develop their own competencies. It is not enough to reduce their current stress; by enhancing their problem-solving skills, we make them better able to meet future challenges. The focus extends from solving presenting problems to preventing future ones. We want to encourage them to anticipate not only how things can go wrong, but how, with their efforts, they can go right.

In resilience-oriented practice, therapists help families to refocus from problems to possibilities. Possibilities are generated as dilemmas are viewed in ways that expand options. Rather than focus on reducing negative behaviors, we are more successful when we help families gain new skills, competence, and confidence. To master the art of the possible, we help families learn from how things have gone wrong and conditions that can't be changed to refocus on how they can succeed and move forward, as in the following case:

> Crystal, age 14, was referred for therapy following her second attempt to run away from home. The therapist learned that she had been sexually abused by her grandfather when she was younger, and just recently by her mother's boyfriend, Rick. Her mother had ended that relationship after the incident, but Crystal angrily blamed her for not having protected her. The therapist, intending to be supportive, joined in faulting the mother, only to find that after the session Crystal took a handful of pills in a suicide attempt.

Family sessions were held, focused on drawing out family resources to handle the current crisis. The mother was genuinely remorseful for not having been aware of the abuse or more tuned in to Crystal's distress. The therapist acknowledged both Crystal's pain and her mother's genuine regret, suggesting that they could learn from those experiences to approach this crisis in a new way. She credited the mother for ending her relationship with Rick, demonstrating that Crystal's well-being came first. They focused on what might be done next. Crystal wanted to have Rick prosecuted. Her mother agreed to press charges. The therapist enlisted Crystal's two older brothers, who lived outside the home, to support Crystal and her mother through the ordeal of the legal maze and the trial ahead.

Over the next 3 months, the therapist tracked and commended the family's progress in doggedly pursuing the case. She supported the mother in remaining firm when Rick tried to get her to back down. The family members pulled together in taking on this challenge and succeeded in winning a conviction. Crystal threw her arms around her mother in the last family session and thanked her mother and brothers: "You really came through for me this time. I feel like we're all really family for the first time."

Families are empowered when they gain access to their power. While acknowledging and honoring trauma and suffering that has occurred, we can put our weight on the side of hope—the potential that things can be changed for the better. We can emphasize positive intentions, tap underutilized strengths, and celebrate progress and successes.

MASTERING PRACTICE CHALLENGES

Reaching Out to Families

Multi-stressed families often become frustrated, wary, and mistrustful of well-intentioned "helpers" because of repeated negative interactions and unhelpful experiences with numerous systems (Boyd-Franklin, 2004). Their guardedness and skepticism can take many forms, from overt anger to missed sessions or lack of follow-through with agreed-upon plans. Their actions may express the attitude "Why bother. Nothing ever works out, workers come and go, and no one really cares." Helping professionals need to understand such learned pessimism and make every effort to connect productively. This demonstrates our commitment to hang in with reluctant family members to gain their trust and acceptance. After a missed appointment, sending a reminder message for the next session communicates our investment and promotes continuity in our working alliance.

Every effort should be made to reach out to reluctant family members, whose participation can contribute to reduce stress, risk, and vulnerability and strengthen family functioning and child well-being. We can best enlist a reluctant father's active involvement in therapy as a caring parent, underscoring his powerful role and pride in helping his children succeed. The unclear role of a parent's cohabiting partner should be explored, assessing any risk factors, but also supporting potential assets to stabilize and strengthen a vulnerable situation.

Searching for Strengths amid Persistent Problems

Some families seem to be in perpetual crisis. Without a systemic frame and clear objectives, therapy sessions may cast about in all directions, reeling from crisis to crisis. With families flooded by problems, it is challenging to resist the pull of pathology and to search for strengths. When families come in crisis, the problematic aspects of their lives stand out, and helping professionals may become as overwhelmed and discouraged as they are. Becoming frustrated, we may pull back from engaging fully with the family or thinking creatively about change. When our clients sense our loss of hope and commitment, they are more likely to give up and drop out of therapy. Gaining an appreciation of their healthy strivings gives us hope, which fuels energy to work with those strengths to overcome the chaos in their lives. When we underestimate our clients, we lose sight of their potential for mastery. There may be truly impossible cases, but that has rarely been my experience, nor that of my strength-oriented colleagues.

Even in the most troubled families, areas of competence can be found and enlarged as sources of pride and accomplishment (Waters & Lawrence, 1993). We are most effective when we encourage family members to develop options and skills rather than dwelling on their limitations. In the unfolding process of therapy, we face constant choices about what to focus on. If we get caught up in a family's hopelessness and helplessness, therapy bogs down. Every maladaptive response also contains the seeds of healthy striving that can be cultivated. Parents may lose control and become abusive *because* they care so much and want so badly for a child to do better. We need continually to emphasize hope, caring, and small gains to enable the parents to hang in and act on their best intentions. Although there is most often caring alongside abuse or neglect, there are some cases (e.g., families with seriously drug-addicted parents) where caring has been extinguished over time and cannot be revived. And yet we should not write off the possibility of change, but make a determined effort to support new beginnings, as we search out positive resources in the kin network.

One of the hardest challenges for therapists is to align empathically with family members who are slow to change. We may also be drawn in to demonize men who have been abusive or mothers who have failed to protect their children. While addressing problem behavior, we need to resist the pull to pathologize the person. We can gain empathy from seeing every person in the context of his or her life struggles: a single parent who is undersupported; a wife whose trust in men has been shattered by past sexual abuse; a father who himself was abused and knows no other way to discipline children. When therapists view entrenched problems as constitutional and inevitable, it may relieve them of a sense of failure for therapeutic gridlock, but they further erode their clients' sense of worth and life chances. We can open possibilities for change by appreciating our clients' struggles and viewing therapeutic impasses as shared challenges, requiring courage, perseverance, and renewed teamwork.

Crisis Intervention and Crisis Prevention

When overwhelmed, some families may view therapy much as they do an emergency room service: they appear in crisis and don't return after things calm down. Therapists, too, can get caught up in a reactive mode: we all become swept up by the latest crisis and its aftermath. One therapist had seen a mother in crisis after being beaten by an abusive boyfriend. The mother canceled the next session, when he was jailed and out of the picture. However, 6 weeks later, the family was in crisis after the mother was battered once again by the boyfriend. The therapist hadn't asked when he was likely to be released and how the mother would deal with his return. Thus, the opportunity was missed to plan ahead and be prepared. Yet many crises can be anticipated and prevented. It's essential to get ahead of the next wave. By structuring family interviews to include a future focus, we can better anticipate problems and increase our ability to prepare clients to manage or avert them.

Creating Problem-Free Zones

Because families come to therapy and counseling to address problems, we need to be careful not to replicate a family's grim experience of life as a barrage of problems. It's important to encourage conversation about nonproblematic and positive areas of life. Faces will light up and conversation will become animated as we show interest in school and activities, highlights of the week, and pleasurable times, however fleeting. It brings welcome relief to laugh together about humorous moments. As we amplify areas of competence and success, it instills hope and encourages family members to see beyond problems. When daily life is consumed by problems, we can help family members to structure problem-free zones: plan a family outing or a "date" for parents to enjoy with problem talk "off limits"; agree on a rule of no fighting at the dinner table or in a couple's bedroom.

In particular, structuring in time and activities for parents to have respite from constant demands enables them to feel nurtured, to "refuel," and then to function more effectively. A single mother can be invited to pick times in the coming week for herself when she is "off duty," and family members can be mobilized to ensure that her time and space are honored. Recruiting extended family members—aunts, uncles—to pitch in periodically, even in small ways, can also relieve the constant stress.

Recruiting Models and Mentors

Models and mentors can be found and involved in even the most troubled family. Older siblings can draw on their abilities to assist younger children who are having difficulties, such as teaching skills or helping with homework, thereby building bonds. In situations where parents are absent or limited by serious mental illness, criminal activity, or substance abuse, it's crucial to engage other members of the extended kin system. In the case of an at-risk youth whose older brother and father were gang involved, we recruited a maternal uncle who had left prison and gang life and turned his life around, who formed a strong mentoring relationship with the boy, supporting his positive pursuits.

The moving story of the life of the poet Maya Angelou reveals the power of kinship bonds in her remarkable resilience in overcoming childhood adversity (Angelou, 2004). Because Maya's divorced parents were heavily involved in an unsafe environment of substance abuse, gambling, and promiscuity, they sent Maya, age 5, and her older brother, Bailey, across the country to their grandmother's care. The strong sibling bond gave each the courage and confidence to overcome many life challenges throughout their lives. Their grandmother provided the stability and security they desperately needed. Living in the segregated rural South, the grandmother sustained her own resilience through her deep faith and personal connection to God, whom she talked to "like a favorite uncle." Every day after school Maya went to the small grocery store run by her uncle Willie, who would grill her on her homework. Uncle Willie, a man of humble means with little formal schooling, was also lame and had a severe speech disability. Yet he valued education and became her mentor and champion. He prodded her to do her best in her studies and to aim high in her life aspirations. She wrote a poem to honor him (Angelou, 2004) and encourage others to seek out their own Uncle Willies in their relational networks who can serve the same function in their lives.

Learning and Growth from Past Trauma

Past crisis situations in one generation may come to the fore in the next, often when a child reaches the same age a parent had been at the time. A mother, worried that her 16-year-old daughter is sexually active and will get pregnant, may herself have become pregnant at 16. Although a family's current stress overload can make history taking challenging, learning about past nodal events often sheds light on immediate concerns.

In an integrative therapeutic approach, work is present- and future-focused, yet is linked to each family's past. It is important to make connections and distinctions between past and present challenges and responses: A father, as a young son, may have lacked his own father's positive involvement or felt powerless to gain his love and approval, but now he can be a loving parent with his children. The therapeutic task is to bring intergenerational patterns and linkages to light, and then to take lessons from painful past experience and seize the opportunity to do things differently with one's partner and children. It can be helpful for children to learn stories of their parents' struggles growing up, and it helps parents to gain empathy for their children's positions. We might ask, "What did you need that your parents were unable to provide?" "Alongside their problems, what positive memories do you have of them and your relationship?" "Now that you're a parent, what can you learn from your experience to better meet your children's needs?" Parents can be commended for caring enough about their children to take steps to prevent a painful history from repeating itself. We can encourage them to act on their best intentions and their yearning to create the strong bonds they themselves longed for.

Combining Therapeutic Modalities

Psychoeducational and support groups are valuable adjuncts to family counseling, helping families decrease isolation and develop a mutual support system. In one housing project, single parents in crisis were seen individually for stress management and parenting issues, but most, after several relocations, were isolated in their apartments and barely acquainted with neighbors. It was a simple matter to set up and facilitate a weekly resilient mothers group in a conference room in the main building where parents could gather to share experiences and strategies for tackling problems.

In another low-income community, an ongoing Spanish-speaking group for Latino mothers has been immensely beneficial: through it they have found mutual empathy, support, and humor, shared stories of their common struggles, and built confidence, competence, and community (Falicov, 2013). Another promising approach involves trained mentor parents who live in the community or come from similar backgrounds. With brief, time-limited programs, monthly support groups are valuable after a program has ended, enabling participants to return for booster sessions.

Treatment models for substance abuse, violence, or sexual abuse, which are beyond the scope of this book, typically employ a multimodality approach (e.g., Barrett & Stone Fish, 2014; Sheinberg & Fraenkel, 2001). Family systems experts in abuse urge a contextual approach and strongly recommend individual or group intervention for offenders, focused on social accountability and on stopping abusive behavior patterns as an immediate priority before couple or family therapy is safely begun (Almeida & Durkin, 1999). Multiple approaches need to be well coordinated, with good communication among the professionals involved.

Ending Our Work but Not Our Caring

When families present multiple, recurrent problems, it is difficult to determine not only where to begin, but also how to end our work. Since they are likely to continue to experience high stress in their lives, their success should be defined not by solving all problems that arise, but by the family's greater ability to deal with problematic situations. We aim for members to gain stronger personal and relational resources to manage and overcome the challenges that lie ahead.

When our therapeutic partnership is meaningful, ending it can reactivate clients' intense feelings from other painful losses. It may stir up memories of past abandonment and beliefs that they were unlovable or drove a parent or partner away. We should anticipate and explore upset and setbacks, and help families not to see them as signs of failure. When a therapist or agency must end contact before a family is ready, it's crucial to clarify that it does not mean we didn't care about them.

In ending, it's important to convey what we most appreciated about each family member and the whole family, citing the progress they have made and the further gains we believe they are capable of making. By normalizing the likelihood that future problems will arise, it's important to emphasize (1) that it doesn't mean our work together failed, and (2) that future contacts with us or other helping professionals could be fruitful in meeting new challenges. If the family is transferred to another therapist or agency, it is important to facilitate a good connection. With vulnerable families, it can be helpful to extend gradually the length of time between sessions. This enables family members to experience some control and predictability in the process and to become increasingly confident in their own abilities, with the therapist still available to help them head off more serious difficulties and sustain their gains. A last session can be marked by a celebration of all the family has accomplished.

Home-Based Services

When families are buffeted by stresses and often commute long distances for jobs, neighborhood and home-based services must be readily accessible (Madsen & Gillespie, 2014). Therapists may need to go the extra distance in scheduling sessions to engage family members and sustain their efforts and gains over time. Home visits show family members that they are worth the effort. They also provide a clear view of both the risks and the potential resources in the family's living situation, as in the following case:

> Jimmy Monroe, age 12, an only child, lived with his mother, Charlayne, and her longtime boyfriend, Al Stevens. Nine months earlier, Jimmy's mother, in an acute psychotic episode, had tried to suffocate him with a pillow in the middle of the night. Jimmy had gone to live with an aunt while she was hospitalized and stabilized on medication, and was now again living at home. Charlayne failed to keep several appointments with Jimmy's new social worker, who then scheduled a home visit. As the worker approached the apartment, the front shade was suddenly pulled down and no one answered her knocking.
>
> In group supervision, the worker was encouraged to set up another home visit later in the day. This time Charlayne opened the door, wearing a bathrobe and somewhat disheveled in appearance, but invited her in. The worker showed her some of Jimmy's artwork, praising his creativity. Charlayne warmed a bit and offered some coffee. In the kitchen a man's voice could be heard. Sensing that they might presume her disapproval of a live-in boyfriend, the worker took the initiative, asking, "Oh, is that Mr. Stevens? Jimmy has told me he thinks the world of him." As Al entered the room hesitantly, the worker greeted him cordially and, with Charlayne's OK, invited him to join their conversation. She began by orienting them to Jimmy's program and her role as a counselor. She explained her reason for meeting them: the program found that kids did best when their families were actively involved in supporting their success. She would set regular meetings to update them on Jimmy's progress, to respond to any concerns they or Jimmy might have, and to work together with

them as a support team. She answered their questions and let them know how to reach her. They were off to a good start. Charlayne thanked the worker for coming back, and Al offered to walk her to the bus stop, saying that the neighborhood could be a little rough toward dusk. She accepted his offer and took the opportunity to get to know him better.

After each session Al walked the worker to the bus stop, at times bringing up concerns about Charlayne. He worked a night shift and worried about her night terror and difficulty sleeping; she often sat up with the TV on until his return and then slept most of the day. First, Charlayne's medication was adjusted to enable her to sleep more soundly at night. The worker explored with Al how he might switch to a morning shift and encouraged his interest in spending time with Jimmy. More regular dinnertime and weekend outings increased their sense of "family."

Conversations then explored future hopes and dreams and ways of moving toward them. Charlayne and Al wished to get a larger apartment on a safer block, but they were financially strapped. Charlayne had dreams of getting a job but said she lacked skills and transportation and felt overwhelmed by the challenge. Together, they brainstormed about possibilities in the neighborhood. Charlayne astonished the worker only a month later by landing a part-time job in a nearby convenience store. Her functioning and sense of worth were enhanced by the job, paycheck, and social contact; as a result, she took better care of herself and Jimmy. Al and Charlayne playfully teased each other about ways to spend her new earnings. With steady progress by Jimmy and his family over the school year, monthly follow-up sessions kept things on track. The family moved into a larger apartment, where Jimmy could play safely outside with friends.

Dogged persistence by a helping professional can be powerful in bringing about crucial structural and interactional changes in a family. In this case, the worker's supportive encouragement by her consultation team bolstered her own perseverance.

Home visits can be more "messy," as Madsen (2011) says, than highly structured office visits. A priority for productive settings is to create a relatively quiet, workable space, setting boundaries to prevent interruption. Enlisting family collaboration in this process sets the stage for therapeutic partnership. We might ask parents to delegate older children to answer the phone or tend to a baby. Structuring a home session establishes a small island of calm in a sea of turmoil. Unlike the artificial setting of a therapist's office, it demonstrates that it is possible to gain more control over the bombardment of stresses in daily life.

Families and Foster Family or Kinship Care: A Collaborative Approach

Foster family and kinship care placement can be essential to protect vulnerable children from imminent danger. Preferably, children are placed with extended family members, most often with grandmothers serving as formal or informal guardians (Engstrom, 2012). Family systems concepts and methods can enable professionals to work more effectively to strengthen family capacities and collaboration across households. A resilience-based reunification program can buffer and lower risks of repeated placements (Thomas, Chenot, & Reifel, 2005).

Collaborative Placement Decisions: Family Meetings

When child placement is considered, a careful systems assessment can determine not only if there is clear and present danger, but also whether extended kin resources can be mobilized to provide essential protection, care, and support. When family members are involved in placement decisions, they are more likely to support the best arrangement for children. The collaborative process reduces the sense that children are being removed by outside forces beyond family control, as well as the risk of arbitrary court decisions. It also promotes the collaboration of family members with an unrelated foster family, their ongoing contact with children, and their investment in a successful placement experience. For children, these continuing bonds, despite living apart, can be a vital lifeline.

In a model program in New Zealand, strongly influenced by Maori culture, a family council is convened, much like a tribal council, rallying the strongest resources in the extended family for their valuable input. Together, the professionals and family members weigh the various options, taking stock of kin and community resources. Any decisions for child placement should be made without robbing parents of humanity, dignity, and hope that they can turn their lives around.

Sustaining Vital Connections

Traditionally, foster care has been viewed as a means of rescuing children from dysfunctional families. This sets up parents and foster caregivers as adversaries, the bad parents versus the good parents. We must see foster and biological families not as adversaries, but instead as collaborators sharing concern for their children's well-being. Maori people have a form of traditional foster care and adoption practiced within extended families, called *whāngai*, literally meaning "to feed." Ties to the biological family are maintained, and many relatives are actively involved in nurturing and mentoring roles (Waldegrave et al., in press).

During placement, maintaining the continuity of significant relationships should be a priority. We can prevent further trauma by not severing all bonds to parents, siblings, and extended family members, a common practice that Salvador Minuchin has decried as "dismembering" families (Minuchin et al., 2007). Successful placement depends on protecting children and sustaining some linkages with their immediate and extended family members, and their community, cultural, and spiritual connections. We need to find ways for children to sustain vital bonds through monitored contact with parents, visits with other relatives, phone calls, cards, and Internet connections. In a model program in California, incarcerated parents sign up for the opportunity to send a video message to their families, which most often elicits heartfelt, loving messages to their children. Even when direct contact isn't possible, it's important for children to have photos and keepsakes and to hear stories of their family history and heritage. A necklace, scarf, or favorite shirt from a parent, older sibling, or grandparent can be a precious "belonging." One girl wore her mother's nightgown wrapped as a scarf to help her sleep well at night. Older children can be encouraged to keep journals or diaries to record their current experiences and past memories, and to voice hopes and dreams for the future.

Addressing Transitional Disruption in Reunification

The transitional challenges when children return home require a systemic lens, as in the following case:

> Eight-year-old Terrell had been seen by an agency for 2 years in individual therapy for "separation anxiety" after he and three siblings were removed from their mother's custody because of cocaine dependence and neglect and were placed in custodial care with their maternal grandmother. The mother left an abusive relationship with her boyfriend as part of her recovery efforts. With the support and encouragement of a drug treatment sponsor, she kept off drugs, got off public assistance and into a job, and recently regained custody of her children.
>
> Over the recent month of transition, Terrell became increasingly agitated. In regaining their mother, the children had now lost their grandmother. The mother, still furious at her for having initiated the court-ordered transfer of the children, cut off their contact. Their loss and conflicted loyalties were more painful and confusing since the

grandmother had just moved to a nearby apartment to maintain close ties.

Terrell's therapist, noticing that his mother looked haggard in the waiting room, asked how she was doing. She said she was "stressed out" and about to quit her demanding job. With difficulty managing, she was at high risk of relapsing and losing her children again. Although overwhelmed and depleted, she declined therapy for herself, saying that she didn't have time.

At this crisis point, I was invited to consult from a family resilience perspective. A systemic approach and some basic structural interventions were needed to guide therapeutic efforts through this transition. The original presenting problem—Terrell's separation anxiety—was clearly intensified by the recent cutoff of contact with the grandmother. His siblings, also suffering from this abrupt loss, were cranky and oppositional toward their mother.

Family interventions first aimed to repair the strained relationship between the mother and grandmother. It was important for both to appreciate the mother's successful efforts in overcoming her past drug problems as well as the grandmother's excellent care of the children during her absence. The current crisis was normalized and contextualized: they were all undergoing a stressful transition with changes in attachments, households, parenting roles, and job demands. Therapy focused on negotiating their changing role relations to enable the children to sustain both attachments, and on supporting the mother's efforts to meet her parenting challenges while managing a full-time job.

The mother and grandmother were helped to shift from competition for the children's love and loyalty, and from a struggle over authority and competence, to a collaborative relationship. The therapist facilitated brainstorming of ways to work together across households, with the mother in charge as primary parent and the grandmother supporting her efforts. Yet for the mother, needing help was viewed as an indication that she'd "messed up" again, and loaded with attributions of failure, blame, and shame. It was crucial to reframe the grandmother's role at this time—not rescuing the kids from a deficient mother, but supporting her daughter's best efforts to succeed with her children and her job. They worked out an arrangement for the grandmother to provide child care after school and for a few hours on weekends, sustaining her bond with the children and giving the mother much needed respite and support.

As this case illustrates, in reunification the transition period should be planned carefully, preparing children and caregivers in both households over the weeks before and after return. Parental visits should be well

structured and gradually increased; emotional upheaval should be anticipated, with troubleshooting for potential crises. Posttransition structural
changes (e.g., shifting household, role relations, and child care arrangements) should be planned to buffer anticipated stresses and then tweaked
to fit each situation. Intensive intervention during the stressful transition
period can be followed by monthly sessions. A range of supportive services may be needed, including parenting groups, education, job training,
and housing referrals. Following an initial "honeymoon" period in family
relationships, risks may heighten with substance abuse relapses, the return
of abusive partners, neglecting behavior, or disillusionment about stressful
family life. Periodic sustaining contacts help to solidify gains and to prevent
crises and further disruptive placements.

Building Therapeutic Partnerships

In work with multi-stressed families, we must re-vision the traditional view
of therapy and our role as helping professionals. When families have been
beaten down, it's important to take an active, mobilizing position instead
of waiting for them to become "motivated." A pragmatic approach that
includes creativity, structured flexibility, and a variety of interventions can
be most useful. We may serve as facilitators, advocates, and allies, as well
as models and nurturing mentors. We can draw from our experiences and
offer examples of others who have prevailed in similar straits to offer new
perspectives and hope.

A collaborative approach is essential although overwhelmed family
members may wish for an expert to solve their problems or rescue them.
While reaching out and actively engaging families, we need to model a
relationship of caring and commitment with realistic limits. Families are
empowered when we help them mobilize potential resources in their own
kin and community networks for support with urgent needs. We all do best
under duress by strengthening real-life connections. Cultural and spiritual
resources can also be wellsprings of resilience.

The general aims of a resilience-oriented approach with vulnerable,
multi-stressed families can be summarized as follows:

- Overcoming the cycle of suspicion, rejection, failure, and withdrawal.
- Forging a trusting partnership through direct, honest, respectful
  communication.
- Helping families to reduce stress and prioritize their many needs
  and goals.

- Believing in each family's potential; instilling hope and confidence that they can improve their situation and overcome long-standing problems.
- Increasing their ability to solve problems, avert crises, and advocate on their own behalf.

To achieve these objectives, we can draw on an array of techniques from strength-based family therapy approaches. The ultimate aim is to enable family members to strengthen their bonds, believe in their competence and worth, and gain the ability to overcome barriers for a better life.

CHAPTER 14

Reconnection and Reconciliation

Healing Relational Wounds

> Our future depends on our ability to build relationships
> and communities that bind us together in common
> aspirations.
> —THE DALAI LAMA, *Harmony in Diversity*

I was often viewed as a resilient person, and came to see myself that way. I accepted the common belief that because I was inherently resilient, I was able to "raise myself up" despite my family's adversities and deficits. Like the resilient individuals from dysfunctional families in many case studies, I followed the conventional wisdom and avoided contact with my family after leaving home. After college, I took the "geographical cure"—traveling halfway around the world, and returning to settle just halfway back, only going home for brief visits. Weekly phone calls were easier, since my father, who never got over the Great Depression, kept an egg timer next to the phone. At 3 minutes he'd announce, "Well, time's up!" and, in midsentence, our conversation was over.

Like many of my peers in clinical training, I went into psychotherapy, which focused on my parents' shortcomings, catalogued and embroidered upon with the therapist exploring the negative connotation of their every word and deed. Only later, gaining new vision through a strengths-oriented systemic lens, did I come to realize that my resilience was forged through the hardships faced by my family and because of its hidden strengths, which were not in my therapy story. Through those challenges, I emerged hardier than I might have if I had grown up in a "normal family" and a placid, "ideal" environment.

Yet the linkage of individual resilience with self-reliance and disconnection from families has been pervasive in the child development and mental health fields. Often encouraged by therapists, recovery movements, or well-meaning friends, many persons avoid contact and assume fixed views of their families as hopelessly dysfunctional and their relationships as beyond repair. The images of their family members become etched in stone as damaged, pathetic, and destructive characters in their early life dramas, as they move on into other relationships. In similar ways, many individuals leave marriages and other significant relationships by casting off old partners, demonizing them, and plunging into new relationships to start afresh.

Some individuals distance from their families as an understandable survival strategy, which may be advisable in cases of persistent strife, abuse, or other extreme situations. Yet in most cases, disconnection is neither a necessary nor optimal pathway for individual resilience—and for the future relationships we build. Like our culture's mistaken view of resilience as simply putting our troubles behind us and moving on, these cut-and-run solutions may bring short-term relief, but they can leave long-term unresolved issues and a pessimism about resolving relational problems, carried along as baggage on life journeys and passed on to the next generation. These disconnections leave a hole in our heart and in the fabric of our lives.

In my experience, we can better gain inner wholeness, deep and lasting bonds, and a compassionate connectedness with the human community through efforts to heal old wounds. In my early research with families of seriously disturbed young adults, I was surprised by the strengths that many so-called "dysfunctional" families revealed in the midst of their adversities. In my practice experience, I found, time and again, that positive changes could occur even in the most troubled relationships and at any time in life. My encouragement of relational repair is based on the conviction (expressed throughout this book) that our resilience is strengthened as we gain a new perspective on past adversity; appreciate the challenges and strengths, as well as the limitations, of those who may have hurt or failed us; make our best efforts to repair bonds; and integrate the whole of this experience into our lives and relationships.

This closing chapter offers guiding principles and case examples demonstrating the possibilities for reconnection and reconciliation. Here, these processes are described in efforts to heal family-of-origin wounds; they also have application in situations involving painful separations and postdivorce family relationships (see Chapter 9). Difficult dilemmas in past grievances are considered. Even when forgiveness and relational repair are not sought or are not possible, the opportunities for personal healing and growth are most often greater than anticipated. Throughout this discussion, I've chosen to speak with a personal voice as well as a professional one, and from an inclusive "we" position, bridging therapists and clients as human beings struggling to come to terms with painful experiences from our past as we move forward and leave our legacies for the future.

THERAPIST, HEAL THY OWN RELATIONSHIPS: PERSONAL JOURNEYS AND REFLECTIONS

If therapists are to help clients overcome pessimism and anxiety about change in long-standing relational patterns, we must have a firm belief that some change is possible in most cases. Such conviction is difficult if we ourselves have given up on change in our own relationships. Similarly, it may be difficult to help partners repair their couple or parent–child bonds while a therapist is stuck, unable to overcome similar impasses or come to terms with situations beyond his or her control. However, therapists can draw on their difficult experience in helpful ways when they have reached a good understanding and reasonable reconciliation following relational breakdown. Curiously, research has not attended to this link between a therapist's own current state of relational repair and the outcome of therapy with couples and families seeking reconciliation of grievances. In the hope that my own personal efforts may inspire others, I offer some of these experiences in coming to know my parents better and in efforts attempting to transform our relationships. As Imber-Black affirms (2012), opening family histories and secrets to the light, despite the anxieties it can raise, can be powerfully healing.

Reconnecting with My Father: Learning about His Adversities, Struggles, and Resilience

Although my early research and practice experiences convinced me that positive changes could occur in even the most troubled relationships, there was one nagging exception: my own relationship with my father, which I had given up on. I felt an uneasy dissonance between the professional and the personal—touting the strengths and possibilities for change in other families, but writing off my father as a hopeless case. For many years I carried disappointment, anger, and shame about my father. He was a shy, unassuming man who walked with a limp. His adage was "Don't get your hopes up too high; then you'll never be disappointed." He made do with little and was looked down upon as a failure by others in our family and community who were impressed by social status and financial success. I took in this view of him and felt his burning shame. Clearly, it was time to work on my own family relationships.

I was fortunate to consult with Murray Bowen, and doubly blessed to be able to process my efforts with my close friend and colleague Monica McGoldrick, who was also working on her family relationships at that time. We shored each other up, with mutual encouragement to stay hopeful and persevere; our own bond was a wellspring for resilience in our change efforts.

I had many opportunities to practice Bowen's reconnection skills as I reengaged with my father. I had not visited him since my mother's death, 4 years earlier. When I phoned to tell him I wanted to fly out to see him, instead of sounding pleased, he gruffly replied, "Well, don't expect me to pay for your airfare." I took a deep breath and assured him I didn't. Indicating no pleasure at the thought of my visit, he replied, "Well, I have a lot of work; I won't have much time to spend with you. And the apartment's a mess." I took a deeper breath and said, "That's OK. I thought I'd stay with a friend. [This was a break with the norm of a home stay.] I could meet you for dinner after work, if you're free." He retorted, "Oh, you mean you're really coming to see your friends." At this point, with my anger mounting, it would have been easy to chalk up another failed attempt and quit. Here I was, making this great effort, and there he was, unappreciative and hopeless. But I tried not to get defensive or annoyed, and reasserted that my main wish was to see him. The call ended with no inkling of encouragement from him, but I went ahead. When my flight arrived at midday, my dad surprised me by being at the gate; he had taken a sick day so that we could spend time together.

We need to stay mindful that in efforts to reconnect, we must take the initiative and not get reactive if the immediate response is disappointing. In Bowen work, we are not trying to change the other person, but to change the way we relate, which most often opens new possibilities in our mutual interactions. It was also crucial for me to try to understand my father's position. I had been working individually toward reconnection for some time. My call came to him out of the blue and he reacted defensively, to protect his feelings. ("If you don't expect too much, you won't be disappointed.") As I came to realize, he had missed me—his only child—terribly, especially now that he was widowed and alone. I tried to put myself in his place: Why was I calling now? Did I want something from him? Was I just being "polite" and really motivated to visit my friends? Aware of my disappointment and discomfort with him over the years, how would he know that I cared about him and might actually want to see him?

My efforts to reconnect with my father reaped benefits far beyond my expectations. Over the next few years, our relationship deepened with each contact, yet not without occasional friction. He was a quiet man who didn't like to talk about problems or painful subjects. He and his family never spoke about his past. It took my genuine interest in hearing more about his life, and my doggedly persistent urging over many visits, for him to share stories of his childhood and reveal the suffering he had endured and his remarkable comebacks.

My father never talked about his limp; my mother gathered it was caused by a sports injury in adolescence. I seized an opportunity to learn more at a family wedding, cornering my uncle, who had had enough champagne to open up. First, he told me that my father had fallen from his high chair as an infant, breaking his hip. (Later, I learned that he was found to have a congenital hip displacement—with the stigma of genetic disabilities, was it easier for my uncle to tell a story of an accident?) That was in 1909, before advances in modern medicine. My father was encased for many months in a plaster cast from waist to foot—three times by the age of 10. Each time, when the cast was removed, his hip slipped out of place again. This ordeal forced him to spend his childhood at home, unable to walk freely, attend school, or play with his brothers or peers. With tremendous support by his parents (who depleted their modest savings), his hip was finally secured, although by then his leg was shorter than the other one. He started school at the age of 11, where, although he was quite bright, the young children in his first-grade class taunted and made fun of him. Awkward and embarrassed, he left school at 14. He later completed his GED on his own and in the 1930s enrolled in a local college to earn a degree in pharmacy, working for a pharmacist to put himself through school. After 3 years, the college went bankrupt and closed, a casualty of the Great Depression. His boss praised my father's hard work and promised to give him the pharmacy at retirement, if he would continue to work for very little pay through those hard times. When my parents married, they were struggling financially, yet hopeful for the future. Despite their best efforts, the pharmacy folded in 1939 and my father's dreams were once again dashed. My parents then started over, moving to a new community where his uncles acquired a small, failed business for my father to try his hand at. They both worked hard; I was born; and just as they seemed to be doing well, a fire in our apartment building wiped out everything they had. It could be said that I was born into adversity, but we also had good fortune: The day of the fire, I was in the hospital having my tonsils out, which saved all our lives.

I pieced together much of this story as my father and I continued our journey of reconciliation. Putting his life into perspective fundamentally altered my view of him and my feelings toward him. My anger and disappointment melted as a compassionate understanding of his life emerged. He was no longer a failure in my eyes, but instead a hero, who had struggled valiantly to overcome the many hardships and cruel disappointments in his life. He was a loner, a misfit, never quite comfortable in social situations or in the company of more financially successful relatives. Yet in many ways he was the strongest, most resilient one in his family. He met his life's adversities with courage. Tested repeatedly, he always rose to meet the challenge. His mother's care through childhood and his loving bond with my mother nourished his resilience.

While I was growing up, my father worked 7 days a week, 12 hours a day—except for the occasional Sunday drive we took, when he put up a sign: "Open every day but not today." He managed to build our small four-room house by teaming up with a neighboring carpenter, plumber, and electrician, who traded services with him. My mother also worked very hard as a music teacher, yet always made time for community service projects. My father worked until, at 70, he could no longer stand on his feet all day. Then, living only on Social Security, he got up each day and did full-time volunteer office work for his Shriner's organization—dedicated to raising money for hospitals serving children with disabilities. In clearing out his apartment at his death, I found many service awards, which in his modesty he had never mentioned. I recalled his love of the circus, his once telling me that he wished he could have been a clown, to make children laugh.

I had never understood my father until I was able to piece together the fragments of his life, gaining a sense of coherence. In the early phase of reconciliation, I experienced tremendous sadness at "time lost," as I regretted all those years when my disappointment and shame at my father's deficits had blinded me to his strengths and blocked our relationship. Those last precious years of discovery and reconnection before his death have been a continual wellspring of love and inspiration in my life.

As McGoldrick reminds us, there are few pure saints or sinners in real families. If we look for redeeming qualities in family members who are seen only as villains or failures, we will begin to see them. Following the wisdom of Native Americans, we may have to believe in those possibilities in order to see them. In the same way, if we can believe that even the most troubled or estranged relationships have the potential for change and growth, we are more likely to act in ways that indeed foster reconnection and reconciliation.

Seizing Opportunities to Reconnect: Learning My Mother's Secrets, Sorrows, and Strengths

My mother had been cut off from her family after leaving the Catholic Church and then converting to Judaism when she married my father. Although we received annual Christmas cards from her brother, I had only met him once briefly. He had turned a cold shoulder when my mother sought his support during hard times: "You made your bed, so you lie in it." Shortly before my mother's death, when I was 27 and eager to know her better in what little time we had, she shared a secret she had kept even from my father: she had been a nun for 17 years. She died before I could ask the many questions I was left with.

Several years later, in the usual holiday card to me from my uncle, he mentioned that he was looking forward to a family reunion. However, he offered no details or invitation. Overcoming my initial anger and identification with my mother's painful exclusion, I decided to take a risk and write back to express my interest and ask if I might attend. He replied immediately with a gracious invitation. I learned that the reunion was in honor of the retirement of Sister Honoria as Mother Superior of her order. She was my mother's cousin and had been her closest confidante through their teen years and early adulthood: as best friends, they had entered the convent together at the age of 16. This reunion was an opportunity I couldn't miss.

I also learned that there were other relatives going to the reunion from Chicago—relatives I didn't even know lived in my city. I found myself more anxious than I had anticipated; these newfound cousins were friendly, yet conversation was superficial and awkward, with no mention of my mother. At the reunion, everyone greeted me warmly, but still no one spoke of my mother. I felt strangely as if I had somehow landed in this family all by myself. And I felt a pang of disloyalty to my mother for wanting to reunite with those who had rejected her.

My family therapy tools of the trade saved the day, relieving my anxiety and helping me make connections. Poring over old photographs, I was eager to hear about the whole cast of characters. Then I sat down at the kitchen table with paper and pencil and began to sketch a genogram, asking questions as I drew. Soon family members gathered around, curious and eager to add their pieces or make corrections: "That's not right at all—don't you remember, he ditched her for her younger sister!" The stories began to flow. As I brought up my desire to hear stories of my mother, and revealed that she had told me she had been a nun, they all opened up and dug out photos of her in her nun's habit; they too had been carrying the secret, unsure whether I knew. Over the next 2 days, relatives kept sharing more stories. I encouraged them to contact others who couldn't be there to "fill in the blanks" and send me any more recollections that might come to them. They eagerly asked me to draw up a complete family genogram and send it to everyone, which I did several months later with a New Year's greeting.

At the reunion, I invited Sister Honoria to go for a walk. She too had hoped for a chance for us to talk. I first wanted to understand how my mother, a good student and gifted pianist, had decided to become a nun. I learned that my maternal grandmother, a deeply religious French Canadian Catholic, had hoped that my mother's brother, whom she favored, would become a priest. When he left the seminary after a year to marry his sweetheart, my mother seized the opportunity to gain her mother's favor by entering the convent.

As I learned about this hidden phase in my mother's life, the discordant parts in my understanding of my mother as a person became more coherent. In her religious life, she earned her college degree, graduating as a Phi Beta Kappa in music, and served as a highly admired teacher, organist, and choir director. But she experienced her deep personal spirituality, humanity, and love of life as increasingly at odds with her hierarchical, ascetic, and cloistered environment. With great anguish, she came to the courageous decision to leave the order for the real world. In that time (the 1930s) such a decision was shame laden and unforgivable. After she left the convent, her mother refused to see her; she died within the year, and my mother was not informed of it until after the funeral. This loss of reconciliation was a deep sadness my mother carried secretly all her life. I now understood the sorrow I had seen in her eyes, the sadness that could find no comfort.

Reaching Out to Widen the Circle

At the family reunion, I felt particularly anxious seeing my mother's cousin Alma. I had a dark memory of her from my childhood, the only time my mother and I visited her. Having married well, she lived in luxury. She received us coldly; my mother said afterward that she thought she was too good for us. Picking up on my mother's embarrassment, I took this to mean that it was my father's fault for being the wrong religion and for our living on the edge of poverty. Seeing her again, I felt intimidated and wary, although she warmed up to me and invited me to visit her.

After the reunion, I kept meaning to visit Alma, but I found myself putting it off. When many months had passed, I finally pushed myself to call and visit. I felt nervous as I approached the house, which looked cold and dark, just as I remembered. Alma greeted me warmly and had a large box of old photographs waiting for me. As she shared memories over the photos, her tears came. She confessed that she had been very jealous of my mother as a child. Her own father had disappeared on a logging job and was presumed dead, although his body was never found. Her mother, left penniless, was forced to work long hours in a laundry and sent Alma to live with my mother's family. Sealing over her losses and grief, she grew aloof and resentful of the loving bond she saw daily between my mother and her father. It was the reactivation of that old pain that had triggered her defensive coldness when my mother and I had visited her. I hugged her with a new affection when this visit ended, treasuring the many photos and new perspectives she gave me.

Three weeks later, a cousin called to tell me that Alma had died in her sleep. I realized that because of my busy schedule and my procrastination, we had nearly missed this transformative connection. Learning from this experience, I now urge my clients and students not to put off acting on good intentions to overcome painful experiences and heal wounded relationships. This is especially urgent with elders and those with life-threatening illnesses. Yet all of our lives are unpredictable, and we should never take time for granted in any relationship. A key to relational resilience is active initiative—seizing the opportunities before us and persevering to create the new relational possibilities we yearn for.

Naming: Bridging the Divide

Naming is often a way of making connections across the generations and joining families through marriage and child rearing. In my own family, naming became a way for my mother to weave together the disparate threads of her life and identity. Her mother, a devout Catholic, named my mother and her brother Mary and Joseph. After Joe left the seminary, my mother not only took his place by entering the convent; she even took his name, becoming Sister Josephine. When she eventually left the religious order to lead a "normal" life, she held on to that part of her identity by changing her name to Mary Jo, preferring to be called simply Jo. (Interestingly, the same year my mother came out into the world, Katharine Hepburn portrayed Jo in a film version of *Little Women*.) When she married my father and converted to Judaism, everyone called her Jo—but she remained Mary to her family. To bridge the cultural and religious divide and to win the approval of her new mother-in-law, she named me after my father's maternal grandmother, Frimid. (My middle name, Carolyn, is her own mother's name.) Only when I reached adulthood did I learn that Froma (Frimid) is derived from the

Jewish name Fruma, meaning "pious" or "spiritual." My name would thus have had special meaning for my mother. Although she chose a secular life, she embraced Judaism—and becoming temple organist. Later, elected B'nai Birth president, one member accused her of not being a "real Jew," cutting her deeply in an old wound. My parents left the congregation, yet remained personally spiritual for the rest of their lives.

THE PROCESS OF RECONCILIATION

All family relationships are bound to have occasional conflict, mixed feelings, or shifting alliances. When conflict has been intense and persistent, when ambivalence is strong, or when bonds have frayed, family therapy offers possibilities for repair and relational growth. Reconciliation is not a hasty peace. Rather, it involves a process of mutual reengagement, requiring a readiness on the part of each person to take the other(s) seriously, to acknowledge violations to the relationship, and to experience the associated pain. Reconciliation is more than righting wrongs; it brings us to a deeper place of trust and commitment.

Seeing Others through New Eyes: Changing Ourselves in Relationships

We tend to see things not as they are, but as we are.

> Roscoe grew up in a very troubled family: his mother suffered chronic depression, and his father, who abused alcohol, was harsh and critical. He came to think of his family as toxic and avoided all contact. Still, thoughts of his parents continually triggered inner turmoil and he found himself becoming harsh and critical with his partner and their children. Expanding his fixed view of his parents was the key to change: "I began to understand that the only way all my relationships could change was for me to see my parents with different eyes."

In the work of reconnection and reconciliation, we need to see and hear in new ways. The most important element is respectful, genuine curiosity about the lives and perspectives of others. One of my psychology professors, Neil Postman, offered this valuable lesson: once you have learned to ask questions—relevant, appropriate, and substantial questions—you have learned how to learn, and no one can keep you from learning whatever you want or need to know.

In family-of-origin work, we first survey the entire extended family field. A genogram and timeline (McGoldrick et al., 2008) are essential tools to diagram the network of relationships and note important information and the timing of nodal events (see Chapter 6). This map guides discussion to explore the meaning and significance of connections. Whereas individual therapy relies on the internalized images and perspectives of the client, which are inherently partial and subjective, family therapists encourage clients to contact extended family members and others in order to clarify obscured information and to gain multiple perspectives on key family members and relationships.

Opportunities can be seized to reconnect with families at holidays and at events marking transitions, such as birthdays, weddings, bar mitzvahs, graduations, and funerals. We can encourage clients to actively plan and shape family gatherings, and to invite family members to bring photos and memorabilia. One client, wishing to repair cutoffs in her family network, decided to organize a "No-Excuses Family Reunion." On the invitation, she drew message bubbles filled with excuses for not attending: "I'm running in a marathon that weekend," "My cat is scheduled for surgery," "Nobody wants to see me anyway." Humor can work wonders.

Setting out to change others is usually doomed. Such failed attempts reinforce feelings of frustration and hopelessness. As Bowen (1978) advised, therapeutic efforts are most fruitfully directed at changing ourselves in relation to other family members. Follow-through is essential to handle the anxiety generated by the process and by the system's initial self-correcting attempts that undermine change. To achieve success, we must deal with our own anxiety, keep from becoming reactive if initial responses are disappointing, and persist in our best efforts. Because of the recursive nature of human systems, if we change our own part in transactions, vicious cycles are interrupted and change by others is more likely to follow over time. Whatever the response, as the process enlarges our own perspective, we gain a more compassionate acceptance of others' strengths and limitations. As McGoldrick observes, we would all like to be ourselves with our family members—to have them accept us as who we are. But we lose sight of the prerequisite: that we understand and accept them for who they really are, and get past the anger, resentments, and regrets of not being an ideal family.

I once worked with Lydia, whose daughter, Amber, age 22, had run off with her boyfriend and cut off from the family 4 years earlier, after her father's death in an auto accident. The harder Lydia pursued Amber, the more she distanced, refusing any visit or phone contact. We considered the vicious cycle that had ensued: The mother's pain and frustration at Amber's estrangement had fueled guilt-inducing complaints that were self-defeating. Amber, further alienated, accused her mother of only needing her to meet her own needs, adding that her therapist agreed (although never having met the mother).

I worked with Lydia's long-standing pain at the double loss of her husband and daughter, and encouraged her own efforts to move on with her life. I supported her efforts to make meaning of Amber's flight—to see it less as a rejection of her mother and to consider other possibilities from a normative, developmental perspective, such as an adolescent's survival strategy at the devastating loss of her father. I helped Lydia sustain hope in the possibility of eventual reconciliation with her daughter, even in the face of repeated rebuffs. I encouraged her to write occasional letters and cards, sending news and photos. It was important to convey the caring yet undemanding message that she loved Amber and was keeping their connection alive and her door open. Lydia called me a year later to tell me that Amber had finally called and then come home for a visit; the healing of their bond was progressing.

The process of reconnection is advanced by redeveloping personal relationships with important family members, repairing cutoffs, detriangling from conflicts, and changing one's own part in emotionally charged vicious cycles. Humor can detoxify emotional situations. In attempting change, Bowen (1978) advised, don't attack, don't withdraw, and don't defend. Clients often ask, "What else is there to do?" The "what else" lies at the heart of effective change: the ability to hold an assertive, centered position, and to express one's own thoughts, feelings, needs, and concerns with respectful consideration of others. This must be accompanied by a genuine effort to understand their positions and to strive for a better relationship (Carter & McGoldrick, 2001).

The use of photos in therapy can help to connect those estranged, as they trigger storytelling about family members, their relationships, and past events. Letter writing and thoughtfully constructed e-mail messages can be another effective aid in reconnecting and in clarifying positions and misunderstandings. Therapists can offer feedback before they are sent, to support clients' best efforts to express their pain, their caring for the other, and their positive aims without attack or defensiveness. Letters, better than e-mail messages, also allow an entire message to be conveyed and considered by recipients without an immediate defensive reply and counterreaction. When a relationship has been strained for a long time, it's wise to proceed slowly, step by step, not expecting too much too soon. We can actively pursue a relationship, but cannot force one. At times, we may need to step back and renew efforts more gradually or take a different tack. Keeping a systemic perspective helps us to anticipate possible setbacks, understand them, and rebound undeterred.

Learning and Expanding Family Stories of Adversity and Resilience

When people have a fixed negative view of parental deficits, it's helpful to look back more broadly in family history to gain a contextual, evolutionary perspective and to search for nuggets of resilience at times of past challenges. I encourage many clients (and students) to explore their families' migration experiences, attending in particular to the trauma and losses suffered, their struggles and triumphs, and the ways they forged resilience to endure hardship and make their way in a new life.

Some have a thin narrative of their family history, with little or no sense of earlier life journeys. Many learn, for the first time, how family members navigated disruptive life transitions. In many ethnic minority families, relatives, when encouraged, share long-buried painful stories: accounts of forced migration; of slavery, racism, or genocide; experiences of trauma and privation in war-torn regions. Some fled political, ethnic, or religious persecution or impoverished conditions. In all cases, it's important to search for resilience in the midst of trauma, loss, and dislocation (see Chapter 11). As we explore the strengths that enabled families to reorient and prevail, the stories themselves are enlarged. Reconnecting with the strengths of our ancestors can be empowering as we realize the courage, perseverance, and inventiveness that enabled them to endure and surmount adversity.

Respectful Confrontation

In seeking reconnection, ways must be found to express anger and disappointment and yet to be respectful and considerate toward others, as the following case illustrates:

> In one Mexican American family, three young adult sons had all become estranged from their parents, but the mother's heart attack led them to seek help from their priest in mending their relationships. The sons held intense anger toward their father for his long-standing harsh and abusive treatment when they failed to meet his expectations. Yet they were reluctant to come for family counseling: they hesitated to confront him because they had been brought up never to show disrespect to their father. They also feared an explosive reaction. Distancing

from the family had been their adaptive strategy. The family counselor, who was also Mexican American, acknowledged his own hesitation in opening up these wounds, since respect toward elders is such a strong value in Mexican culture. The therapeutic challenge was to face these sensitive issues in a respectful rather than an attacking way, with the goal of reconciliation.

The father, José, pained by his sons' estrangement, was quite open to family sessions to heal the wounds. With the counselor's facilitation, the sons talked about how it had felt to receive his harsh treatment and about their belief that they could never please him. The father hung his head, remaining silent. The counselor asked what was going through his mind. He said that he himself had suffered beatings and humiliation by his father and fled through immigration, never again seeing his father.

José had never spoken about this experience and became tearful in realizing how he had turned into his father, driving his sons away. This acknowledgment led him to make a heartfelt apology. The sons were deeply moved by their father's account and his genuine remorse. Still, at the following session they were uneasy about how to move forward and what to do with lingering feelings about the past. The counselor noted that the family members had mentioned the importance of their Catholic faith but hadn't all gone to church together in years. He asked whether this might be a resource. The mother suggested that they all go to mass the next Sunday and pray for guidance in healing their bonds. After the mass, the oldest son invited them all to his house for tamales (an old family tradition on Sundays), where José met his grandchildren for the first time. The healing had begun.

Weaving Strands into a Larger Whole

The process of reconciliation involves attempts to incorporate disparate aspects of experience into a larger whole while giving each its place. The understanding of diverse aspects of our relationships as parts of a larger whole offers a path out of irreconcilable polarities (e.g., "How could my father have loved me if he hurt me so badly?" "Was it a loving or destructive romance?"). It requires a shift in our perspective from a split view to a larger, holistic perspective—from an "either–or" stance to a "both–and" inclusive position. A parent may be both loving and harsh; a romantic relationship may be both passionate and destructive.

The Courage to Reach Out

Our families build our physical, emotional, and relational resilience through love and trust. I was most fortunate; despite my parents' persistent hardships and the toll these took on our lives, I never doubted their love and trustworthiness. In many families those resources have been depleted by hurtful actions, such as neglect, long-standing addictions, or physical, emotional, or sexual abuse. When an individual is harmed or violated by a loved one, family transactions—powerful beliefs, patterns of organization, and communication processes—may allow the abuse to be denied or perpetuated. Individuals often distance and cut off altogether from the family when contact reactivates destructive transactional patterns and pain. Yet they carry disappointment, anger, and mistrust with them on their life journeys. Self-doubt and blame can permeate other relationships with partners and children.

Attempting reconciliation takes enormous courage because we may reenter relationships or reach out to others, only to find that they rebuff our efforts or still betray our trust. The work involves both risk and opportunity: the risk of reexperiencing hurt and no change; the opportunity to experience new relational possibilities. The challenge is to reconcile grievances and forgive injuries to the fullest extent possible. When others are unable to respond as we would wish, we have still gained in generosity, and gained a sense that we've done all we could. This facilitates greater acceptance and enables us to embrace life with fuller integrity.

Even in cases of serious past injury or injustice, relationships can be reconciled and past emotional damage healed through work toward reconciliation, as Hargrave et al. (2007) has found in helping people journey toward forgiveness by building love, justice, and trust. His approach involves four intertwined "stations" focused on insight, understanding, providing the opportunity for compensation, and the overt act of forgiving. This work can be painful and difficult. In the course of seeking understanding, we may get in touch with rage and sorrow, or a threatening image of an abuser. Yet when this work is carefully guided, it can be unexpectedly fruitful because it deals with a powerful vortex where past and future relationships can be changed simultaneously.

Creating Rituals for Healing and Reconciliation

Active involvement in meaningful rituals can be valuable in healing strained relationships after family trauma, as in the following case:

> Raymundo, a trainee in our program, told of his powerful experience of a "family healing ceremony" held by a pastoral counselor for him and members of his family of origin. With the family seated around a table, the pastoral counselor first helped them to construct a large genogram and place it in the center of the table. Family members were

invited to tell their own stories of suffering—from drinking problems to intense conflict and abuse. The counselor then asked for accounts of strength and resilience to rebalance their stories, identify potential resources, and generate hope for positive change. He asked each family member to specify the relational impasses they most hoped to heal, and to point out the relevant parts of the genogram. All family members were encouraged to contribute to this healing conversation from their own positions, expressing both their worries and their hopes. As each spoke in turn, the others were asked to listen attentively. Then they were each asked three questions: Did they desire reconciliation? Would they be willing to own accountability for their part in problems? Would they share in responsibility for improving relations? Each in turn affirmed a commitment to these vows and to working together in family therapy to achieve them. In conclusion, the pastoral counselor led a silent meditation for the success of family reconciliation, lighting a candle with all holding hands. For Raymundo and his family, this experience was quite profound and marked a turning point in healing their relationships.

It is never too late for rituals that honor loved ones and foster connection. On the 20th anniversary of my mother's death, I wanted to mark the event in a meaningful way with my husband and small daughter, who had never known her. Inspired by her love of music, I arranged a short memorial concert of carillon bells at my university. This summer, in remembrance of my mother's beloved father, whom she lost at 19 (in a tragic train crash) I'm flying to his hometown for the first time, to lay flowers on his grave.

Time Can Heal Old Wounds: Reconciliation between Adults and their Elders

Fitting the adage that "you can't teach an old dog new tricks," most young people expect that older adults are set in their ways, so relationships with them can't change. However, research advances in human development and neuroscience reveal the potential for growth and change throughout middle and later life (see Chapter 9). As Bateson (1994) observes, in response to new circumstances, individuals can (and may be forced to) reinvent themselves many times over. With life experience and the wisdom that comes with aging, people can and do change their ways. As older adults seek meaning and coherence to their lives, many attempt to come to terms with problematic and regrettable aspects of their relationships and look for new opportunities to repair frayed bonds. This involves accepting what cannot be changed in the past, developing new perspectives on experiences, putting regrets in their place, and celebrating the successes.

Caregiving for an older parent can be complicated by an adult child's lingering anger and pain at not having received good care from that parent in childhood. Unresolved issues from the past can block the ability to see and respond to aging parents as persons facing their own ongoing challenges.

At various phases in the life course, different issues come to the fore and others recede. As we change and grow through our experiences, our remembrance of the past and current feelings about past events and relationships are altered. A conflict over autonomy and control that flared with burning intensity between an adolescent son and his father may no longer be relevant when the son is more secure in his identity in midlife and the father has mellowed with age. Likewise, the impact of past traumatic events may be altered with subsequent experience. A woman's mothering of a newborn is influenced less by her own early relationship with her mother than by the degree of resolution she has achieved in that relationship over time.

Adult development thus presents new possibilities for healing of old intergenerational wounds. In early and middle adulthood, such relationships continue to be renegotiated on an adult-to-adult basis. Rapprochement commonly occurs with such transitions as parenthood, when those in the younger generation directly experience the challenges involved in child rearing and begin to gain empathy for their own parents. As we age, we may find an increasing number of things we need to learn from and can appreciate in our elders. We may discover that our parents, like Mark Twain's father, become wiser every year.

Seeing Relational Issues in Current Context

Many relationships become frozen at an earlier period of conflict or cutoff, as if time stood still. In interviews with troubled families, I was struck how often reactivity to old patterns of interaction could be aroused decades later, keeping us from understanding and appreciating what is happening in a current situation.

> Charleen, a 35-year-old single parent, was furious with her father. He left an abrupt phone message saying that he would not come for Easter dinner because she wasn't planning to serve ham, the traditional dinner her mother had always prepared. Charleen was incensed; he knew full well that she was a vegetarian and that she was going to great lengths to prepare a no-meat feast for their extended family. She heard his refusal to attend as a ploy to control her, just as she had always felt controlled by him as a child. She would not give in to him and serve ham!

Charleen's therapist helped to calm her reactivity and, after hearing more about their past interactions, suggested that she take a breath from that childhood experience and try to understand the immediate situation in context—particularly in light of her mother's death a year earlier. Charleen knew that her father had recently retired, but, busy with her own life, she knew little about it. Her therapist encouraged her to call her brother, who was close to their father, and get his ideas on what might have triggered their father's abrupt behavior. She was shocked to learn that her father had been forced to retire. Shortly before his call to her, he had gone in to work the last day and found that his name had already been removed from the door, his office cleared out, and his belongings piled in the hallway.

Charleen's perspective shifted. She had framed the incident, as she usually did, in the context of their old parent–child dynamics—her father's need to wield authority over her. Each time that old drama was reactivated, she rebelled angrily against feeling controlled and manipulated. Now she saw his recent actions in new light: he was recently widowed, living alone, and in a devastating life crisis of forced retirement. She went to see him and found him jolted by the cruel way in which he was terminated and by feelings that he had lost control over his own life. His work world, his identity, his future security, and his dignity were suddenly shattered—and he was alone, missing his wife more than ever. For the first time, Charleen felt truly like an adult with compassion for her elder parent, who was facing losses all around him. She could appreciate her father's urgent need for continuity with his past. She lovingly included her mother's recipe for ham in the Easter dinner preparations.

Healing Sibling Bonds

Sibling bonds can be vital sources in resilience, but can be torn apart by old rivalries and grievances from childhood.

Jimmy, age 34, sought therapy to improve his relationships with his two sisters. They had been estranged since the sudden death of both parents in a car crash 2 years earlier. Old sibling rivalries had pitted them against one another since childhood. Their father had been remote and their mother chronically depressed, with the siblings competing fiercely for the little attention they received. In an attempt to reconnect, Jimmy invited his sisters for dinner, but it was disastrous. His sister Carmen saw a treasured photo of their mother on the mantel and was furious with him for failing to make a copy for her, as he had promised at their parents' funeral. Defensively, Jimmy snapped, "Get off my case!" Carmen lashed out at him for being a "self-centered mama's boy." He retorted that she was a "spiteful old nag" who stole all their mother's jewelry. Enraged, she grabbed the photo and tore it up; as they struggled he knocked her down, causing a nosebleed. The other sister, Dara, settled things down. But in ensuing weeks, the hostilities escalated: Carmen hired a lawyer to sue Jimmy for damages, and he refused to apologize, blamed the incident on her, and threatened to countersue. Dara sided with Carmen against him. Jimmy's wife berated him for his "childish" plans for revenge.

Intense family triangles can entangle helpers: when the therapist questioned Jimmy's proposed counterattack, he accused her of siding with his sister and wife against him. She clarified her position: She was not colluding with them against him; rather, she was trying to align with his better self. She knew him to be a decent and generous man, and she believed that deep down, he knew he had played a part in the conflict and might have some regrets. He put his head in his hands, sighed deeply, and nodded. They now more calmly reflected on the chain of events and the relational significance of the incident: keeping for himself—or, from his sister's perspective, withholding from her— the photo of their deceased mother, who hadn't been available when they had most needed her as children. Jimmy agreed to take responsibility for his own procrastination, since he knew how much the photo meant to Carmen. The therapist also helped him to see that no matter what his sister had done that had provoked him, he was accountable for his own violent reaction and harm to her. His therapist appealed to his better nature, urging him to apologize for his actions and to cease litigation, which would undermine his aim of improving his sibling relationships. She affirmed his idea to have enlarged copies made and framed for each of them. A later session including all siblings enabled each one to be heard and better understood. The therapist, knowing they enjoyed cooking, offered the suggestion that, in the spirit of reconciliation, they might plan a potluck dinner together, each contributing a favorite dish. At a follow-up session, Jimmy brought photos of them celebrating their reunion.

Serious Illness and Threatened Loss: Time Sensitive Dilemmas

Terminal illness and threatened loss can spark urgency in making amends for past relational grievances before it is too late. Yet, heart-wrenching dilemmas can complicate the situation.

Diane came to see me in an urgent family crisis. She and her husband and their 16-year-old son had a "perfect" family life that now could be shattered. She recounted that she had become pregnant with Jason in a past relationship. Her boyfriend, Ron, had left town, saying he was sorry but he wasn't ready for marriage or parenthood. She never heard from him again. In despair, she'd married Dwayne, a good friend who knew the baby wasn't his but gladly accepted paternity. Jason had grown up believing that Dwayne was his biological father. Now, out of the blue, Ron had called her from California, saying that he had terminal cancer and wanted to see Jason before he died. She wanted me to advise her: what she should do?

A wise therapist doesn't solve such dilemmas for clients, but helps them survey their situation and options as fully as possible to come to their best decision. First we explored the case for not telling: She worried that the news would be too upsetting for Jason, who was doing well. Her catastrophic fear was that his psychological adjustment and school achievements would plummet. Further, she worried that it could be devastating for her husband, who was such a kind and loving father to Jason, and would risk shattering their stable family unit. She also feared that Jason would hate her for keeping the truth from him and living a lie all his life. I also asked about Diane's own complex feelings. She was enraged that Ron had abandoned her and their son and over the years had never expressed the slightest interest in Jason or contributed to his support. What right did he have to disrupt their lives now?

I suggested that in the next session we explore the other side of the dilemma, and consider the ramifications if she decided *not* to tell her son. On further reflection, she didn't want Jason to learn the truth somehow later on from others. For instance, what if Ron's other children, his half siblings, ever contacted him? He would hate her for lying, and more so for denying him his only chance to know his birth father. After deep soul searching, she decided that Jason had a right to know about Ron and to meet him if he chose to do so. She believed she needed to summon the courage to trust in her son and in the strong bonds their family had forged over the years. We considered how this secret might best be revealed. She decided to first discuss it with her husband, who was very supportive. They agreed to tell Jason together and to hold each other through any upheaval. To be prepared, I asked how they anticipated Jason might react. She thought he might run off, but wouldn't do something destructive and would likely return. I encouraged her to keep a supportive openness to "hang in" with him through an immediate turbulent period.

Jason initially was disbelieving, then enraged at both parents. As predicted, he stormed out of the house. They called his best friend's parents and were reassured that he was there for the night. The next day he returned but refused to talk to them. The following day he asked for Ron's phone number. The parents told him they would support whatever decision he made. Jason decided to go to meet his father.

The visit was short but meaningful. Ron showed sincere remorse for having been so scared and immature in running out on Jason and his mother. He revealed, tearfully, that a day had not passed without his thoughts of Jason. He was also ashamed that he had not sent money for Jason's support. He wanted Jason to know that he had just signed over half of his pension to Jason for college. He said he knew he couldn't change the past and that this wouldn't make up for the lost years, but he wanted to do what he could now. After returning home, Jason was very grateful for his parents' trust in him. I applauded them for their generosity in giving Jason and his father this opportunity. Several months later, at his father's death, Jason went to his funeral, where he began to connect with his half siblings. Through this process, contrary to Diane's fear of losing their "intact" family, their bonds, while expanded, were strengthened.

Healing a Relationship Long after a Death

"Death ends a life, but not a relationship, which struggles on in the survivor's mind, seeking some resolution which it may never find." This opening line in Anderson's (1968) play *I Never Sang for My Father* conveys the protracted anguish experienced when relational wounds were not reconciled before a death. Much of my clinical work involves helping clients find healing, even many years after a loss.

Lena, age 43, came for therapy to explore painful issues around the loss of her mother when she was 9. She had now reached the age at which her mother had died, and she was experiencing a pervasive sense of emptiness in her life. Lena had few memories of her mother, and had always believed that she had been cold and distant and had never loved her. I asked her to bring in old family photos; she had very few. As her mother's health deteriorated, she hadn't wanted to be photographed. In one photo, Lena and several friends were in costumes for a school musical, with her mother to the side. I commented on how struck I was by her mother's fond gaze at her in the photo. She had never noticed that before but could see it at once. She reported at our next session that she'd kept the photo with her all week, looking at it over and over, her eyes brimming with tears each time. She recalled that the photo was taken less than a year before her mother's death, when she was in great pain and limited in what she could do. Nevertheless, she had volunteered to make costumes for Lena and her classmates. Now, seeing evidence of her mother's deeply caring attachment, new memories flowed out of the past darkness, and she began to revise her beliefs and stories to incorporate her mother's love. She realized that she, too, had withdrawn as her mother's illness progressed, protecting herself from unbearable sadness in her loss.

Lena also realized that because of the long illness, she'd barely known her mother. I urged her to contact her aunt to learn more about her mother as a child and a young woman. Her aunt sent photos and invited her to visit. There she saw her mother's childhood home, heard poignant and funny stories about her mother's life, and learned how high-spirited she had been before her illness. Her aunt gave her a letter written by her mother shortly before her death, confiding that her greatest regret was not being there for Lena and sharing her sorrow that the illness had robbed her of strength to do all she might have for her. Lena's enlarged view of her mother and their relationship, and new connection with her aunt and hometown, were enormously healing. Single with no children, she was a talented schoolteacher, yet had kept to herself, cool and aloof. She now felt more "full of life" and became more engaged in her community, with new spirit in her work and in her connections to students.

Couples on the Brink of Divorce

In every couple relationship, there are troubled times and tensions that can escalate to disconnection. For couples today, the stresses of job and family demands and changing gender role relations heighten the need to negotiate and reconcile differences. Partners from different cultural, racial, and religious backgrounds may bring different values and expectations to their relationship that first attract them to each other but later can fuel conflict. We expect more from marriage than ever before, leading to greater frustration and disappointment when unrealistic dreams and incompatibilities collide. If we can help each partner value the uniqueness of the other and honor the differences, these can add to the richness of the relationship.

Couple therapists, for all our experience, cannot reliably predict which couples will stay together and which will ultimately split up. Some couples come to therapy hoping that we will tell them what they should do or confirm their belief that their situation is hopeless. A partner may consider leaving as the only option when feeling powerless to change things. Therapists can understand their pessimism and yet encourage them not to walk away without assessing with their partners the possibilities for relational healing. Some ruminate over whether to stay or to go, viewing their situation in a "stick with it or leave it" manner; staying means accepting the status quo, which may be intolerable. Couple consultations can help both partners identify and communicate changes needed for them to reinvest in the relationship and work toward shared aims in therapy. Partners can be helped to reframe accusations and complaints in terms of their own needs for a satisfying relationship, and to clarify positive aims to work toward. The possibility of reconciliation for a couple, as for a family-of-origin relationship, depends most on the depth of the will to reconcile. It requires a readiness to take the other person seriously, acknowledge violations, and make amends for the pain suffered.

A strong relationship is a loving collaboration that requires flexibility, mutual accommodation, and shared commitment. Because partners and circumstances inevitably change, all enduring relationships require regeneration, updating, and renegotiation of bonds and mutual expectations (the relational "quid pro quo"). Anderson (2007) proposed the ritual of "promising again," an intentional, mutual renewal of vows requiring that each partner actively choose the other again. Such rituals can be meaningful within or outside religious structures, especially at a transition or crisis. Recommitment—including vows of needed change—is necessary when promises have been broken. The renewal expresses the choice of hope over despair, promoting a vital reconnection to sustain and strengthen a relationship over its life course. Reconciliation, catalyzing needed change, brings partners to a deeper place of trust and commitment.

TRANSCENDING TRAUMA: LESSONS FOR THE FUTURE

Resilience can be forged out of the cauldron of past trauma as we strive to integrate those painful experiences into the fabric of our lives and our relationships. We can seize opportunities for transformation and growth in our personal lives, our wider communities, and our global connections. Reconciliation is a process of moving toward mutual acceptance and developing a vision of peaceful coexistence (Staub, 2013).

In one of the most painful and enduring photo images of the Vietnam War, 9-year-old Phan Thi Kim Phuc was running naked, her arms outstretched, screaming in agony and terror as napalm seared her body. She endured a score of surgical procedures and became a political symbol of the horror of war. By her mid-30s, she felt she was finally living a "normal, happy life" with her husband and small son in an Asian neighborhood in Toronto. In an act of reconciliation nearly 25 years after her ordeal, she went to Washington, D.C., to lay a wreath at the Vietnam Veterans Memorial on Veterans Day. Speaking before a large audience, she told them:

I have suffered a lot from both physical and emotional pain. Sometimes I could not breathe. But God saved my life and gave me faith and hope. Even if I could talk face to face with the pilot who dropped the bombs, I would tell him, "We cannot change history, but we should try to do good things for the present and for the future to promote peace." (quoted in Sciolino, 1996, p. A1)

As shown by generations of Vietnamese, we can suffer brutal atrocities and yet not be locked into a perpetual struggle as wounded victims. Avoiding the trap of a victimized life stance is within our power. Instead, we forge resilience by rising above the trauma, transforming the experience to galvanize our determination to make significant changes for the better.

Expanding Possibilities for Forgiveness

In fostering healing and resilience, traumatic events in the past are not erased, but perceptions and feelings concerning them can be fundamentally altered, as well as their implications for our lives going forward. In exploring possibilities for forgiveness, we can encourage clients to shift from endless condemnation of the offender to learn how patterns of harm or injustice evolved and view them in social and historical context. When a relational injustice has occurred in a couple, a family, a community, or between ethnic, political, or religious groups, it's reasonable and just to expect the offenders to be held accountable. Forgiveness and reconciliation are facilitated when wrongdoers accept responsibility for the injustice and resulting harm and vow never again to repeat it. Forgiveness is also fostered by meaningful compensation for past injustices and by trustworthy actions in the future.

In many cultural and religious traditions, forgiveness does not require acknowledgment or compensatory efforts by the offender (Hargrave et al., 2009). In the Hindu Bhagavad Gita, it is said that if you want to see the brave, look at those who can forgive. It involves taking a courageous position that frees those who forgive from hatred and bitterness and opens pathways for healing and transcendence. Studies find that the process can reduce health risks and promote resilience in those who forgive (Worthington & Scherer, 2004). As we saw in Chapter 11, when a teenage son was killed, the mother began her journey of forgiveness primarily for her own and her family's healing. As the effects of her positive actions spiraled outward, this also contributed to a remarkable transformation for the offender. The incarcerated youth rose above his initial self-pity to take accountability, convey genuine remorse to the bereaved family, and devote his full efforts to turning his life around. The compassion shown between parents of the victim and those of the offender fostered mutual healing.

Essentially, forgiving a loved one involves relational transformation. The process balances the personal need to maintain integrity and protection with efforts to tap family resources of love and trust that will strengthen the individual and bear fruit in other relationships. Reconciliation may—or may not—involve forgiveness for the part of the relationship that was a violation. Without forgiving that part, one can forgive the person and heal the relationship. Doing so honors the hurtful experience while keeping it in its place so that it doesn't destroy the whole.

Forgive and Remember

Contrary to the popular saying "Forgive and forget," forgiveness does not mean that the slate is wiped clean or that harmful actions should be forgotten. The pain attached to past injustices does tend to fade with time if reconciliation and forgiveness are achieved, especially when love and trust are rebuilt (Flaskas, McCarthy, & Sheehan, 2007). However, if we forget the damage that occurred, we may not learn from it to take the steps necessary to prevent such actions from happening again in the future. Trust is best restored not when family members (or a society) act as if no violation occurred, but rather when they remain mindful of past injustice and strive to relate differently. New terms for the relationship must be set to ensure that such damage never again occurs.

In the family, understanding how past traumas contributed to parental vulnerabilities and limitations does not excuse violations. Family members must be held accountable for their motives, actions, and consequences. To explore possibilities, as therapists we might ask clients: "Are there any parts of the experience that can be forgiven? What might make it possible for you to forgive the person, if not the actions? Would it be possible to forgive the person if he or she made an effort to change and were able to acknowledge and apologize with genuine remorse? To demonstrate genuine interest in you and your well-being?"

Can or should the wounded forgive those who were abusive or destructive? It is not for therapists to make that decision for any individual or family. Although it can be enormously fruitful, the decision is up to each person who has been offended. One woman, understandably, could never forgive her father for killing her mother. Different paths may be taken in varied situations. Forgiveness is complex and may involve violations at multiple system levels. When a priest has sexually abused children he has betrayed his religious vows and the trust of the faith community and also committed criminal acts. When a powerful position is abused, seriously harms another, and violates trust, it must be weighed quite seriously. If some form of abuse continues to be a threat, the abused person might run an unwise risk in pursuing a forgiving relationship with the offender. Some individuals may decide that forgiveness is not possible for them. In each case, emotional, relational, and ethical dilemmas must be grappled with. As therapists we can try to help clients to gather information, deal with intense emotions, and weigh various perspectives to make events, relationships, and actions more comprehensible as they come to their own decisions.

Intrafamilial relational violations are among the most devastating. In families where there has been abuse, neglect, or other destructive behavior, therapists can strive to help clients reach a position of holding those family members accountable for their behavior. In many cases, therapy can attempt to increase understanding of formative experiences that shaped the vulnerabilities and limitations of offending persons without excusing the deplorable acts, yet gaining empathy for their experiences of suffering. We can encourage clients' refusal to spend their own lives immersed in accusation and bitterness. Above all, this entails our compassionate response to those who have suffered, and yet also extends compassion to parents or other offenders for their hardship and suffering. In many cases, offenders also need therapists' help in forgiving themselves for past wrongs or shameful actions.

The ability of resilient individuals and families to emerge from traumatic situations strong and healthy should not imply that they are weak and deficient if they are more deeply wounded and less hardy in recovery. Judith Herman (1992) has stressed the importance of "moral solidarity," with respect for those struggling with trauma because they are most in need of hope and least in need of another reason to make them feel bad about themselves.

Truth Telling and Justice

In rebalancing stories and legacies of our history to highlight heroes and positive models, we must be careful not to tilt to the other extreme, airbrushing atrocities to reveal only the inspiring. We have to face the unpleasant as well as the affirmative side of the human story, including our own stories as a nation and our own stories of our peoples. Our history as a society, like history in families, is too easily written in the voice of its dominant members, with the experiences of the marginalized and vulnerable silenced (Hernandez, 2002). In many cases, we must have the ugly facts in order to challenge the official view of reality. Sadly, great nations, like our own, too often have difficulty acknowledging and repairing past injustices and harm, from slavery and the genocide of native peoples to the destruction and dehumanization of wars.

Truth is required of justice when human rights have been violated, whether in a family, a community, or a nation. The Truth and Reconciliation Commission, formed in South Africa to investigate human rights violations under apartheid, was a unique experiment in gathering facts and publishing historical records about past atrocities. Those who committed crimes were obliged, at the very least, to acknowledge their deeds publicly as a necessary condition of a plan for amnesty. Amnesty was then considered and offered on a case-by-case basis. In one situation, for instance, a police captain who had killed 13 women and children admitted his actions and apologized to the victims' families, asking them "to consider" forgiving him. It was then the families' decision as to whether their forgiveness was possible (Gobodo-Madikizela, 2002).

Compensation can often further a sense of justice. Yet in some situations, survivors may feel that horrific crimes are beyond compensation. Even when survivors are unable to forgive, telling and learning the truth about past atrocities is important for a brutalized individual, group, or society to bind up wounds. It offers details about what happened and more catharsis for those who have suffered. Making some meaning of the senseless helps to render the horrific intelligible. The ambitious South African experiment was fraught with dilemmas, as many perpetrators seeking amnesty were accused of distorting or covering up facts to deny or minimize their role. Yet in an imperfect world, such societal efforts to resist revenge and retribution and instead to seek a healing justice can foster vital transformation, as has been seen more recently in Rwanda. Reviving trauma can initially increase pain and conflict, especially if the cold facts are brutal. Yet the ability to integrate painful experience and move on with life is furthered by the whole truth, including its comprehension within the context of its time and place. In the words of Martin Luther King Jr., "the truth will set you free."

Learning from History: Informing and Inspiring Our Best

History is essential to our ongoing understanding of ourselves, our families, and our culture. Humans have a deep need to be connected to our larger community and to our own history. As Griffin (1993) asserts, all history, including the histories of our families, is part of us, such that when we hear terrible secrets revealed, about a grandparent or an uncle, or about our society's past injustices, our lives are made clearer to us, as "the heaviness of unspoken truth" is dispersed. Lifting this heaviness is part of the process of opening communication across the generations and in our social world.

History tends to be written by the most powerful, to support their privilege and legitimize their actions. We need to expand the power of history to people who have been unjustly or brutally treated and marginalized, either within their families or by societies, so that all of us are empowered to use our understanding of the past to inform and inspire our best actions in the present and the future.

Spirit with a Broken Heart

In Ken Burns's powerful video documentary *The West* (Ives, Abramson, & Kantor, 1996), Albert White Hat, a Lakota native teacher and mentor, tells of his struggle to come to terms with the genocidal atrocities committed against his tribe over more than 150 years, which churned inside his entire being:

> "I grew up with a lot of the older people, listened to the stories. The stories were inside of me. I went into a boarding school system and they killed those stories in that system. I came to be ashamed of who I am, what I am.
>
> "In the late '60s I returned to the culture, let my hair grow, and started speaking the language. I did the Vision Quest for 5 years; I fasted. . . . One of those times, it was a beautiful night, the stars were out, it was calm, and around midnight I got up and I prayed and sat there a while. Then all of a sudden I had these flashbacks—of Sand Creek, Wounded Knee—and every policy, every law that was imposed on us hit me one at a time and how it affected my life. And as I sat there I got angrier and angrier, till it turned to hatred. And I looked at this whole situation, the whole history, and there was nothing I could do. It was too much. The only thing I could do, to me, was: 'When I come off that hill I'm going to grab a gun and I'm going to start shooting; and then maybe my grandfathers will honor me if I go that route.'
>
> "I got up and I turned around and faced the East and it was beautiful; there was dawn light. Right above that blue light in the darkness was the sliver of the moon in the morning. And I wanted to live. I wanted to live and be happy. I feel I deserve it. But the only way I was going to do that was if I forgive. And I cried that morning because I had to forgive.
>
> "Since then I work every day on that commitment. Now, I don't know how many people feel that way, but every one of us, if you're a Lakota, you have to deal with this at some point in your life. You have to address that and you have to make a decision. If you don't, you're going to die on the road someplace, either from being too drunk or from putting a bullet in your head. So this isn't history; it's still with us. What has happened in the past will never leave us. The next 100 years it will be with us. And we have to deal with it every day."

As Albert White Hat realized, if we are consumed by rage, however justified, it can enslave our present and our future to past horrors, and preclude our having a decent life.

We may be drawn to the wish-fulfilling fantasy of a time machine that will allow us to go back to the past so that we can change it. Although we can't change the past in that way, we can revise and enlarge our perspectives on that past, learn from it, and vow to live and relate differently. This involves mastering the art of the possible, a core process in resilience.

We can strive to make meaning of past hurt and injustice, and then draw upon our inner resources and bonds with loved ones, our larger communities, and transcendent values in order to live and love to our fullest potential and to leave positive legacies for the future. As children in our families and communities, we had little control over traumatic events; as adults and parents, we have the power and opportunity to do better—with our own children and with all others in our lives. Our shared future will be promising if we can come to understand our lives, gain compassion for the struggles of others, and take up our responsibilities to all living things.

APPENDIX 1

Walsh Family Resilience Questionnaire©

Directions: We are interested in your family's experience with your highly stressful situation. Please share your view on how your family deals with crises and ongoing challenges. Read each statement below and circle a number, 1–5, to indicate how much this is true for your family.

Rarely/Never (1); Not Often (2); Sometimes (3); Often (4); Almost Always (5)

Respondent(s):

	Rarely/Never	Infrequent	Sometimes	Often	Almost Always
1. Our family faces difficulties together as a team, rather than individually.	1	2	3	4	5
2. We view distress with our situation as common, understandable.	1	2	3	4	5
3. We approach a crisis as a challenge we can manage and master with shared efforts.	1	2	3	4	5
4. We try to make sense of stressful situations and focus on our options.	1	2	3	4	5
5. We keep hopeful and confident that we will overcome difficulties.	1	2	3	4	5
6. We encourage each other and build on our strengths.	1	2	3	4	5
7. We seize opportunities, take action, and persist in our efforts.	1	2	3	4	5
8. We focus on possibilities and try to accept what we can't change.	1	2	3	4	5
9. We share important values and life purpose that help us rise above difficulties.	1	2	3	4	5
10. We draw on spiritual resources (religious or nonreligious) to help us cope well.	1	2	3	4	5
11. Our challenges inspire creativity, more meaningful priorities, and stronger bonds.	1	2	3	4	5
12. Our hardship has increased our compassion and desire to help others.	1	2	3	4	5

13. We believe we can learn and become stronger from our challenges.	1	2	3	4	5
14. We are flexible in adapting to new challenges.	1	2	3	4	5
15. We provide stability and reliability to buffer stresses for family members.	1	2	3	4	5
16. Strong leadership by parents/caregivers provides warm nurturing, guidance, and security.	1	2	3	4	5
17. We can count on family members to help each other in difficulty.	1	2	3	4	5
18. Our family respects our individual needs and differences.	1	2	3	4	5
19. In our immediate and extended family, we have positive role models and mentors.	1	2	3	4	5
20. We can rely on the support of friends and our community.	1	2	3	4	5
21. We have economic security to be able to get through hard times.	1	2	3	4	5
22. We can access community resources to help our family through difficult times.	1	2	3	4	5
23. We try to clarify information about our stressful situation and our options.	1	2	3	4	5
24. In our family, we are clear and consistent in what we say and do.	1	2	3	4	5
25. We can express our opinions and be truthful with each other.	1	2	3	4	5
26. We can share difficult negative feelings (e.g., sadness, anger, fears).	1	2	3	4	5
27. We show each other understanding and avoid blame.	1	2	3	4	5
28. We can share positive feelings, appreciation, humor, and fun and find relief from difficulties.	1	2	3	4	5
29. We collaborate in discussing and making decisions, and we handle disagreements fairly.	1	2	3	4	5
30. We focus on our goals and take steps to reach them.	1	2	3	4	5
31. We celebrate successes and learn from mistakes.	1	2	3	4	5
32. We plan and prepare for the future and try to prevent crises.	1	2	3	4	5

What family beliefs and/or practices are especially helpful in dealing with your stressful situation?

Comment: _____

358

Developing Resilience-Based Genograms

Outline and Sample Questions

GRYD[1] FAMILY TRAINING, 2011–2012
JOHN ROLLAND, MD, AND FROMA WALSH, PhD

Guiding Principles

- All families, individuals, and communities have the inherent capacity to transform themselves and change the narrative of their lives.
- The concept of family is defined through the broad lens of multiple generations, including grandparents, aunts, uncles, cousins, etc.
- The concept of "caregivers" is reflective of key relationships dominant in a youth's life, particularly for youth living in foster homes and/or group home situations.
- It is as important to identify and affirm the strengths of a community, family, peer group, and/or an individual as it is to identify areas of deficits.
- It is preferable to view a functional and/or dysfunctional range of behaviors in the context of a youth's living situation, which includes consideration of both family and peer environments.
- The genogram is a tool to map family processes, a graphic representation that charts interactional processes over at least three generations.

[1]Designed and conducted for the Gang Reduction and Youth Development Program of the Los Angeles Mayor's Office; Deputy Mayor Guillermo Cespedes, MSW; Research Director Denise Herz, PhD; and program managers Perla Aragon, MSW, and Maryum Ali. Coordinated by Miguel Leon, MSW, prevention team leader. Genogram format based on McGoldrick, Gerson, and Petry (2008).

General Guidelines: Genogram Information Gathering

1. Convey the value in doing a genogram—not just filling out a form. Don't expect to complete the genogram in one meeting. Aim to engage the youth's and family's interest in learning more about their relationships and their history. The goals are:
   - To increase understanding and positive connections with the family's history and network of relationships. This will strengthen positive youth identity and differentiation from negative influences.
   - To identify and recruit family members who can be "relational lifelines" for positive youth development: emotional support and problem solving to support youth efforts to decrease problem behaviors, resist gang involvement, and strive toward a positive future life vision.

2. Gather information in an affirming and supportive tone. Our resilience-oriented approach does not ignore youth or family problems. We address those most relevant to GRYD prevention program goals by identifying and drawing on family strengths and resources and by supporting their problem-solving efforts.
   - Listen with compassion to accounts of problem behavior, suffering, and/or struggle of youth and their families so they feel you understand their situation and concerns. Avoid scapegoating or pathologizing persons by focusing on the behavior and interactions of greatest concern.
   - Draw out and affirm the youth and family's positive intentions, behaviors, and coping strategies alongside the problems (e.g., faith, endurance, tenacity, mutual support, caring).

3. Normalize or contextualize distress by, for example, acknowledging how the family's frustration is understandable in their situation. This reduces blame and shame. *Never affirm or normalize harmful behavior.* You might affirm a person's caring intentions or upset feelings, while being clear that you do not endorse risky or destructive behavior. You can help them find better ways to handle their issues or link them with appropriate resources if the issue is beyond the scope of your GRYD work.

4. Some information may be emotionally loaded. Do ask relevant questions, yet respect clients' reluctance to discuss highly sensitive information in the initial stages. You can acknowledge it as a painful or difficult issue. If relevant to GRYD aims, it can be explored later in an individual session and you can decide with parents whether and how to share the information with youth.

5. In starting this process you have been asked to visit the family's relational network and history. Work diligently to strengthen their connections and affirm their history.

Getting Started

1. Start where the family's comfort is.
2. Go from the immediate household to the extended family and broader social systems, including peer networks.
3. Go from the present family situation to significant past family events.

Immediate Household Questions (Sample)

4. Who lives in the household (name, age, gender)? How long? Any recent changes?
5. Indicate how all are related.
6. Ask about functional, informal, or chosen kin (not biologically or legally related, e.g., godparents, parent's live-in boyfriend or best friend, like an "auntie").
7. Does the youth currently live in more than one household (e.g., divides time between mom's and dad's house, grandparent's house)?

On the genogram, draw a dotted line around household members.

Timeline

Use together with genogram.
An easy way to diagram the timing of major events, milestones, stressors, or cluster of events.

Genogram Interview: Explanation to Parents, Youth, and Other Family Members (Suggested Language)

"We ask that parents and family members help us draw a genogram, a diagram like a family tree, using symbols to see everyone and their relationships in one picture. We will start it together and explain what the symbols mean. Because you are the experts on your family relationships and history, it is important for you to build it. The more you can teach your son/daughter about the long line of people he/she comes from, the more family medicine you will be able to provide to help counteract the challenges he/she is facing."

Suggested Demographic Questions

Begin with Mom's or Dad's family of origin.
- "When and where were your grandparents born?"
- "What are their names?"

- "Are they still alive? If so, where are they living now?"
- "If deceased, when did they die, at what age, and what was the cause?"
- "What kind of work do or did they do?"
- "Did they remain together? If separated or divorced, what were their ages?"
- "What is/was their ethnic/racial background? Religious affiliation?"
- "Is there any other information that comes to mind when you think about them?"
- "How many children did they have?" (Diagram the parent and his/her siblings, older to younger, left to right.)
- "How many brothers and sisters?" (Diagram older to younger.)

Repeat for the other parent's family of origin.

Examples of Relationship Resilience–Based Questions

- "As we look at the folks who are drawn here, who would you say you are real close with? What do you value or appreciate most in that relationship?"
- "Who would you like to know better, or get closer to? What draws you to that person?"
- "In every family there are people we may not have much or any connection to. Maybe we don't even know them. Who are those folks in your family?"
- "Who are the people you have a good relationship with, but you don't get to spend time together?"
- "Who is looked up to as a role model in the family?"
- "Who has been a source of inspiration?"
- "Can you share a story about that person and what strengths you admire?"
  - Overcoming adversity (e.g., migration challenges, economic hardship, disability).
  - Resisting or leaving gang involvement; turning their life around after addiction or incarceration.
- "Who can you turn to in times of trouble for practical support? For emotional support?"
- "Who contributes to joy in your life? In what ways? What do you do together?"
- "Can you recall a particular fun memory with any family members in your genogram so far?"
- "Is there something else any family members did that has been important to you?"

Sample Questions about Culture and Spirituality: Important Beliefs and Practices

- "What ethnic or racial group, religious group, or faith community do you consider yourself part of?"

- "What beliefs [e.g., religious], values, and traditions are most important to you and your family"
- "How do they help strengthen and sustain your family?"
- "You are here because of ancestors who had great strength and courage. What do you think are some of the strengths you got from them that sustain you now?"
- "What do you think they would want for you and your family now?"

Mentoring

- "Who has been or could be a mentor for positive development [e.g., school achievement, relationship skills, interest or skill building]"?
  - Identify family members and teacher, coach, priest/pastor, etc.
  - Consider how older siblings, nonresidential parent, and extended family members can play a role: grandparents, godparent, aunts/uncles, cousins, and informal kin, etc. (e.g., older sibling help with reading, homework).
- "Which of that person's qualities or abilities do you most admire?"
- "If someone has been a mentor, tell me a little about your relationship to him/her. How and when did it start and develop, and are you still connected to the person? If not, what happened?"

Before Ending the Family Meeting

Commend family on at least two strengths or resources you have observed or heard during the meeting or that they have reported since the last session. Link your commendation to a concrete behavior or example, not just a generality that might sound like empty praise. For example:

- "Your family is showing a great deal of courage in tackling the challenges you describe."
- "Your efforts this week show you really care about each other in spite of the disappointments and despair that you have often struggled with."

Homework and Coaching

1. *Learning more about family.* Gaps in the genogram or chronology are often a useful place to start. More information expands perspective and facilitates relationship change in the family system.
2. *Supporting youth steps to reduce identified risks and increase positive development.* Identify key persons and relationships that have potential to help the client take positive steps and reduce targeted problem behaviors.
   - Initially, prioritize one relationship based on its relevance and chances of helping a youth.

- Identify specific strengths/resources of this family member that can be helpful.
- In what specific ways can this person and relationship benefit the youth in relation to problem behaviors?
- Identify any barriers that need to be overcome for that positive potential to emerge.
- Coach the adult on how to address barriers.
- Decide what actions will be carried out by the helping family member and the youth before the next session.
- Decide on a primary goal as you plan a particular conversation with this person.
- Coach and rehearse your strategy for approach and conversation.
    - Decide: Where? When? Who should be present?
    - If safety is an issue: Discuss in the presence of a trusted family member (e.g., grandparents).

INFORMATION TO COLLECT
FOR A STRENGTHS-BASED GENOGRAM

Household

Circle members living together.

Demographic Information

- Name and age.
- Birth year and place.
- Marital status.
- Line of work/employment status.
- If deceased, note year, age, cause.
- Ethnicity/race.
- Religion.
- Current living location/recent changes/other involved households.
- Immigration.

Interactional/Relationship Information

- Positive.
- Very close.
- Cutoff/cutoff repaired.
- Hostile/conflictual.
- Close/conflictual.

- Physical, emotional, or sexual abuse.
- Caretaker.

Positive or Potential Resources to Reduce Youth Risks and Problem Behaviors and Increase Positive Development

- Mentoring for youth.
- Role model for positive youth aspirations.
- Emotional support (e.g., provide comfort, understanding for youth or parent challenges).
- Practical support (e.g., provide help/respite for overburdened parent; swapping child care; rides to/from school; after-school, evening, or weekend supervision).
- Peer and social network.
- Cultural and/or Spiritual (values, practices, community).

Problems of Family Members That May Increase Youth Risks and Problem Behaviors

- Addiction/substance abuse.
- Serious physical or mental illness.
- Gang affiliation, association, or involvement.
- Incarceration.
- English language difficulty.

APPENDIX 3

Exploring the Spiritual Dimension in Family Life

Sources of Distress and Resources for Well-Being, Healing, and Resilience

START BY GROUNDING IN INDIVIDUAL, COUPLE, AND FAMILY EXPERIENCE OF RELIGION/SPIRITUALITY

1. *Religious identification, affiliation* organized, institutionalized faith system—personal beliefs, practices; relationship to higher power; congregational involvement.
2. *Spirituality:* personal faith, transcendent values, practices within and/or outside formal religion (e.g., through prayer, meditation, nature, creative arts, service/activism). Include cultural influences (e.g., indigenous spiritual beliefs and practices).
   - "What role do religion and/or spirituality play in your life?"
     - Importance in daily living; shared in couple/family practices?
     - In dealing with life challenges?
     - In the past? In family of origin?
     - Desire for greater spiritual dimension in life?
   - "How are couple or family religious/spiritual differences handled and accepted?"

EXPLORE RELIGIOUS/SPIRITUAL SOURCES OF DISTRESS

- Is there couple/family conflict or cutoff over spiritual matters (e.g., interfaith marriage and/or conversion; marriage or family standards; divorce, abortion, end-of-life decisions)?
- Have religious/spiritual convictions contributed to suffering (e.g., concerns about sin, punishment, afterlife, karma)? Experienced as oppressive, harmful (e.g., sexist or heterosexist dogma, devaluation, abuse, or condemnation)?
- Has adversity, trauma, or injustice wounded the spirit; alienation or anger at God?
- Has a spiritual void or a cutoff from spiritual roots increased suffering or isolation?

IDENTIFY SPIRITUAL RESOURCES
(RELIGIOUS AND/OR NONRELIGIOUS)

- "How do you find spiritual nourishment, connection, strength, meaning, inspiration?"
- How might current, past, or potential spiritual resources support personal and relational well-being, healing, and resilience? Consider:
  - Moral compass; humanistic values
  - Personal faith; intimate bonds
  - Relationship with God, Higher Power, Universal Spirit, Creator
  - Contemplative practices (e.g., prayer, meditation, rituals)
  - Faith community: connection, involvement (worship, programs), support
  - Spiritual guidance, counsel (by clergy, pastoral counselor, chaplain)
  - Communion with nature
  - Creative arts, music, literature (expression, appreciation)
  - Service to benefit others, activism

THERAPISTS

Explore own spiritual journey; examine values, biases; learn about other faiths. Take care not to impose own values or assume clients follow all doctrines of their faith. Build links with pastoral care professionals, congregations: consultation, referral, collaboration.

References

Ahrons, C. (2004). *We're still family*. New York: HarperCollins.

Aisenberg, E., & Herrenkohl, T. (2008). Community violence in context: Risk and resilience in children and families. *Journal of Interpersonal Violence, 23*(3), 296–315.

Almeida, R., & Durkin, T. (1999). The cultural context model: Therapy for couples with domestic violence. *Journal of Marital and Family Therapy, 25,* 313–324.

American Psychiatric Association. (2013). *Diagnostic and statistical manual of mental disorders* (5th ed.). Arlington, VA: Author.

American Psychological Association. (2010). *The road to resilience*. Washington, DC: Author.

Anderson, C. M. (1986). The all-too-short trip from positive to negative connotation. *Journal of Marital and Family Therapy, 12,* 351–354.

Anderson, C. M. (2012). The diversity, strengths, and challenges of single-parent households. In F. Walsh (Ed.), *Normal family processes: Growing diversity and complexity* (4th ed., pp. 128–148). New York: Guilford Press.

Anderson, C. M., Reiss, D., & Hogarty, G. (1986). *Schizophrenia and the family.* New York: Guilford Press.

Anderson, H. (2007). A spirituality for family living. In F. Walsh (Ed.), *Spiritual resources in family therapy* (2nd ed., pp. 194–211). New York: Guilford Press.

Angelou, M. (1993, January 20). "On the pulse of morning." Poem delivered at the inauguration of President Bill Clinton, Washington, DC.

Angelou, M. (2004). *The collected autobiographies of Maya Angelou.* New York: Modern Library Edition.

Anthony, E. J. (1987). Risk, vulnerability, and resilience: An overview. In E. J. Anthony & B. Cohler (Eds.), *The invulnerable child* (pp. 3–48). New York: Guilford Press.

Antonovsky, A. (1998). The sense of coherence: An historical and future perspective. In H. McCubbin, E. Thompson, A. Thompson, & J. Fromer (Eds.), *Stress, coping and health in families: Sense of coherence and resiliency* (pp. 3–20). Thousand Oaks, CA: Sage.

Antonovsky, A., & Sourani, T. (1988). Family sense of coherence and family adaptation. *Journal of Marriage and Family, 50,* 79–92.

Aponte, H. (1994). *Bread and spirit.* New York: Norton.

Aponte, H. (2009). The stresses of poverty and the comfort of spirituality. In F. Walsh (Ed.), *Spiritual resources in family therapy* (2nd ed., pp. 125–140). New York: Guilford Press.

Barnes, G. G. (1999). Divorce transitions: Identifying risk and promoting resilience for children and their parental relationships. *Journal of Marital and Family Therapy, 25*(4), 425–444.

Barrett, M. J., & Stone Fish, L. (2014). *Treating complex trauma.* New York: Springer.

Barton, W. H. (2005). Methodological challenges in the study of resilience. In M. Ungar (Ed.), *Handbook for working with children and youth: Pathways to resilience across cultures and contexts* (pp. 135–147). Thousand Oaks, CA: Sage.

Bateson, G. (1979). *Mind and nature: A necessary unity.* New York: Dutton.

Bateson, M. C. (1989). Composing a life. New York: HarperCollins.

Bateson, M. C. (1994). *Peripheral visions.* New York: HarperCollins.

Bayat, M. (2007). Evidence of resilience in families of children with autism. *Journal of Intellectual Disabilities Research, 5,* 702–714.

Beardsley, W. R. (2013). Military and veteran family-centered preventive interventions and care: making meaning of experiences over time. *Clinical Child and Family Psychology Review, 16,* 341–343.

Beavers, W. R., & Hampson, R. B. (2003). Measuring family competence: The Beavers systems model. In F. Walsh (Ed.), *Normal family processes* (3rd ed., pp. 549–580). New York: Guilford Press.

Beck, A. T., Rush, A. J., Shaw, B. F., & Emory, G. (1979). *Cognitive therapy of depression.* New York: Guilford Press.

Becker, C., Sargent, J., & Rolland, J. (2000). Kosovar Family Professional Education Collaborative. *American Family Therapy Academy Newsletter, 80,* 26–30.

Becvar, D. S. (Ed.). (2013). *Handbook of family resilience.* New York: Springer.

Bellah, R., Madsen, R., Sullivan, W., Swidler, A., & Tipton, S. (1985). *Habits of the heart: Individualism and commitment in American life.* Berkeley: University of California Press.

Bengston, V. G. (2001). Beyond the nuclear family: The increasing importance of multigenerational bonds. *Journal of Marriage and Family, 63,* 1–16.

Berg, I. (1997). *Family-based services: A solution-focused approach.* New York: Norton.

Berger, R., & Weiss, T. (2009). The posttraumatic growth model: An expansion to the family system. *Traumatology, 15,* 63–74.

Betancourt, T. S., & Kahn, K. T. (2007). The mental health of children affected by armed conflict: Protective processes and pathways to resilience. *International Review of Psychiatry, 20*(3), 317–328.

Bianchi, S. B., & Milkie, M. A. (2010). Work and family research in the first decade of the 21st century. *Journal of Marriage and Family, 72,* 705–725.

Biblarz, T., & Savci, E. (2010). Lesbian, gay, bi-sexual, and transgender families. *Journal of Marriage and Family, 72,* 480–497.

Black, K., & Lobo, M. (2008). A conceptual review of family resilience factors. *Journal of Family Nursing, 14,* 33–55.

Bogenschneider, K., & Corbett, T. (2010). Family policy: Becoming a field of inquiry and subfield of social policy. *Journal of Marriage and Family, 72,* 783–803.

Bonanno, G. A. (2004). Loss, trauma, and human resilience: Have we underestimated the ability to thrive after extremely aversive events? *American Psychologist, 59,* 20–28.

Boss, P. (1999). *Ambiguous loss.* Cambridge, MA: Harvard University Press.

Boss, P. (2006). *Loss, trauma, and resilience: Therapeutic work with ambiguous loss.* New York: Norton.

Boss, P., Beaulieu, L., Weiling, E., Turner, W., & LaCruz, S. (2003). Healing loss, ambiguity, and trauma: A community-based intervention with families of union workers missing after the 9/11 attack in New York City. *Journal of Marital and Family Therapy, 29*(4), 455–467.

Boszormenyi-Nagy, I. (1987). *Foundations of contextual family therapy.* New York: Brunner/Mazel.

Bowen, M. (1978). *Family therapy in clinical practice.* New York: Jason Aronson.

Bowlby, J. (1988). *A secure base: Parent–child attachment and healthy human development.* New York: Basic Books.

Boyd-Franklin, N. (2004). *Black families in therapy: A multisystems approach* (2nd ed.). New York: Guilford Press.

Boyd-Franklin, N. (2010). Families affected by Hurricane Katrina and other disasters: Learning from the experiences of African American survivors. In P. Dass-Brailsford (Ed.), *Crisis and disaster counselling: Learning from Hurricane Katrina and other disasters* (pp. 67–82). Thousand Oaks, CA: Sage.

Boyd-Franklin, N., & Karger, M. (2012). Intersections of race, class, and poverty: Challenges and resilience in African American families. In F. Walsh (Ed.), *Normal family processes* (4th ed., pp. 273–296). New York: Guilford Press.

Brody, E. M. (2004). *Women in the middle: Their parent-care years* (2nd ed.). New York: Springer.

Brody, G. (2004). Siblings' direct and indirect contributions to child development. *Current Directions in Psychological Science, 13,* 124–126.

Bronfenbrenner, U. (1979). *The ecology of human development.* Cambridge, MA: Harvard University Press.

Bruner, J. (1986). *Actual minds, possible worlds.* Cambridge, MA: Harvard University Press.

Brunner, E. (1984). *Revelation and reason.* Raleigh, NC: Stevens Book Press.

Burton, L. M., Bonilla-Silva, E., Ray, V., Buckelew, R., & Freeman, E. H. (2010). Critical race theories, colorism, and the decade's research on families of color. *Journal of Marriage and Family, 72,* 420–439.

Byng-Hall, J. (1995). Creating a secure family base: Some implications of attachment theory for family therapy. *Family Process, 34*(1), 45–58.

Byng-Hall, J. (2004). Loss and family scripts. In F. Walsh & M. McGoldrick (Eds.), *Living beyond loss: Death in the family* (pp. 85–98). New York: Norton.

Cacioppo, J., Reis, H., & Zautra, A. (2011). Social resilience. *American Psychologist*, *66*, 43–51.

Calhoun, L. G., & Tedeschi, R. G. (2013). *Posttraumatic growth in clinical practice*. New York: Routledge.

Campbell, J. (1988). *The power of myth*. New York: Doubleday.

Campbell, T. (2003). The effectiveness of family interventions for physical disorders. *Journal of Marital and Family Therapy*, *29*(2), 263–281.

Card, N., & Barnett, M. (2015). Methodological considerations in studying individual and family resilience. *Family Relations*, *64*(1), 120–133.

Carr, D., & Springer, K. W. (2010). Advances in families and health research in the 21st century. *Journal of Marriage and Family*, *72*(3), 743–761.

Carter, B., & McGoldrick, M. (2001). Advances in coaching: Family therapy with one person. *Journal of Marital and Family Therapy*, *27*, 281–300.

Catherall, D. R. (Ed.). (2004). *Handbook of stress, trauma, and the family*. New York: Brunner-Routledge.

Cederblad, M., & Hansson, K. (1996). Sense of coherence: A concept influencing health and quality of life in a Swedish psychiatric at-risk group. *Journal of Medical Science*, *32*, 194–199.

Central Conference of American Rabbis. (1992). *Gates of prayer for weekdays and at a house of mourning: A gender-sensitive prayerbook*. New York: Author.

Chapin, M. (2011). Family resilience and the fortunes of war. *Social Work in Health Care*, *50*(7), 527–542.

Cherlin, A. (2010). Demographic trends in the United States: A review of research in the 2000s. *Journal of Marriage and Family*, *72*, 403–419.

Cicchetti, D. (2010). Resilience under conditions of extreme stress: A multilevel perspective. *World Psychiatry*, *9*, 145–154.

Cohen, O., Slonim, I., Finzi, R., & Leichtentritt, R. (2002). Family resilience: Israeli mothers' perspectives. *American Journal of Family Therapy*, *30*, 173–187.

Cohler, B. (1991). The life story and the study of resilience and response to adversity. *Journal of Narrative and Life History*, *1*, 169–200.

Cohler, B. J., & Galatzer-Levy, R. M. (2000). *The course of gay and lesbian lives: Social and psychoanalytic perspectives*. Chicago: University of Chicago Press.

Coleman, M., Ganong, L., & Russell, L. (2013). Resilience in stepfamilies. In D. Becvar (Ed.), *Handbook of family resilience* (pp. 85–104). New York: Springer.

Conger, R. D., & Conger, K. J. (2002). Resilience in Midwestern families: Selected findings from the first decade of a prospective, longitudinal study. *Journal of Marriage and Family*, *64*(2), 361–373.

Conger, R.D., Conger, K. J., & Martin, M. (2010). Socioeconomic status, family process, and individual development. *Journal of Marriage and Family*, *72*, 685–704.

Cooke, L. P., & Baxter, J. (2010). "Families" in international context: Comparing institutional effects across Western societies. *Journal of Marriage and Family*, *72*, 516–536.

Coontz, S. (2005). *The history of marriage*. New York: Viking.

Coulter, S. (2011). Systemic psychotherapy as an intervention for post-traumatic stress responses: An introduction, theoretical rationale, and overview of developments in an emerging field of interest. *Journal of Family Therapy*, *41*(3), 502–519.

Courtois, C. A. (2004). Complex trauma, complex reactions: Assessment and treatment. *Psychotherapy: Theory, Research, Practice, and Training, 41,* 412–425.

Cousins, N. (2001). *Anatomy of an illness as perceived by the patient: Reflections on healing and regeneration.* New York: Norton. (Original work published 1979)

Cowan, P. A., & Cowan, C. (2012). Normative family transitions, couple relationship quality, and healthy child development. In F. Walsh (Ed.), *Normal family processes,* (4th ed., pp. 428–451). New York: Guilford Press.

Coyle, J. P., Nochajski, T., Maguin, E., Safyer, A., DeWitt, A., & MacDonald, S. (2009). An exploratory study of the nature of family resilience in families affected by parental alcohol abuse. *Journal of Family Issues, 30,* 1606–1623.

Cozolino, L. (2014). *The neuroscience of human relationships.* New York: Norton.

Dalai Lama. (2009). *Harmony in diversity: How to move from conflict to compassion* [DVD]. New York: GAIAM Conscious Media.

D'Amore, S., & Scarciotta, L. (2011). Los(t)s in transitions: How diverse families are grieving and struggling to achieve a new identity. *Journal of Family Psychotherapy, 22,* 46–56.

Danieli, Y. (1985). The treatment and prevention of long-term effects and intergenerational transmission of victimization: A lesson from Holocaust survivors and their children. In C. R. Figley (Ed.), *Trauma and its wake* (pp. 295–313). New York: Brunner/Mazel.

Dattilio, F. M. (2005). The restructuring of family schemas: A cognitive-behavioral perspective. *Journal of Marital and Family Therapy, 31*(1), 15–30.

DeFrain, J., & Asay, S. (2007). Strong families around the world: The family strengths perspective. *Marriage and Family Review, 41*(1–2), 1–10.

Delage, M. (2008). *La résilience familiale.* Paris: Odile Jacob.

Denborough, D. (2006). *Trauma: Narrative responses to traumatic experience.* Adelaide, Australia: Dulwich Centre.

DeSilva, C. (Ed.). (1996). *In memory's kitchen: A legacy from the women of Terezin.* New York: Jason Aronson.

Dobbs, S. (2014, March 3). Tribute for Sandy Hook victim. *Democrat and Chronicle.* Retrieved from *www.democratandchronicle.com/story/news/2014/03/02/catherines-peace-team-plans-living-tribute/5956621.*

Doherty, W. (2013). *Take back your marriage.* New York: Guilford Press.

Doka, K. (2002). *Disenfranchised grief.* Champaign, IL: Research Press.

Dolan, P. (2008). Prospective possibilities for building resilience in children, their families and communities. *Child Care in Practice, 14,* 83–91.

D'Onofrio, B. M., & Lahey, B. B. (2010). Biosocial influences on the family: A decade review. *Journal of Marriage and Family, 72*(3), 762–782.

Driver, J., Tabares, A., Shapiro, A., & Gottman, J. (2012). Interaction in happy and unhappy marriages: Gottman Laboratory studies. In F. Walsh (Ed.), *Normal family processes* (4th ed., pp. 57–77). New York: Guilford Press.

Dugan, T., & Coles, R. (Eds.). (1989). *The child in our times: Studies in the development of resiliency.* New York: Brunner/Mazel.

Dunst, C. J., & Trivette, C. M. (2009). Capacity-building family-systems intervention practices. *Journal of Family Social Work, 12,* 119–143.

Dura-Vila, G., Dein, S., & Hodes, M. (2010). Children with intellectual disability: A gain, not a loss: Parental beliefs and family life. *Clinical Child Psychology and Psychiatry, 15,* 171–184.

Ehrenreich, B. (2009). *Bright-sided: How the relentless promotion of positive thinking has undermined America.* New York: Metropolitan Books.

Elder, G. H., & Shanahan, M. J. (2006). The life course and human development. In R. M. Lerner & W. Damon (Eds.), *Handbook of child psychology* (6th ed., Vol. 1, pp. 665–715). Hoboken, NJ: Wiley.

Emmerik, A., Kamphuis, A., Hulsbosch, P., & Emmelkamp, P. (2002). Single session debriefing after psychological trauma: A meta-analysis. *Lancet, 360,* 766–771.

Engstrom, M. (2012). Family processes in kinship care. In F. Walsh (Ed.), *Normal family processes* (4th ed., pp. 196–221). New York: Guilford Press.

Epston, D. (2012). The corner: Mother appreciation parties. *Journal of Systemic Therapies, 31,* 74–81.

Falicov, C. J. (Ed.). (1988). *Family transitions: Continuity and change over the life cycle.* New York: Guilford Press.

Falicov, C. J. (2007). Working with transnational immigrants: Expanding meanings of family, community and culture. *Family Process, 46,* 157–172.

Falicov, C. J. (2012). Immigrant family processes: A multidimensional framework. In F. Walsh (Ed.), *Normal family processes* (4th ed., pp. 297–323). New York: Guilford Press.

Falicov, C. J. (2013). *Latino families in therapy: A guide to multicultural practice* (2nd ed.). New York: Guilford Press.

Feder, A., Nestler, E. J., & Charney, D. S. (2009). Psychobiology and molecular genetics of resilience. *Nature, 10,* 1–12.

Felsman, J. K., & Vaillant, G. (1987). Resilient children as adults: A 40-year study. In E. J. Anthony & B. Cohler (Eds.), *The invulnerable child* (pp. 289–314). New York: Guilford Press.

Fiese, B. H. (2006). *Family routines and rituals.* New Haven, CT: Yale University Press.

Figley, C. R. (1998). *The traumatology of grieving.* San Francisco: Jossey-Bass.

Figley, C. R. (Ed.). (2002). *Treating compassion fatigue.* New York: Brunner-Routledge.

Figley, C. R., & McCubbin, H. (Eds.). (1983). *Stress and the family: Coping with catastrophe.* New York: Brunner-Mazel.

Fincham, F. D., & Beach, S. R. (2010). Marriage in the new millennium: A decade in review. *Journal of Marriage and Family, 72,* 630–649.

Fishbane, M. (2013). *Loving with the brain in mind.* New York: Norton.

Flaskas, C. (2007). Holding hope and hopelessness: Therapeutic engagements with the balance of hope. *Journal of Family Therapy, 29*(2), 186–202.

Flaskas, C., McCarthy, I., & Sheehan, J. (2007). *Hope and despair in narrative and family therapy: Adversity, forgiveness, and reconciliation.* London: Routledge.

Fomby, P., & Cherlin, A. J. (2007). Family instability and child well-being. *American Sociological Review, 72*, 181–204.

Fowers, B., Lyons, E. M., & Montel, K. H. (1996). Positive illusions about marriage: Self-enhancement or relationship enhancement? *Journal of Family Psychology, 10*, 192–208.

Fraenkel, P. (2006). Engaging families as experts: Collaborative family program development. *Family Process, 45*, 237–257.

Fraenkel, P., & Capstick, C. (2012). Two-parent families: Navigating work and family challenges. In F. Walsh (Ed.), *Normal family processes* (4th ed., pp. 78–101). New York: Guilford Press.

Fraenkel, P., Hameline, T., & Shannon, M. (2009). Narrative and collaborative practices in work with families who are homeless. *Journal of Marital and Family Therapy, 35*, 1–18.

Frances, A. (2013). *Saving normal: An insider's revolt against out-of-control psychiatric diagnosis, DSM-5, Big Pharma, and the medicalization of ordinary life.* New York: HarperCollins.

Frankl, V. (1984). *Man's search for meaning.* New York: Simon & Schuster. (Original work published 1946)

Fredrikson, B. L. (2003). The value of positive emotions. *American Scientist, 91*, 330–335.

Freedman, J., & Combs, G. (1996). *Narrative therapy: The social construction of preferred realities.* New York: Norton.

Garbarino, J. (1997). *Raising children in a socially toxic environment.* San Francisco: Jossey-Bass.

Garmezy, N. (1991). Resiliency and vulnerability to adverse developmental outcomes associated with poverty. *American Behavioral Scientist, 34*, 416–430.

Gawande, A. (2014). *Being mortal: Medicine and what matters in the end.* New York: Henry Holt.

Geertz, C. (1986). Making experiences, authoring selves. In V. Turner & E. Bruner (Eds.), *The anthropology of experience* (pp. 373–380). Chicago: University of Chicago Press.

Gergen, K. (1991). *The saturated self: Dilemmas of identity in contemporary life.* New York: Basic Books.

Gewirtz, A., Forgatch, M., & Wieling, E. (2008). Parenting practices as potential mechanisms for child adjustment following mass trauma. *Journal of Marital and Family Therapy, 34*, 177–192.

Gobodo-Madikizela, P. (2002). Remorse, forgiveness, and rehumanization: Stories from South Africa. *Journal of Humanistic Psychology, 42*, 7–32.

Goldberg, A. E. (2010). *Lesbian and gay parents and their children: Research on the family life cycle.* Washington, DC: American Psychological Association Press.

Goldenberg, H., & Goldenberg, I. (2013). *Family therapy: An overview* (8th ed.). Belmont, CA: Brooks/Cole.

Gonzalez, S., & Steinglass, P. (2002). Application of multifamily groups in chronic medical disorders. In W. F. McFarlane (Ed.), *Multifamily groups in the treatment of severe psychiatric disorders* (pp. 315–340). New York: Guilford Press.

Gorell Barnes, G. (1999). Divorce transitions: Identifying risk and promoting resilience for children and their parental relationships. *Journal of Marital and Family Therapy, 25,* 425–441.

Gorman-Smith, D., Henry, D., & Tolan, P. (2004). Exposure to community violence and violence perpetration: The protective effects of family functioning. *Journal of Clinical Child and Adolescent Psychology, 33,* 439–449.

Grandin, T., & Johnson, C. (2004). *Animals in translation: Using the mysteries of autism to decode animal behavior.* New York: Scribner.

Greeff, A. P., & Human, B. (2004). Resilience in families in which a parent has died. *American Journal of Family Therapy, 32*(1), 27–42.

Greeff, A. P., & Joubert, A.-M. (2007). Spirituality and resilience in families in which a parent has died. *Psychological Reports, 100*(3), 897–900.

Greeff, A. P., & Nolting, C. (2013). Resilience in families of children with developmental disabilities. *Families, Systems and Health, 31,* 396–405.

Greeff, A. P., & Van der Merwe, S. (2004). Variables associated with resilience in divorced families. *Social Indicators Research, 68*(1), 59–75.

Greeff, A. P., & Van der Walt, K. J. (2010). Resilience in families with an autistic child. *Education and Training in Autism and Developmental Disabilities, 45,* 347–355.

Greeff, A. P., Vansteenwegen A., & Gillard, J. (2012). Resilience in families living with a child with a physical disability. *Rehabilitation Nursing, 37,* 97–104.

Greeff, A. P., Vansteenwegen, A., & Herbiest, T. (2011). Indicators of family resilience after the death of a child. *Omega, 63,* 343–358.

Green, R.-J. (2012). Gay and lesbian couples and families. In F. Walsh (Ed.), *Normal family processes* (4th ed., pp. 172–195). New York: Guilford Press.

Green, R.-J., & Werner, P. D. (1996). Intrusiveness and closeness–caregiving: Rethinking the concept of family enmeshment. *Family Process, 35,* 115–136.

Greene, S., Anderson, E., Forgatch, M. S., DeGarmo, D. S., & Hetherington, E. M. (2012). Risk and resilience after divorce. In F. Walsh (Ed.), *Normal family processes* (4th ed., pp. 102–127). New York: Guilford Press.

Griffin, S. (1993). *A chorus of stones.* New York: Anchor.

Grinker, R. R., & Spiegel, J. (1945). *Men under stress.* Philadelphia: Blakiston.

Hadley, T., Jacob, T., Milliones, J., Caplan, J., & Spitz, D. (1974). The relationship between family developmental crises and the appearance of symptoms in a family member. *Family Process, 13,* 207–214.

Hansson, K., & Cederblad, M. (2004). Sense of coherence as a meta-theory for salutogenic family therapy. *Journal of Family Psychotherapy, 15,* 39–54.

Hardy, K., & Laszloffy, T. A. (1995). The cultural genogram: Key to training culturally competent family therapists. *Journal of Marital and Family Therapy, 21*(3), 227–237.

Hargrave, T., Froeschle, J., & Castillo, Y. (2009). Forgiveness and spirituality: Elements of healing in relationships. In F. Walsh (Ed.), *Spiritual resources in family therapy* (pp. 301–322). New York: Guilford Press.

Harris, I. B. (1996). *Children in jeopardy: Can we break the cycle of poverty?* New Haven, CT: Yale Child Study Center.

Hartman, A. (1995). Diagrammatic assessment of family relationships. *Families in Society, 76,* 111–122.

Harvey, A. R., & Hill, R. B. (2004). Africentric youth and family rites of passage program: Promoting resilience among at-risk African-American youths. *Social Work, 49*(1), 65–74.

Hauser, S. (1999). Understanding resilient outcomes: Adolescent lives across time and generations. *Journal of Research on Adolescence, 9,* 1–24.

Hawley, D. R. (2013). The ramifications for clinical practice of a focus on family resilience. In D. Becvar (Ed.), *Handbook of family resilience* (pp. 31–49). New York: Springer.

Hawley, D. R., & DeHaan, L. (1996). Toward a definition of family resilience: Integrating life-span and family perspectives. *Family Process, 35,* 283–298.

Hayslip, B., & Kaminski, P. (2005). Grandparents raising their grandchildren: A review of the literature and suggestions for practice. *Gerontologist, 45,* 262–269.

Henggeler, S., Cunningham, P., Schoenwald, S., & Borduin, C. (2009). *Multisystemic therapy for antisocial behavior in children and adolescents* (2nd ed.). New York: Guilford Press.

Herman, J. (1992). *Trauma and recovery.* New York: Basic Books.

Hernandez, P. (2002). Resilience in families and communities: Latin American contributions from the psychology of liberation. *Journal of Counseling and Therapy for Couples and Families, 10*(3), 334–343.

Hernandez, P., Engstrom, D., & Gangsei, D. (2010). Exploring the impact of trauma on therapists: Vicarious resilience and related concepts in training. *Journal of Systemic Therapies, 29,* 67–83.

Hernandez, P., Gangsei, D., & Engstrom, D. (2007). Vicarious resilience: A new concept in work with those who survive trauma. *Family Process, 46,* 229–241.

Heru, A. (2013). *Working with families in medical settings: A multidisciplinary guide for psychiatrists and other health professionals.* New York: Routledge.

Hess, G., & Handel, G. (1959). *Family worlds: A psychological approach to family life.* Chicago: University of Chicago Press.

Hetherington, E. M. (2003). Intimate pathways: Changing patterns in close personal relationships across time. *Family Relations, 52,* 318–331.

Hetherington, E. M., & Kelly, J. (2002). *For better or for worse: Divorce reconsidered.* New York: Norton.

Higgins, G. O. (1994). *Resilient adults: Overcoming a cruel past.* San Francisco: Jossey-Bass.

Hill, R. (1949). *Families under stress.* New York: Harper.

Hodge, D. (2005). Spiritual assessment in marital and family therapy: A methodological framework for selecting from among six qualitative assessment tools. *Journal of Marital and Family Therapy, 31*(4), 341–356.

Hoffman, L. (1990). Constructing realities: An art of lenses. *Family Process, 29,* 1–12.

Imber-Black, E. (1998). *The secret life of families.* New York: Bantam Books.

Imber-Black, E. (2012). The value of rituals in family life. In F. Walsh (Ed.), *Normal family processes* (4th ed., pp. 483–497). New York: Guilford Press.

IRIN News Service. (2009, January 16). New tool to measure resilience. Retrieved from *www.irinnews.org/Report.aspx?ReportId=82434.*

Ives, S., Abramson, J., & Kantor, M. (Producers). (1996). *The West* [Videocassettes, 9 vols.]. Alexandria, VA: PBS Home Video.

Janoff-Bulman, R. (1992). *Shattered assumptions: Towards a new psychology of trauma.* New York: Free Press.

Johnson, S. (2002). *Emotionally focused couples therapy for trauma survivors.* New York: Guilford Press.

Jordan, D. (1996). *Family first.* New York: HarperCollins.

Jordan, J. (1992, April). *Relational resilience.* Paper presented at the Stone Center Colloquium Series, Wellesley College, Wellesley, MA.

Jordan, K. (2004). The color-coded timeline trauma genogram. *Brief Treatment and Crisis Intervention, 1,* 57–70.

Kabat-Zinn, J. (2003). Mindfulness-based interventions in context: Past, present, and future. *Clinical Psychology: Science and Practice, 10*(2), 144–156.

Kagan, J. (1984). *The nature of the child.* New York: Basic Books.

Kagan, S., & Weissbourd, B. (1994). *Putting families first.* San Francisco: Jossey-Bass.

Kamya, H. (2009). Healing from refugee trauma: The significance of spiritual beliefs, faith community, and faith-based service. In F. Walsh (Ed.), *Spiritual resources in family therapy* (2nd ed., pp. 286–300). New York: Guilford Press.

Kaplan, L., & Girard, J. (1994). *Strengthening high-risk families.* New York: Lexington Books.

Kaufman, J., & Zigler, E. (1987). Do abused children become abusive parents? *American Journal of Orthopsychiatry, 57,* 186–192.

Kazak, A. (2006). Pediatric Psychosocial Preventative Health Model (PPPHM): Research, practice and collaboration in pediatric family systems medicine. *Families, Systems and Health, 24,* 381–395.

Keller, H. (1968). *Midstream: My later life.* New York: Greenwood. (Original work published 1929)

Kelley, J. B. (2007). Children's living arrangements following separation and divorce: Insights from empirical and clinical research. *Family Process, 46,* 35–52.

Kelly, M. S., Bluestone-Miller, R., Mervis, B., & Fuerst, R. (2012). The Family and School Partnership Program: A framework for professional development. *Children and Schools, 34*(4), 249–252.

Kilmer, R., Gil-Rivas, V., Tedeschi, R., & Calhoun, L. (Eds.). (2010). *Helping families and communities recover from disaster.* Washington, DC: American Psychological Association.

Kim-Cohen, J., & Turkewitz, R. (2012). Resilience and measured gene–environment interactions. *Development and Psychopathology, 24,* 1297–1306.

King, D. A., & Wynne, L. C. (2004). The emergence of "family integrity" in later life. *Family Process, 43*(1), 7–21.

Kirmayer, L. J., Dandeneau, S., Marshall, E., Phillips, M. K., & Williamson, K. J. (2011). Rethinking resilience from indigenous perspectives. *Canadian Journal of Psychiatry, 56,* 84–91.

Kirmayer, L. J., Sehdev, M., Whitley, R., Dandeneau, S., & Isaac, C. (2009).

Community resilience: Models, metaphors, and measures. *Journal of Aboriginal Health, 5,* 62–117.

Kleinfeld, N. R. (2014, January 24). After a son's death, parents channel grief into activism. Retrieved from *www.nytimes.com/2014/01/26/nyregion/after-a-sons-death-parents-turn-their-grief-to-activism.html?hp&_r=0.*

Kleinman, A. (1988). *Illness narratives: Suffering, healing, and the human condition.* New York: Basic Books.

Kliman, G., Oklan, E., Wolfe, H., & Kliman, J. (2005). *My Hurricane Katrina workbook.* San Francisco: Children's Psychological Health Center.

Knestricht, T., & Kuchey, D. (2009). Welcome to Holland: Characteristics of resilient families raising children with severe disabilities. *Journal of Family Studies, 15,* 227–244.

Knowles, R., Sasser, D., & Garrison, M. E. B. (2010). Family resilience and resiliency following Hurricane Katrina. In R. Kilmer, V. Gil-Rivas, R. Tedeschi, & L. Calhoun (Eds.), *Helping families and communities recover from disaster* (pp. 97–115). Washington, DC: American Psychological Association.

Knudsen-Martin, C. (2012). Changing gender norms in families and society. In F. Walsh (Ed.), *Normal family processes* (4th ed., pp. 324–346). New York: Guilford Press.

Koenig, H. (2012). Religion, spirituality, and health: The research and clinical implications. *International Scholarly Research Network (ISRN) Psychiatry,* Vol. 2012, Article ID 278730.

Kramer, L. (2010). The essential ingredients of successful sibling relationships: An emerging framework for advancing theory and practice. *Child Development Perspectives, 4,* 80–86.

Landau, J. (2007). Enhancing resilience: Families and communities as agents for change. *Family Process, 46*(3), 351–365.

Landau, J., Mittal, M., & Wieling, E. (2008). Linking human systems: Strengthening individuals, families, and communities in the wake of mass trauma. *Journal of Marital and Family Therapy, 34,* 193–209.

Landau, J., & Saul, J. (2004). Family and community resilience in response to major disaster. In F. Walsh & M. McGoldrick (Eds.), *Living beyond loss: Death in the family* (2nd ed., pp. 285–309). New York: Norton.

Lansford, J. E., Ceballo, R., Abby, A., & Stewart, A. J. (2001). Does family structure matter?: A comparison of adoptive, two-parent biological, single-mother, stepfather, and stepmother households. *Journal of Marriage and Family, 63,* 840–851.

LaSala, M. (2010). *Coming out, coming home: Helping families adjust to a gay or lesbian child.* New York: Columbia University Press.

Lattanzi-Licht, M., & Doka, K. (Eds.). (2003). *Living with grief: Coping with public tragedy.* Washington, DC: Hospice Foundation of America.

Lavee, Y., McCubbin, H. I., & Olson, D. H. (1987). The effect of stressful life events and transitions on family functioning and well-being. *Journal of Marriage and Family, 49,* 857–873.

Lazarus, R., & Folkman, S. (1984). *Stress, appraisal, and coping.* New York: Springer.

Lebow, J. (2012). Common factors, shared themes, and resilience in families and family therapy. *Family Process, 51,* 159–162.

Lebow, J. (2013). *Couple and family therapy: An integrative map of the territory.* New York: Routledge.

Lebow, J., & Stroud, C. (2012). Assessment of couple and family functioning: Useful models and instruments. In F. Walsh (Ed.), *Normal family processes* (4th ed., pp. 501–528). New York: Guilford Press.

Lefley, H. P. (2009). *Family psychoeducation for serious mental illness.* Thousand Oaks, CA: Sage.

Lerner, R. M., Agans, J. P., Arbeit, M. R., Chase, P. A., Weiner, M. B., Schmid, K. L., et al. (2013). Resilience and positive youth development: A relational developmental systems model. In S. Goldstein & R. B. Brooks (Eds.), *Handbook of resilience in children* (2nd ed., pp. 293–308). New York: Springer.

Levine, K. A. (2009). Against all odds: Resilience in single mothers of children with disabilities. *Social Work in Health Care, 48,* 402–419.

Liddle, H. (2013). Multidimensional family therapy for adolescent substance abuse: A developmental approach. *Interventions for Addictions, 3.*

Lietz, C. A. (2006). Uncovering stories of family resilience: A mixed methods study of resilient families: Part 1. *Families in Society, 87*(4), 575–558.

Lietz, C. A. (2007). Uncovering stories of family resilience: A mixed methods study of resilient families: Part 2. *Families in Society, 88*(1), 147–155.

Lietz, C. A. (2011). Empathic action and family resilience: A narrative examination of the benefits of helping others. *Journal of Social Service Research, 37,* 254–265.

Lietz, C. A. (2013). Family resilience in the context of high-risk situations. In D. Becvar (Ed.), *Handbook of family resilience* (pp. 153–172). New York: Springer.

Lietz, C. A., & Strength, M. (2011). Stories of successful reunification: A narrative study of family resilience. *Families in Society, 92*(2), 203–210.

Lifton, R. J. (1979). *The broken connection: On death and the continuity of life.* New York: Simon & Schuster.

Lifton, R. J. (1993). *The protean self: Human resilience in an age of fragmentation.* New York: Basic Books.

Litz, B. T. (2004). *Early intervention for trauma and traumatic loss.* New York: Guilford Press.

Lucksted, A., McFarlane, W., Downing, D., Dixon, L., & Adams, C. (2012). Recent developments in family psychoeducation as an evidence-based practice. *Journal of Marital and Family Therapy, 38,* 101–121.

Luthar, S., & Brown, P. (2007). Maximizing resilience through diverse levels of inquiry: Prevailing paradigms, possibilities, and priorities for the future. *Development and Psychopathology, 19,* 931–955.

Luthar, S. S. (2006). Resilience in development: A synthesis of research across five decades. In D. Cicchetti & D. J. Cohen (Eds.), *Developmental psychopathology: Risk, disorder, and adaptation* (pp. 740–795). New York: Wiley.

MacDermid, S. M. (2010). Family risk and resilience in the context of war and terrorism. *Journal of Marriage and Family, 72,* 537–556.

MacDermid, S. M., Sampler, R., Schwartz, R., Nishida, J., & Nyarong, D. (2008). *Understanding and promoting resilience in military families.* West Lafayette, IN: Military Family Research Institute at Purdue University.

Maddi, S. (2002). The story of hardiness: Twenty years of theorizing, research, and practice. *Consulting Psychology, 54,* 173–185.

Madsen, W. C. (2009). Collaborative helping: A practice framework for family-centered services. *Family Process, 48,* 103–116.

Madsen, W. C. (2011). Collaborative helping maps: A tool to guide thinking and action in family-centered services. *Family Process, 50,* 529–543.

Madsen, W. C., & Gillespie, K. (2014). *Collaborative helping: A strengths framework for home-based services.* New York: Wiley.

Mahoney, A. (2010). Religion in the home 1999 to 2009: A relational spirituality perspective. *Journal of Marriage and Family, 72,* 805–827.

Markman, H., Stanley, S., & Blumberg, S. (2010). *Fighting for your marriage.* New York: Wiley.

Marks, L. (2006). Religion and family relational health: Overview and conceptual model. *Journal of Religion and Health, 45*(4), 603–618.

Masten, A., & Monn, A. R. (2015). Child and family resilience: A call for integrating science, practice, and training. *Family Relations, 64*(1), 5–21.

Masten, A. S. (2013). Risk and resilience in development. In P. D. Zelazo (Ed.), *Oxford handbook of developmental psychology: Self and other* (Vol. 2, pp. 579–607). New York: Oxford University Press.

Masten, A. S. (2014). *Ordinary magic: Resilience in development.* New York: Routledge.

Masten, A. S., & Narayan, A. J. (2012). Child development in the context of disaster, war and terrorism: Pathways of risk and resilience. *Annual Review of Psychology, 63,* 227–257.

Masten, A. S., & Obradovic, J. (2008). Disaster preparation and recovery: Lessons from research on resilience in human development. *Ecology and Society, 13*(1), article 9. Retrieved from *www.ecologyandsociety.org/vol13/iss1/art9.*

McCubbin, H. I., & Patterson, J. M. (1983). The family stress process: The Double ABCX model of adjustment and adaptation. *Marriage and Family Review, 6*(1–2), 7–37.

McCubbin, L. D., & McCubbin, H. I. (2013). Resilience in ethnic family systems: A relational theory for research and practice. In D. Becvar (Ed.), *Handbook of family resilience* (pp. 175–196). New York: Springer.

McCubbin, M. A., & McCubbin, H. I. (1993). Families coping with illness: The resiliency model of family stress, adjustment, and adaptation. In C. B. Danielson, B. Hammel-Bissel, & P. Winsted-Fry (Eds.), *Families, health, and illness: Perspectives on coping and intervention* (pp. 21–63). St. Louis, MO: Mosby.

McCubbin, M. A., Balling, K., Possin, P., Friedrich, S., & Bryne, B. (2002). Family resiliency in childhood cancer. *Family Relations, 51,* 103–111.

McDaniel, S., Doherty, W., & Hepworth, J. (2013). *Medical family therapy and integrated care* (2nd ed.). Washington, DC: American Psychological Association.

McFarlane, W. (Ed.). (2002). *Multifamily groups in the treatment of severe psychiatric disorders.* New York: Guilford Press.

McGoldrick, M., Anderson, C., & Walsh, F. (Eds.). (1989). *Women in families: A framework for family therapy*. New York: Norton.

McGoldrick, M., Garcia Preto, N., & Carter, B. (Eds.). (2016). *The expanded family life cycle: Individual, family, and social perspectives* (5th. ed.). New York: Pearson.

McGoldrick, M., Gerson, R., & Petry, S. (2008). *Genograms: Assessment and intervention* (3rd ed.). New York: Norton.

Miklowitz, D. (2010). *Bipolar disorder: A family-focused treatment approach* (2nd ed.). New York: Guilford Press.

Miller, J. (2012). *Psychosocial capacity building in response to disasters*. New York: Columbia University Press.

Minuchin, P., Colapinto, J., & Minuchin, S. (2007). *Working with families of the poor* (2nd ed.). New York: Guilford Press.

Minuchin, S. (1974). *Families and family therapy*. Cambridge, MA: Harvard University Press.

Minuchin, S., Lee, W.-Y., & Simon, G. (2005). *Mastering family therapy: Journeys of growth and transformation* (2nd ed.). New York: Wiley.

Mollica, R. (2006). *Healing invisible wounds: Pathways to hope and recovery in a violent world*. New York: Harcourt.

Mueller, M. M., & Elder, G. H., Jr. (2003). Family contingencies across the generations: Grandparent–grandchild relationships in holistic perspective. *Journal of Marriage and Family, 65*(2), 404–417.

Murphy, L. (1987). Further reflections on resilience. In E. J. Anthony & B. Cohler (Eds.), *The invulnerable child*. New York: Guilford Press.

Nadeau, J. W. (1997). *Families making sense of death*. Thousand Oaks, CA: Sage.

Nadeau, J. W. (2008). Meaning-making in bereaved families: Assessment, intervention, and future research. In M. Stroebe, R. Hansson, H. Schut, & W. Stroebe (Eds.), *Handbook of bereavement research and practice: 21st century perspectives* (pp. 511–530). Washington, DC: American Psychological Association.

Nash, W. P., & Litz, B. T. (2013). Moral injury: A mechanism for war-related trauma in military family members. *Clinical Child and Family Psychology Review, 16*, 365–375.

Neimeyer, R. A. (Ed.). (2001). *Meaning reconstruction and the experience of loss*. Washington, DC: American Psychological Association.

Neugarten, B. (1976). Adaptation and the life cycle. *Counseling Psychologist, 6*, 16–20.

Norris, F. H., & Alegria, M. (2005). Mental health care for ethnic minority individuals and communities in the aftermath of disasters and mass violence. *CNS Spectrums, 10*(2), 132–140.

Norris, F. H., Stevens, S. P., Pfefferbaum, B., Wyche, K. F., & Pfefferbaum, R. L. (2008). Community resilience as a metaphor, theory, set of capacities, and strategy for disaster readiness. *American Journal of Community Psychology, 41*, 127–150.

Oliver, L. (1999). Effects of a child's death on the marital relationship: A review. *Omega, 39*(3), 197–227.

Olson, D. H., & Gorall, D. M. (2003). Circumplex model of marital and family systems. In F. Walsh (Ed.), *Normal family processes* (3rd ed., pp. 514–548). New York: Guilford Press.

Olson, D. H., Gorall, D. M., & Tiesel, J. W. (2006). *FACES IV package*. Minneapolis, MN: Life Innovations.

Orthner, D. K., Jones-Sanpei, H., & Williamson, S. (2004). The resilience and strengths of low-income families. *Family Relations, 53,* 159–167.

Oswald, R. F. (2002). Resilience within the family networks of lesbians and gay men: Intentionality and redefinition. *Journal of Marriage and Family, 64*(2), 374–383.

Pargament, K. I. (2007). *Spiritually integrated psychotherapy: Understanding and addressing the sacred.* New York: Guilford Press.

Pasley, K., & Garneau, C. (2012). Remarriage families and stepparenting. In F. Walsh (Ed.), *Normal family processes* (4th ed., pp. 149–171). New York: Guilford Press.

Patterson, J. M. (2002). Integrating family resilience and family stress theory. *Journal of Marriage and Family, 64,* 349–360.

Patterson, J. M., & Garwick, A. W. (1994). Levels of family meaning in family stress theory. *Family Process, 33,* 287–304.

Perry, A., & Rolland, J. (2009). Benefits of a justice-seeking spirituality: Empowerment, healing, and hope. In F. Walsh (Ed.), *Spiritual resources in family therapy* (2nd ed., pp. 379–396). New York: Guilford Press.

Pertman, A. (2011). *Adoption nation: How the adoption revolution is transforming families and America* (2nd ed.). New York: Basic Books.

Pinderhughes, E. (2004). The multigenerational transmission of loss and trauma: The African-American experience. In F. Walsh & M. McGoldrick (Eds.), *Living beyond loss: Death in the family* (2nd ed., pp. 161–181). New York: Norton.

Pulleyblank-Coffey, E., Griffith, J., & Ulaj, J. (2006). The first family-focused community mental health center in Kosovo. In A. Lightburn & P. Session (Eds.), *Handbook of community-based clinical practice* (pp. 514–528). New York: Oxford University Press.

Qualls, S., & Zarit, S. (Eds.). (2009). *Aging families and caregiving.* New York: Wiley.

Rampage, C., Eovaldi, M., Ma, C., Weigel-Foy, C., Samuels, G. M., & Bloom, L. (2012). Adoptive families. In F. Walsh, (Ed.), *Normal family processes* (4th ed., pp. 222–246). New York: Guilford Press.

Reiss, D. (1981). *The family's construction of reality.* Cambridge, MA: Harvard University Press.

Repetti, R., Wang, S., & Saxbe, D. (2009). Bringing it all back home: How outside stressors shape families' everyday lives. *Current Psychological Directions in Science, 18,* 106–111.

Retzlaff, R., Hornig, S., Müller, B., Gitta, R., & Pietz, J. (2006). Family sense of coherence and resilience: A study of families with children with mental and physical disabilities. *Praxis der Kinderpsychologie und Kinderpsychiatrie, 55,* 36–52.

Risman, B. (Ed.). (2010). *Families as they really are.* New York: Norton.

Robbins, R., Robbins, S., & Stennerson, B. (2013). Native American family resilience. In D. S. Becvar (Ed.), *Handbook of family resilience* (pp. 197–213). New York: Springer.

Rolland, J. S. (1994). *Families, illness, and disability: An integrative treatment model.* New York: Basic Books.

Rolland, J. S. (2012). Mastering family challenges in illness, disability, and genetic conditions. In F. Walsh (Ed.), *Normal family processes,* (4th ed., pp. 452–482). New York: Guilford Press.

Rolland, J. S. (in press). *Mastering family challenges with illness and disability: An integrative practice model.* New York: Guilford Press.

Rolland, J. S., McPheters, J., & Carbonell, E. (2008). *Resilient partners: A collaborative project with the MS Society.* Paper presented at the 10th annual conference of the Collaborative Family Healthcare Association, Denver.

Rolland, J. S., & Walsh, F. (2005). Systemic training for healthcare professionals: The Chicago Center for Family Health approach. *Family Process, 44*(3), 283–301.

Rolland, J. S., & Walsh, F. (2006). Facilitating family resilience with childhood illness and disability. *Pediatric Opinion, 18,* 1–11.

Rolland, J. S., & Weine, S. (2000). Kosovar Family Professional Educational Collaborative. *American Family Therapy Academy Newsletter, 79,* 34–36.

Rolland, J. S., & Williams, J. K. (2005). Toward a biopsychosocial model for 21st century genetics. *Family Process, 44,* 3–24.

Rosenblatt, P. C. (2013). Family grief in cross-cultural perspective. *Family Science, 4*(1), 12–19.

Rubin, S. S., Malkinson, R., & Witzum, E. (2012). *Working with the bereaved: Multiple lenses on loss and mourning.* New York: Routledge.

Rutter, M. (1987). Psychosocial resilience and protective mechanisms. *American Journal of Orthopsychiatry, 57,* 316–331.

Ryan, C., Epstein, N. B., Keitner, G., Miller, I. W., & Bishop, D. S. (2005). *Evaluating and treating families: The McMaster approach.* New York: Routledge.

Ryan, C., Huebner, D., Diaz, R., & Sanchez, J. (2009). Family rejection as a predictor of negative outcomes in white and Latino lesbian, gay, and bisexual young adults. *Pediatrics, 123,* 346–352.

Saltzman, W. R., Lester, P., Beardslee, W. R., Layne, C. M., Woodward, K., & Nash, W. P. (2011). Mechanisms of risk and resilience in military families: Theoretical and empirical basis of a family-focused resilience enhancement program. *Clinical Child and Family Psychology Review, 14,* 213–230.

Saltzman, W. R., Lester, P., Pynoos, R., & Beardslee, W. (2012). *FOCUS Family Resilience Training Manual.* Los Angeles: University of California at Los Angeles.

Saltzman, W. R., Pynoos, R. S., Lester, P., Layne, C. M., & Beardsley, W. R. (2013). Enhancing family resilience through family narrative co-construction. *Clinical Child and Family Psychology Review, 16,* 294–310.

Sameroff, A. (2010). A unified theory of development: A dialectic integration of nature and nurture. *Child Development, 81,* 6–22.

Samuels, G. M. (2010). Building kinship and community: Relational processes of bicultural identity among adult multiracial adoptees. *Family Process, 49,* 26–42.

Sanders, G., & Krall, I. T. (2000). Generating stories of resilience: Helping gay and lesbian youth and their families. *Journal of Marital and Family Therapy, 26*(4), 433–442.

Sassler, S. (2010). Partnering across the life course: Sex, relationships, and mate selection. *Journal of Marriage and Family, 72,* 557–575.

Satir, V. (1988). *The new peoplemaking.* Palo Alto, CA: Science & Behavior Books.

Saul, J. (2013). *Collective trauma, collective healing: Promoting community healing in the aftermath of disaster.* New York: Routledge.

Sciolino, E. (1996, November 11). A painful road from Vietnam to forgiveness. *New York Times,* pp. A1, A8.

Seccombe, K. (2002). "Beating the odds" versus "changing the odds": Poverty, resilience, and family policy. *Journal of Marriage and Family, 64*(2), 384–394.

Seligman, M. E. P. (1990). *Learned optimism.* New York: Random House.

Sexton, T. L. (2011). *Functional Family Therapy in clinical practice: An evidence-based treatment model for working with troubled adolescents.* New York: Taylor & Francis.

Shapiro, E. R. (2012). Nurturing family resilience in response to chronic illness: An integrative approach to health and growth promotion. In D. Becvar (Ed.), *Handbook of family resilience* (pp. 385–408). New York: Springer.

Shefsky, J. (2000). *A justice that heals* [Documentary film]. Chicago: Window to the World Communications.

Sheinberg, M., & Fraenkel, P. (2001). *The relational trauma of incest: A family-based approach to treatment.* New York: Guilford Press.

Siegel, D. (2012) *The developing mind: How relationships and the brain interact to shape who we are* (2nd ed.). New York: Guilford Press.

Simon, J., Murphy, J., & Smith, S. (2005). Understanding and fostering family resilience. *Family Journal, 13,* 427–436.

Sitterle, K. A., & Gurwitch, R. H. (1999). The terrorist bombing in Oklahoma City. In E. S. Zinner & M. B. Williams (Eds.), *When a community weeps: Case studies in group survivorship* (pp. 160–189). New York: Brunner/Mazel.

Skinner, H., Steinhauer, P., & Sitarenios, G. (2000). Family Assessment Measure (FAM) and process model of family functioning. *Journal of Family Therapy, 22,* 190–210.

Sluzki, C. (1983). Process, structure, and worldviews in family therapy: Toward an integration of systemic models. *Family Process, 22,* 469–476.

Sotomayor, S. (2013). *My beloved world.* New York: Vintage Books.

Southwick, S. M., & Charney, D. S. (2012). *Resilience: The science of mastering life's greatest challenges.* New York: Cambridge University Press.

Spotts, E. (2012). Unraveling the complexity of gene–environmental interplay and family processes. In F. Walsh (Ed.), *Normal family processes* (4th ed., pp. 529–552). New York: Guilford Press.

Sprenkle, D., Davis, S., & Lebow, J. (2009). *Common factors in couple and family therapy.* New York: Guilford Press.

Stacey, J. (1990). *Brave new families.* New York: Basic Books.

Staub, E. (2013). Building a peaceful society: Origins, prevention, and reconciliation after genocide and other group violence. *American Psychologist, 68,* 576–589.

Steinberg, L., Blatt-Eisengart, I., & Cauffman, E. (2006). Patterns of competence and adjustment among adolescents from authoritative, authoritarian,
indulgent, and neglectful homes: A replication in a sample of serious juvenile
offenders. *Journal of Research on Adolescence, 16,* 47–58.

Steinglass, P. (1998). Multiple family discussion groups for patients with chronic
medical illness. *Families, Systems, and Health,* 16(1–2), 55–71.

Stillman, J. R., & Erbes, C. R. (2012). Speaking two languages: A conversation
between narrative therapy and scientific practices. *Journal of Systemic Therapies, 31,* 74–88.

Stinnett, N., & DeFrain, J. (1985). *Secrets of strong families.* Boston: Little, Brown.

Stone, E., Gomez, E., Hotzoglou, D., & Lipnitsky, J. (2005). Transnationalism as
a motif in family stories. *Family Process, 44,* 381–398.

Stroebe, M., & Schut, H. (2010). The dual process model of coping with bereavement: A decade on. *Omega: Journal of Death and Dying,* 61(4), 273–289.

Stroebe, M., Schut, H., & Boerner, K. (2010). Continuing bonds in adaptation
to bereavement: Toward theoretical integration. *Clinical Psychology Review,
30,* 259–268.

Swadener, B. B., & Lubeck, S. (Eds.). (1995). *Children and families "at promise":
Deconstructing the discourse of risk.* Albany: State University of New York
Press.

Taylor, S. (1989). *Positive illusions: Creative self-deception and the healthy mind.*
New York: Basic Books.

Taylor, S., Kemeny, M., Reed, G., Bower, J., & Gruenwald, T. (2000). Psychological
resources, positive illusions, and health. *American Psychologist,* 55(1), 99–109.

Tedeschi, R. G., & Calhoun, L. G. (2004). Posttraumatic growth: Conceptual
foundations and empirical evidence. *Psychological Inquiry, 15,* 1–18.

Tedeschi, R. G., & Kilmer, R. P. (2005). Assessing strengths, resilience, and growth
to guide clinical interventions. *Professional Psychology, Research and Practice,* 36(3), 230–237.

Tedeschi, R. G., Park, L. C., & Calhoun, L. G. (1996). The Posttraumatic Growth
Inventory: Measuring the positive legacy of trauma. *Journal of Traumatic
Stress, 9,* 455–471.

Terkel, S. (2000). *Will the circle be unbroken?: Reflections on death, rebirth, and
hunger for faith.* New York: Norton.

Terkel, S. (2003). *Hope dies last: Keeping the faith in troubled times.* New York:
Norton.

Thody, P. (Ed.). (1970). *Albert Camus: Lyrical and critical essays.* New York: Vantage Books.

Thomas, M., Chenot, D., & Reifel, B. (2005). A resilience-based model of reunification and reentry: Implications for out-of-home care services. *Families in
Society,* 86(2), 235–243.

Tienari, P., Wynne, L. C., Sorri, A., Lahti, I., Laksy, K., Moring, J., et al. (2004).
Genotype–environment interaction in schizophrenia-spectrum disorder. *Brit-
ish Journal of Psychiatry, 184,* 216–222.

Ungar, M. (2004). The importance of parents and other caregivers to the resilience
of high-risk adolescents. *Family Process,* 43(1), 23–41.

Ungar, M. (2010). Families as navigators and negotiators: Facilitating culturally and contextually specific expressions of resilience. *Family Process, 49*, 421–435.

U.S. Census Bureau. (2014). Retrieved June 17, 2014, from *www.census.gov/population/projections/data/national/2014/summarytables.html*.

Vaillant, G. (2002). *Aging well*. Boston: Little Brown.

Valdez, C. R., Abegglen, J., & Hauser, C. (2013). Fortalezas Familiares Program: Building sociocultural and family strengths in Latina women with depression and their families. *Family Process, 52*(3), 378–393.

Valdez, C. R., Padilla, B., Moore, S. M., & Magana, S. (2013). Feasibility, acceptability, and preliminary outcomes of the Fortalezas Familiares intervention for Latino families facing maternal depression. *Family Process, 52*, 394–410.

Valladares, B. A., & Moore, K. A. (2009). *The strengths of poor families*. Washington, DC: Child Trends.

van der Kolk, B. A., McFarlane, A. C., & Weisaeth, L. (Eds.). (2006). *Traumatic stress: The effects of overwhelming experience on mind, body, and society* (2nd ed.). New York: Guilford Press.

von Bertalanffy, L. (1968). *General system theory: Foundation, development, application*. New York: George Braziller.

Waldegrave, C., King, P., Maniapoto, M., Tamasese, T. K., Parsons, T. L., & Sullivan, G. (in press). Resilience in sole parent families: A qualitative study of relational resilience in Maori, Pacific and Pakeha Families. *Family Process*.

Waller, M. R. (2012). Cooperation, conflict, or disengagement?: Coparenting styles and father involvement in fragile families. *Family Process, 51*, 325–342.

Walsh, F. (1983). The timing of symptoms and critical events in the family life cycle. In H. Liddle (Ed.), *Clinical implications of the family life cycle* (pp. 120–133). Rockville, MD: Aspen.

Walsh, F. (1989). Reconsidering gender in the marital quid pro quo. In M. McGoldrick, C. Anderson, & F. Walsh (Eds.), *Women in families: A framework for family therapy* (pp. 267–285). New York: Norton.

Walsh, F. (1996). The concept of family resilience: Crisis and challenge. *Family Process, 35*, 261–281.

Walsh, F. (2002a). A family resilience framework: Innovative practice applications. *Family Relations, 51*(2), 130–137.

Walsh, F. (2002b). Bouncing forward: Resilience in the aftermath of September 11, 2001. *Family Process, 41*(1), 34–36.

Walsh, F. (2003). Family resilience: A framework for clinical practice. *Family Process, 42*(1), 1–18.

Walsh, F. (2006). The clinical value of a family resilience framework. In R. Welter-Enderlin & B. Hildenbrand (Eds.), *Resilienz: Gedeihen trotz widriger Umstände* [Resilience: Thriving despite adversity] (pp. 43–79). Heidelberg, Germany: Carl-Auer Verlag.

Walsh, F. (2007). Traumatic loss and major disasters: Strengthening family and community resilience. *Family Process, 46*(2), 207–227.

Walsh, F. (2009a). Human–animal bonds: I. The relational significance of companion animals. *Family Process, 48*(4), 462–480.

Walsh, F. (2009b). Human–animal bonds: II. The role of pets in family systems and family therapy. *Family Process, 48*(4), 481–499.

Walsh, F. (2009c). Integrating spirituality in family therapy: Wellsprings for health, healing, and resilience. In F. Walsh (Ed.), *Spiritual resources in family therapy* (2nd ed., pp. 31–61). New York: Guilford Press.

Walsh, F. (Ed.). (2009d). *Spiritual resources in family therapy* (2nd ed.). New York: Guilford Press.

Walsh, F. (2010). Spiritual diversity: Multifaith perspectives in family therapy. *Family Process, 49*, 330–348.

Walsh, F. (2011). Family resilience: A collaborative approach in response to stressful life challenges. In S. Southwick, D. Charney, B. Litz, & M. Freedman (Eds.), *Resilience and mental health: Challenges across the life span* (pp. 149–161). New York: Cambridge University Press.

Walsh, F. (2012a). Family resilience: Strengths forged through adversity. In F. Walsh (Ed.), *Normal family processes* (4th ed., pp. 399–427). New York: Guilford Press.

Walsh, F. (2012b). Successful aging and family resilience. In B. Haslip & G. Smith (Eds.), *Annual review of gerontology and geriatrics: Vol. 32* (pp. 153–172). New York: Springer.

Walsh, F. (2012c). The "new normal": Diversity and complexity in 21st-century families. In F. Walsh (Ed.), *Normal family processes* (4th ed., pp. 4–27). New York: Guilford Press.

Walsh, F. (2012d). The spiritual dimension of family life. In F. Walsh (Ed.), *Normal family processes* (4th ed., pp. 347–372). New York: Guilford Press.

Walsh, F. (2013a). Community-based practice applications of a family resilience framework. In D. Becvar (Ed.), *Handbook of family resilience* (pp. 65–82). New York: Springer.

Walsh, F. (2013b). Religion and spirituality: A family systems perspective in clinical practice. In K. Pargament, A. Mahoney, & E. Shafranske (Eds.), *APA handbook of psychology, religion, and spirituality* (Vol. 2, pp. 189–205). Washington, DC: American Psychological Association.

Walsh, F. (2014a). Conceptual framework for family bereavement care: Strengthening resilience. In D. Kissane (Ed.), *Bereavement care for families* (pp. 17–29). New York: Routledge.

Walsh, F. (2014b). Family therapy: Systemic approaches to practice. In J. Brandell (Ed.), *Essentials of clinical social work* (pp. 160–185). Thousand Oaks, CA: Sage.

Walsh, F. (2016a). A family developmental framework: Challenges and resilience across the life cycle. In T. Sexton & J. Lebow (Eds.), *Handbook of family therapy* (4th ed.). New York: Routledge.

Walsh, F. (2016b). Families in later life: Challenges, opportunities, and resilience. In M. McGoldrick, B. Carter, & N. Garcia Preto (Eds.), *The expanded family life cycle* (5th ed.). Boston: Allyn & Bacon.

Walsh, F. (2015). Family transitions: Challenges and resilience. In M. Dulcan (Ed.), *Textbook of child and adolescent psychiatry* (2nd ed.). Washington, DC: American Psychiatric Association.

Walsh, F., & Anderson, C. M. (Eds.). (1988). *Chronic disorders and the family*. New York: Haworth Press.

Walsh, F., Jacob, L., & Simons, V. (1995). Facilitating healthy divorce processes:

Therapy and mediation approaches. In N. Jacobson & A. Gurman (Eds.), *Clinical handbook of couple therapy* (2nd ed., pp. 340–362). New York: Guilford Press.

Walsh, F., & McGoldrick, M. (Eds.). (2004). *Living beyond loss: Death in the family* (2nd ed.). New York: Norton.

Walsh, F., & McGoldrick, M. (2013). Bereavement: A family life cycle perspective. *Family Science, 4,* 20–27.

Waters, D., & Lawrence, E. (1993). *Competence, courage, and change.* New York: Norton.

Watzlawick, P., Beavin, J., & Jackson, D. (1967). *Pragmatics of human communication.* New York: Norton.

Webb, N. B. (Ed.). (2003). *Mass trauma and violence: Helping families and children cope.* New York: Guilford Press.

Weihs, K., Fisher, L., & Baird, M. (2001). Families, health, and behavior: A section of the commissioned report for the Institute of Medicine, National Academy of Sciences. *Families, Systems, and Health, 20*(1), 7–47.

Weil, A. (1994). *Spontaneous healing.* New York: Knopf.

Weine, S. (2006). *Testimony after catastrophe: Narrating the traumas of political violence.* Evanston, IL: Northwestern University Press.

Weine, S. (2011). Developing preventive mental health interventions for refugee families in resettlement. *Family Process, 50,* 410–430.

Weine, S., Knafi, K., Feetham, S., Kulauzavic, Y., Klebec, A., Sclove, S., et al. (2005). A mixed methods study of refugee families engaging in multiple-family groups. *Family Relations, 54,* 558–568.

Weine, S., Muzurovic, N., Kulauzovic, Y., Besic, S., Lezic, A., Mujagic, A., et al. (2004). Family consequences of refugee trauma. *Family Process, 43*(2), 147–160.

Weingarten, K. (2004). Witnessing the effects of political violence in families: Mechanisms of intergenerational transmission of trauma and clinical interventions. *Journal of Marital and Family Therapy, 30*(1), 45–59.

Weingarten, K. (2010). Reasonable hope: Construct, clinical applications, and supports. *Family Process, 49,* 5–25.

Werner, E. E., & Smith, R. S. (2001). *Journeys from childhood to midlife: Risk, resilience, and recovery.* Ithaca, NY: Cornell University Press.

Whitaker, C., & Keith, D. (1981). Symbolic–experiential family therapy. In A. Gurman & D. Kniskern (Eds.), *Handbook of family therapy* (pp. 187–225). New York: Brunner/Mazel.

White, M. (2007). *Maps of narrative practice.* New York: Norton.

White, M., & Epston, D. (1990). *Narrative means to therapeutic ends.* New York: Norton.

Wiesel, E. (1995). *All rivers run to the sea: Memoirs.* New York: Knopf.

Windle, G., Bennett, K. M., & Noyes, J. (2011). A methodological review of resilience measurement scales. *Health and Quality of Life Outcomes, 9*(8), 1–18.

Wolin, S., Muller, W., Taylor, F., Wolin, S., Ranganathan, S., Saymah, D., et al. (2009). Religious perspectives on resilience: Buddhism, Christianity, Judaism, Hinduism, and Islam. In F. Walsh (Ed.), *Spiritual resources in family therapy* (2nd ed., pp. 103–124). New York: The Guilford Press.

Wolin, S., & Wolin, S. (1993). *The resilient self: How survivors of troubled families rise above adversity.* New York: Villard.

Worden, J. W. (2008). *Grief counseling and grief therapy* (4th ed.). New York: Springer.

World Health Organization. (2011, October). Mental health: A state of well-being. Retrieved from *www.who.int/features/factfiles/mental_health/en/index.html.*

Worthington, E. L., Jr., & Scherer, M. (2004). Forgiveness is an emotion-focused coping strategy that can reduce health risks and promote health resilience: Theory, review, and hypotheses. *Psychology and Health, 19,* 385–406.

Wortman, C., & Silver, R. (1989). The myths of coping with loss. *Journal of Counseling and Clinical Psychology, 57,* 349–357.

Wright, L. M. (2009). Spirituality, suffering, and beliefs: The soul of healing with families. In F. Walsh (Ed.), *Spiritual resources in family therapy* (2nd ed., pp. 65–80). New York: Guilford Press.

Wright, L. M., & Bell, J. M. (2009). *Beliefs and illness: A model for healing.* Calgary, Alberta, Canada: 4th Floor Press.

Wuerffel, J., DeFrain, J., & Stinnett, N. (1990). How strong families use humor. *Family Perspective, 24,* 129–142.

Yang, O.-K., & Choi, M.-M. (2001). Koreans' Han and resilience: Application to mental health social work. *Mental Health and Social Work, 11*(6), 7–29.

Zinner, E. S., & Williams, M. B. (Eds.). (1999). *When a community weeps: Case studies in group survivorship.* New York: Brunner/Mazel.

Index

The letter *f* following a page number indicates figure; the letter *t* indicates table.